LEFT BRAIN, RIGHT BRAIN

LEFT BRAIN, RIGHT BRAIN
Fourth Edition

Sally P. Springer
University of California, Davis
Georg Deutsch
University of Alabama, Birmingham

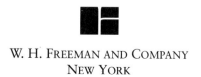

W. H. FREEMAN AND COMPANY
NEW YORK

Library of Congress Cataloging-in-Publication Data

Springer, Sally P.,
    Left brain, right brain / Sally P. Springer and Georg Deutsch. —
4th ed.
        p.   cm.
    Includes bibliographical references and index.
    ISBN 0-7167-2372-7. — ISBN 0-7167-2373-5 (pbk.)
    1. Cerebral dominance. 2. Brain—Localization of functions.
    3. Left and right (Psychology) I. Deutsch, Georg. II. Title.
    QP385.5.S67 1993
    612.8'25—dc20   93-21642
                                                                          CIP

Printed in the United States of America

    2 3 4 5 6 7 8 9 0   VB   7 6 5 4   089

To the memory of
Peter Deutsch
and
Fanny Margulies, Lilyan Margulies,
and Nathaniel Margulies

CONTENTS

3

ASYMMETRIES IN THE NORMAL BRAIN   65

4

MEASURING THE BRAIN AND ITS ACTIVITY: Physiological Correlates of Asymmetry   89

5
THE PUZZLE OF THE LEFT-HANDER 125

6
FURTHER EVIDENCE FROM THE CLINIC:
Aphasia, Apraxia, Agnosia 147

10
ASYMMETRY'S ROLE IN DEVELOPMENTAL DISABILITIES AND PSYCHIATRIC ILLNESS 253

11
HEMISPHERICITY, EDUCATION, AND ALTERED STATES 271

12
CONCLUDING HYPOTHESES AND SPECULATIONS 289

APPENDIX 325

NOTES 335

INDEX 361

PREFACE
to the Fourth Edition

The fourth edition of *Left Brain, Right Brain* is the first to appear in the 1990s, the decade the U.S. Congress has declared the "Decade of the Brain." This designation recognizes the importance, to individuals and to society as a whole, of research on the brain. It is our hope that the new edition of *Left Brain, Right Brain* provides readers with a clear and accurate understanding of research into cerebral hemispheric function as well as conveys some of the excitement surrounding scientific inquiry into the brain.

As in previous editions, we first present basic findings on asymmetry in brain-damaged, split-brain, and normal subjects and then consider special topics such as left handedness, sex differences in brain asymmetry, and the development of asymmetry. In providing an overview of the left brain and the right brain, we have tried to separate what is reasonably established as fact from what is purely speculative, without sacrificing the intrigue of either. In addition, we have sought wherever possible to identify potential explanations for inconsistent findings. We have also tried to show how the investigation of hemispheric asymmetry has yielded important insights about brain function in general. Studying the left brain and the right brain is but one approach to brain research. We hope that this book conveys the sense in which it is a fruitful one.

The fourth edition is updated throughout, particularly in areas that have undergone the most rapid development. The reader familiar with previous editions will find many new references throughout the book to the fascinating ways in which modern brain imaging techniques have been brought to bear on key issues. The reader will also note greater emphasis on the conceptual underpinnings of cognitive neuropsychology and the way in which such concepts have influenced how investigators look at problems and interpret their data.

We continue to write for a relatively broad audience, with the book providing coverage at several levels on most topics. We strive to be as clear as possible without compromising accuracy or the complexity of the issues we present. The book will be of interest to the general reader who wishes to go beyond oversimplified and exaggerated popular accounts of brain asymmetry; it is also designed to serve as a text in a wide variety of courses.

We are indebted to many colleagues and friends for their contributions to *Left Brain, Right Brain* over four editions. Valuable comments and suggestions on previous editions were provided by Alan Rubens, Chuck Hamilton, Phil Bryden, Morris Moscovitch, Barry Lorinstein, Nick Goldberg, Andy Papanicolaou, and Peter Shulman. Many of them contributed to the fourth edition as well. In addition, for the fourth edition Eran Zaidel and Michael Gazzaniga shared their insights into what was new and important with us. James Mountz, Donald Tweig, and Hoby Hetherington kindly provided us with some of the brain scan images used in this edition. We are grateful to many others who graciously sent us preprints of their work that was not yet published.

We have had the privilege of working with exceptional senior editors at W. H. Freeman and Company over the period of the four editions — W. Hayward Rogers, now retired, Jonathan Cobb, and most recently, Susan Brennan. We have also been fortunate to have had excellent project editors: Judith Wilson and Jim Maurer for the first and second editions, respectively; and Diane Maass for the third and fourth editions. The fourth edition was the first one to be published electronically. A special word of thanks goes to Jim Whatley at UC Davis for positioning us to take advantage of the computer technology to make it all possible.

Our spouses, Håkon Hope and Martha Pezrow, deserve our gratitude for the understanding and support they provided during the long revision process. Both made substantial and sustained sacrifices so that the project could be completed.

July 1993
Sally P. Springer
Georg Deutsch

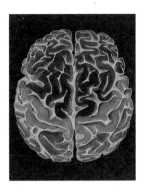

Early Evidence
from the Clinic:
The Discovery of Asymmetry

In 1836, Marc Dax, an obscure country doctor, read a short paper at a medical society meeting in Montpellier, France. Dax had not been a frequent contributor to medical conferences. In fact, this paper was his first and only scientific presentation.

During his long career as a general practitioner, Dax had seen many patients suffering from loss of speech—known technically as aphasia—following damage to the brain. This observation in itself was not new. Cases of sudden, permanent disruption of the ability to speak coherently had been reported by the ancient Greeks. Dax, however, was struck by an association between loss of speech and the side of the brain where the damage had occurred. In more than 40 patients with aphasia, Dax had found signs of damage to the left half of the brain. He was unable to find a single case that involved damage to the right side alone. In his paper to the medical society, he summarized these observations and presented his conclusions: Each half of the brain controls different functions; speech is controlled by the left half.

The paper was an unqualified flop. It aroused little interest among those who heard it and was soon forgotten. Dax died the following year, unaware that he had anticipated one of the most exciting and active areas of scientific inquiry of the second half of the twentieth century—the investigation of the differences between the left brain and the right brain.

Although most of us think of the brain as a single structure, it is actually divided into halves. These two parts, or hemispheres, are tightly packed together inside the skull and are linked by several distinct bundles of nerve fibers that serve as channels of communication between them.

Anatomically, each hemisphere appears to be approximately a mirror image of the other, very much in keeping with the general left-right symmetry of the human body. Functionally, control of the body's basic movements and sensations is evenly divided between the two cerebral hemispheres. This control occurs in a crossed fashion: The left hemisphere controls the right side of the body (right hand, right leg, and so on), and the right hemisphere controls the left side. Figure 1.1 shows this arrangement.*

The left-right physical symmetry of the brain and body does not imply, however, that the right and left sides are equivalent in all respects. We have only to examine the abilities of our two hands to note asymmetry of function. Few people are truly ambidextrous; most have a dominant hand. (In many instances a person's handedness can be used to predict a great deal about the organization of higher mental functions in her or his brain. In right-handers, for example, it is almost always the case that the hemisphere that controls the dominant hand is also the hemisphere that controls speech.)

And differences in the abilities of the two hands are but one manifestation of basic asymmetries in the functions of the two cerebral hemispheres. A great deal of evidence has accumulated in recent years showing that the left brain and the right brain are not identical in their capabilities or organizations.

The earliest and most dramatic evidence of functional asymmetries came from observations of the behavior of individuals with brain damage. Data of this type are known as clinical data because they are based

---

* A brief overview of neuroanatomy may be found in the Appendix.

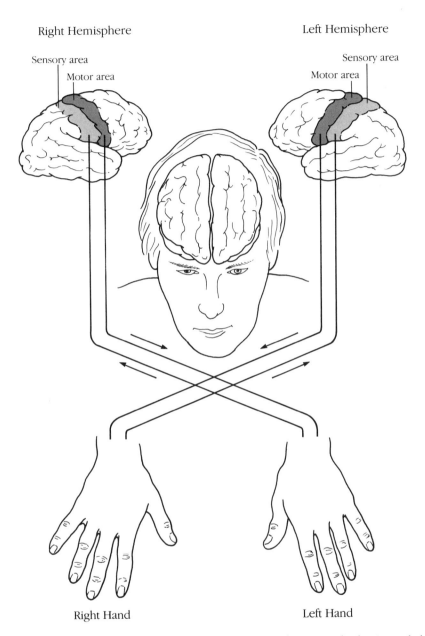

FIGURE 1.1   Motor control and sensory pathways between the brain and the rest of the body are almost completely crossed. Each hand is served primarily by the cerebral hemisphere on the opposite side.

on the study of patients with brain damage. Marc Dax's conclusion about the link between damage to the left hemisphere and loss of speech is an example of the use of clinical data. Later observations in the clinic led to the discovery of still other asymmetries.

In contrast with people who experience speech problems because of damage to the left hemisphere, patients with certain kinds of right-hemisphere damage are much more likely to have perceptual and attentional problems. These include serious difficulties in spatial orientation and memory for spatial relationships. For example, a patient may have great difficulty learning his or her way around a new building or may even be disoriented in familiar surroundings. Other patients may have difficulty recognizing familiar faces. Damage to the right hemisphere can also result in a problem called neglect. A patient experiencing the neglect syndrome pays no attention to the left side of space and sometimes pays no attention to the left side of the body. In many cases the patient will not eat food on the left side of the dinner plate and may refuse to acknowledge a paralyzed left arm as being his or her own. Surprisingly, similar damage to the left hemisphere usually does not produce such severe and long-lasting neglect of the right side of space.

Although clinical data pointing to brain asymmetries have been available for over 100 years, current interest in the left brain and the right brain is traceable to recent work involving so-called split-brain patients. For medical reasons, these patients have undergone surgery to cut the cortical pathways that normally connect the cerebral hemi-spheres. Figure 1.2 shows the corpus callosum, the major pathway involved. To the untrained observer, this radical surgery seems to do little to interfere with the patient's normal functioning. To the inquisitive scientist, however, it affords an unparalleled opportunity to study the abilities of each hemisphere separately within the same head.

Special techniques make it possible to confine detailed sensory information to just one hemisphere. The limiting of stimuli to one hemisphere is often called lateralization. One way to accomplish lateralization is to let a blindfolded patient feel an object with only one hand. A split-brain patient who does this with the right hand (which is controlled principally by the left hemisphere) will have no difficulty naming the object. But if the procedure is repeated with the left hand, the patient will be unable to name the object. Apparently, information about the object does not get through to the speech centers located in the left hemisphere. Nevertheless, the patient can easily use his or her left hand to retrieve the object from a number of other objects hidden from sight. A casual onlooker might conclude that the patient's left hand knew and remembered what it held earlier even though the patient did not.

By using other techniques that confine visual and auditory information to one hemisphere at a time, researchers have demonstrated sig-

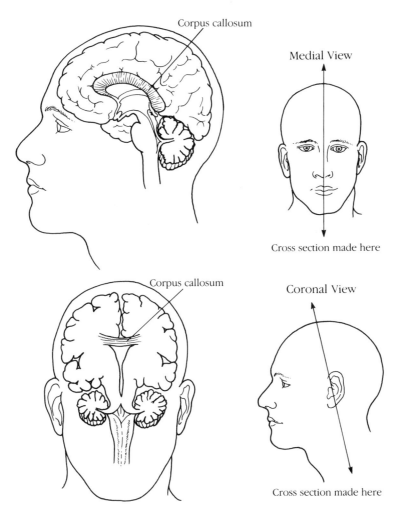

FIGURE 1.2   Two views of the cerebral hemispheres and the corpus callosum, the major nerve-fiber tract connecting them.

nificant differences in the capabilities of the two hemispheres in split-brain patients. The left hemisphere has been found to be predominantly involved with analytic processes, especially the production and understanding of language, and it appears to process input in a sequential manner. The right hemisphere appears to be responsible for certain spatial skills and musical abilities and to process information simultaneously and holistically.

Encouraged by discoveries with brain-damaged and split-brain patients, investigators have sought ways to study hemispheric differences in neurologically normal subjects. Do the differences between the functions of the left brain and the right brain noted in brain-damaged patients have any consequences for the functions of the normal brain? Techniques developed to answer this question have shown that they do.

Split-brain studies have shown that, although each half of the brain is capable of perceiving, learning, remembering, and feeling independently of the other, some differences exist in the way in which each hemisphere deals with incoming information. Roger Sperry, winner of the 1981 Nobel Prize in Physiology or Medicine for his pioneering work with split-brain patients, has proposed that an independent stream of consciousness resides in each of the separate hemispheres.[1] He has suggested that surgical division of the brain divides the mind into two distinct realms of consciousness. This model leads to speculation about dual consciousness in the intact, normal brain under certain conditions.

Other investigators have emphasized the significance of the differences between the hemispheres, even claiming that these differences clearly reflect the traditional dualisms of intellect versus intuition, science versus art, and the logical versus the mysterious. According to psychologist Robert Ornstein, brain research shows that these distinctions are not simply a reflection of culture or philosophy.[2] The old belief in distinct Eastern and Western forms of consciousness, he argued, now has a physiological basis in the differences between the two hemispheres.

It has also been suggested that lawyers and artists use different halves of the brain in their work and that the differences between the halves show up in activities not related to their work.[3] Others have extended this idea further and have claimed that everyone may be classified as either a right-hemisphere person or a left-hemisphere person, depending on which hemisphere guides the bulk of an individual's behavior.[4]

Recent interest in brain asymmetries has sparked concern with the general issue of handedness. Studies have shown differences between left-handers and right-handers in the way the brain is organized. What are the effects, if any, of these differences on intelligence and creativity? What factors produce left-handedness in the first place? Genes? Experience? Minor brain damage? These and other questions related to handedness have been the subject of intensive study in the last 20 years.

Various other issues have been studied in connection with hemispheric asymmetry. Diverse problems such as learning disabilities, stuttering, and schizophrenia have been attributed to abnormalities in the division of labor between the two hemispheres. Joseph Bogen, a neurosurgeon involved in split-brain research, has suggested that research on hemispheric differences has important implications for education.[5] He argued that the current emphasis on the acquisition of verbal skills and the development of analytic thought processes neglects the development of important nonverbal abilities. As a result, he claimed, "we are starving" one-half of the brain and ignoring its potential contribution to the whole person.

From its modest beginnings in 1836, research on the left brain and the right brain has gone on to capture the imaginations of scientists and laypersons alike. Few areas of scientific inquiry have generated so much interest from so diverse an audience. This attention has had both good and bad effects. On the positive side, vast quantities of new data have been collected in a short period of time, and investigators are hard at work considering the implications of their findings for human behavior. On the negative side, there is a tendency to interpret every behavioral dichotomy, such as rational versus intuitive and deductive versus imaginative, in terms of left brain and right brain. This occupational hazard has been named "dichotomania" by some. In addition, the dividing line between fact and fantasy has often been blurred, making it difficult for nonspecialists to know what is speculation and what has been established firmly as fact.

Undoubtedly, however, important insights into brain function and its relation to behavior have resulted from the study of the left brain and the right brain, and many more important discoveries remain to be made. The goals of this book are to survey the current state of knowledge, to draw conclusions where possible, and to point out the gaps in knowledge that still exist. We shall begin with an account of some of the clinical data that have given rise to current ideas concerning the left brain and the right brain.

·········

LOSS OF SPEECH AND RIGHT-SIDED WEAKNESS:
Long-overlooked evidence of asymmetry

Anyone walking through a stroke ward in a hospital can see that patients are fairly evenly distributed between two groups: those with paralyzed left sides and those with paralyzed right sides. A stroke generally involves a stoppage of the blood supply to part of the brain and results in damage to the affected region. Because blood is supplied to each hemisphere separately, a stroke usually affects only one-half of the brain. Because each half controls the opposite side of the body, paralysis of the right side indicates a stroke in the left hemisphere, and left-sided paralysis indicates a stroke in the right hemisphere.

Throughout the long history of medicine, the clinical combination of speech disturbances with weakness or paralysis of the right half of the body has been reported again and again. These observations should have suggested a link between loss of speech and damage to the left hemisphere of the brain. The significance of the relationship, however, was not appreciated by the medical community as a whole until the second half of the nineteenth century.

It is perhaps not surprising that this evidence of hemispheric asymmetry was overlooked for so long. Early anatomical studies showed that the halves of the brain were mirror images of each other, roughly equal in size and weight. Also, most scientists firmly believed that the brain functioned as a whole unit and, thus, the scientists were not predisposed to "see" evidence that suggested otherwise.

By the first decades of the nineteenth century, however, serious attention was being given to the idea that particular functions could be assigned to specific regions of the brain. The notion that one could study the role of specific regions became known as the doctrine of cerebral localization.

...

The Doctrine of Cerebral Localization

Franz Gall, a German anatomist, was the first to propose that the brain is not a uniform mass and that various mental faculties can be localized to different parts of the brain. The faculty of speech, he believed, is located in the frontal lobes, the part of each hemisphere closest to the front of the head. Unfortunately, Gall also claimed that the shape of the skull reflects the underlying brain tissue and that an individual's mental and emotional characteristics can be determined through a careful study of bumps on the head.

In many scientific circles, Gall was dismissed as a quack on the grounds that no good evidence existed to show that skull shape can be used reliably to predict anything about the person whose head is being measured. The basic idea that different functions are controlled by different regions within the brain, however, did attract many followers. Among them was Jean Baptiste Bouillaud, a French professor of medicine. Bouillaud was so certain Gall was correct in localizing speech to the frontal lobes that he offered 500 francs (a considerable sum at the time) to anyone who could produce a patient with damage to the frontal lobes that was unaccompanied by loss of speech.[6]

For many years, most scientists quietly aligned themselves with one of the two sides of this issue. One group firmly believed that speech is controlled by the frontal lobes; the other side argued that particular functions cannot be localized to specific regions of the brain. At that time, there was little in the way of new data to change anyone's mind, and each group held firmly to its position in the absence of compelling evidence to the contrary. It was in this scientific climate that Marc Dax presented his work to the medical community in Montpellier in 1836. As we have seen, his observations pointing to a special role for the left hemisphere in speech were essentially ignored.

···

A Turning Point: The Findings of Paul Broca

The stalemate ended in 1861. At a meeting of the Society of Anthropology in Paris, Bouillaud's son-in-law, Ernest Auburtin, repeated Bouillaud's claim that the center controlling speech is in the frontal lobes. His remarks impressed Paul Broca, a young surgeon who was present at the meeting.

A few days before the meeting, an old man suffering from a serious leg infection had been admitted to Broca's service at a local hospital. The infection was recent, but the patient had for many years suffered from loss of speech as well as from paralysis of one side of his body (hemiplegia). After the meeting, Broca approached Auburtin and suggested it might be useful for them to examine this patient together.

A day or so after their examination, the man died. Broca performed a postmortem examination of the patient's brain and found a region of damaged tissue, or lesion, in part of the left frontal lobe. At the next meeting of the Society, Broca brought the brain and pointed out his findings. But no one seemed to pay much attention to his comments.

A few months later, Broca again reported to the Society that he had observed a similar lesion at autopsy in a second patient suffering from loss of speech. What changed the minds of the Society of Anthropology members is not clear, but this time Broca's report was received with great excitement and touched off heated debate and controversy. Broca soon found himself viewed as the chief proponent of cerebral localization of function.

His new evidence did not convince everyone, however. Die-hard critics of the concept of localization directed their attacks at him. If speech is localized in the frontal lobes, he was challenged, why is it that monkeys with large frontal-brain areas do not possess the ability to speak? Similarly, how can one account for the occasional case of extensive frontal-lobe damage that does not produce loss of speech?

Even Broca's terminology came under fire. He had been careful to differentiate between loss of speech due to simple paralysis of the muscles used to produce speech and loss of speech in his brain-damaged patients—he called the latter condition aphemia. One critic, M. Trousseau, claimed that the word *aphemia* was derived from a Greek root meaning "infamous" and was not appropriate in this context. Trousseau suggested that aphasia was a better term to use when referring to loss of speech. Although Broca ably defended his choice of words, investigators had already begun to use Trousseau's terminology, which has survived to the present day.

Broca was an unwilling participant in the controversy generated by his work. He later stated that his two reports to the Society of Anthropology were simply an attempt to bring to the attention of others a curious fact that he had observed by chance and that he did not desire to be involved in debates about the localization of speech centers. Despite his protests, Broca continued to figure centrally in the controversy. He went on to collect data from additional cases and was able to pinpoint more precisely the area of the brain involved in instances of speech loss. Figure 1.3 shows the location of this region, which has since become known as Broca's area. This figure also illustrates the division of a hemisphere into four lobes: frontal, parietal, occipital, and temporal.

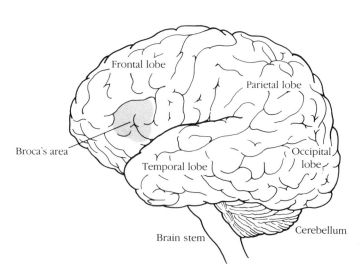

FIGURE 1.3   The location of Broca's area in the left cerebral hemisphere.

...

Recognizing the Role of the Left Hemisphere

Although his two earliest cases had involved lesions of the frontal lobe of the left hemisphere, Broca did not immediately see the link between speech loss and the side of the lesion. For two years, he made no attempt to explain this coincidence. In commenting on other cases showing the same relationship, he noted: "Here are eight cases where the lesion is situated in the posterior portion of the third frontal convolution and a thing most remarkable in all of these patients [is that] the lesion is on the left side. I do not attempt to draw a conclusion and I await new findings."[7]

By 1864, however, Broca had become convinced of the importance of the left hemisphere in speech:

> I have been struck with the fact that in my first aphemics the lesion always lay not only in the same part of the brain but always the same side—the left. Since then, from many postmortems, the lesion was always left sided. One has also seen many aphemics alive, most of them hemiplegic, and always hemiplegic on the right side. Furthermore, one has seen at autopsy lesions on the right side in patients who had shown no aphemia. It seems from all this that the faculty of articulate language is localized in the left hemisphere, or at least that it depends chiefly upon that hemisphere.[8]

This important insight embroiled Broca in yet another controversy, this time over who had priority in the discovery of this fundamental brain asymmetry. Shortly after learning of Broca's work, Gustav Dax, a physician and the son of Marc Dax, wrote a letter to the medical press claiming that Broca had willfully ignored his father's earlier paper showing that lesions affecting speech always occur in the left half of the brain. Broca replied, protesting that he had never heard of Dax or his work and could find no record of a paper by Dax having been delivered in 1836. (Historians disagree about whether Broca was aware of Marc Dax's work at the time he published his own, and they probably will never resolve this question.) Meanwhile, Gustav Dax located and proceeded to publish the text of his father's original talk in order to establish the elder Dax's priority.

Eventually, Broca presented a considerably more impressive argument for the association between aphasia and damage to the left hemisphere than had Dax. Dax's cases lacked verification of the location of damage and complete clinical histories. Broca's work, in contrast, contained extensive anatomical findings and information about the nature of the speech problems present.

Broca also went on to consider the relationship between handedness and speech. He suggested that both speech and manual dexterity are attributable to the inborn superiority of the left hemisphere in right-handers. "One can conceive," he speculated, "that there may be a certain number of individuals in whom the natural pre-eminence of the convolutions of the right hemisphere reverses the order of the phenomenon which I have just described."[9] These individuals, of course, are left-handers. Broca's "rule" that the hemisphere controlling speech is on the side opposite the preferred hand was influential well into the twentieth century.

Broca may be properly credited with being the first person to bring to the attention of the medical community the asymmetry of the human brain with regard to speech. He was also the first to link that asymmetry with hand preference.

·········

THE CONCEPT OF CEREBRAL DOMINANCE

Within ten years of the publication of Broca's initial observations, the concept now known as cerebral dominance began to emerge as the major view of the relationship between the two hemispheres of the brain. In 1864 the great British neurologist John Hughlings Jackson wrote, "Not long ago, few doubted the brain to be double in function as well as physically bilateral; but now that it is certain from the researches of Dax, Broca, and others, that damage to one lateral half can make a man entirely speechless, the former view is disrupted."[10]

In 1868 Jackson proposed his idea of the "leading" hemisphere—a notion that may be viewed as the precursor of the idea of cerebral dominance. "The two brains cannot be mere duplicates," he wrote, "if damage to one alone can make a man speechless. For these processes [of speech], of which there are none higher, there must surely be one side which is leading." Jackson further concluded "that in most people the left side of the brain is the leading side—the side of the so-called will, and that the right is the automatic side."[11]

By 1870 other investigators began to realize that many types of language disorders could result from damage to the left hemisphere. Early work concentrating on speech production problems that resulted from injury to the left hemisphere had overlooked the fact that these same patients frequently had difficulty understanding the speech of others. Karl Wernicke, a German neurologist, is credited with showing that damage to the back part of the temporal lobe of the left hemisphere could produce difficulties in understanding speech.

Similarly, problems in reading and writing were identified in some patients and were shown to result from damage to the left hemisphere, not from damage to the right. Clearly, the picture emerging by the end of the nineteenth century was one in which the left hemisphere played a role of great importance in language functions in general and not just in speech per se. It had also become apparent that different kinds of language problems resulted from damage to different areas within the left hemisphere.

Further evidence supporting the notion that the left hemisphere possesses functions not shared by the right came from Hugo Liepmann's studies of *apraxia.* This disorder is generally defined as the inability to perform purposeful movements on command.*An apraxic patient might have no difficulty brushing his or her teeth in the context of a normal bedtime routine, but he or she would be unable to reproduce the same movements when instructed to pretend to brush in an unrelated context.

Liepmann had shown that, although such deficits are not due to a general inability to understand speech, they are associated with injury to the left hemisphere. He concluded that the left hemisphere controls "purposeful" movements as well as language but that the specific areas of the left hemisphere involved are different in the two cases.

Taken together, these findings formed the basis of a widely held view of the relationship between the two hemispheres. One hemisphere, usually the left in right-handers, was seen as the director of speech and other higher functions; the right, or "minor," hemisphere, was without special functions and subordinate to control by the "dominant" left. The origin of the term *cerebral dominance* is obscure, but it captures nicely the idea of one-half of the brain directing behavior. Although the concept originally associated with this term underestimates the role of the right hemisphere, cerebral dominance is still widely used today.

....

THE RIGHT BRAIN:
The neglected hemisphere

Almost as soon as the concept of cerebral dominance became popular, evidence began to appear suggesting that the right, or minor, hemi-

---

* Apraxia and other clinical disorders considered in this chapter are discussed in more detail in Chapter 6.

sphere also possesses specialized abilities. John Hughlings Jackson's notion of the left hemisphere as "leading" was the intellectual grandparent of the idea of dominance. Interestingly, Jackson was also one of the first to consider that an extreme, one-sided view of the way mental functions are localized in the brain was wrong. "If then," he wrote in 1865, "it should be proven by wider experience that the faculty of expression resides in one hemisphere, there is no absurdity in raising the question as to whether perception—its corresponding opposite—may be seated in the other."[12]

This speculation took more concrete form 11 years later when Jackson argued that the lobes at the rear of the brain are the seat of visual ideation or thought and that "the right posterior lobe is the leading side, the left the more automatic."[13] Jackson based this proposal on his observation of a patient who had a tumor in the right hemisphere and experienced difficulty recognizing objects, persons, and places.

Like Dax's important insight 40 years earlier, Jackson's idea was way ahead of its time. Although other reports of a similar nature occasionally appeared, little attention was paid to Jackson's evidence. Investigators concerned themselves with localizing various functions within the left hemisphere and essentially ignored the right. By the 1930s, however, more data showing specialized roles for the right hemisphere had been collected, and scientists began to reconsider their ideas about the functions of the minor half of the brain.

...

Visuospatial Abilities in the Right Hemisphere

One important development was the discovery of significant and fairly consistent differences in the way subjects with left-hemisphere damage and those with right-hemisphere damage performed on standard psychological tests. The tests were originally developed to study and compare normal subjects along such dimensions as verbal ability, appreciation of spatial relationships, and ability to manipulate forms.

The first large-scale effort using these measures to study the effects of brain damage involved over 200 patients and more than 40 different tests—an average of 19 hours of testing per patient.[14] The results of this and subsequent studies were impressive. It was found, as a general rule, that damage to the left, or dominant, hemisphere results in poor performance on the tests that emphasize verbal ability. Although this finding was not too surprising, it was also found that patients with damage to the right hemisphere consistently do more poorly on nonverbal tests involving the manipulation of geometric figures, puzzle assembly, completion of missing parts of patterns and figures, and other tasks involving form, distance, and space relationships. (Two visuospatial tasks are shown in Figure 1.4.)

The most striking evidence for specialized right-hemisphere function comes from direct observations of the patients themselves, who often display profound disturbances in orientation and awareness. Such patients can be so disoriented in space that they are unable to find their way around a house in which they have lived for many years. Some show neglect, or hemispatial inattention: They consistently miss objects or events on their left.

Certain *agnosias*—disturbances in the recognition or perception of familiar information—are also associated with damage to the right hemisphere. Spatial agnosia is a disorientation with respect to locations and spatial relationships. Some right-hemisphere patients have deficits in their ability to comprehend depth and distance relationships or to deal with mental images of maps and forms.

One of the most interesting forms of agnosia is facial agnosia. A patient with this condition is unable to recognize familiar faces and sometimes cannot discriminate between people in general. The deficit is

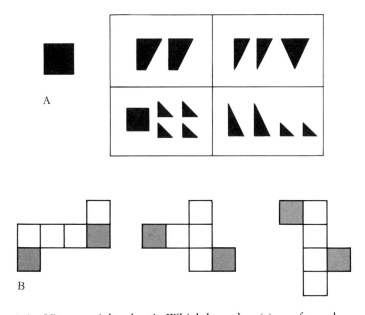

FIGURE 1.4   Visuospatial tasks. A. Which boxed set(s) can form the square on the outside? B. If you fold these patterns into cubes, in which cube(s) will the dark sides meet at one edge?

quite specific. Recognition of scenes and objects, for example, may not be impaired. This problem has been found in cases where there was damage to both halves of the brain, although several investigators have argued for the importance of right-hemisphere lesions in this disorder.[15]

...

The Role of the Right Hemisphere in Music

Additional evidence pointing to the specialization of the right hemisphere came from the observation that the ability to sing is frequently unaffected in patients suffering from severe speech disturbances. One of the earliest recorded cases of this type was described in 1745:

> He had an attack of a violent illness which resulted in a paralysis of the entire right side of the body and complete loss of speech. He can sing certain hymns, which he had learned before he became ill, as clearly and distinctly as any healthy person. . . Yet this man is dumb, cannot say a single word except "yes" and has to communicate by making signs with his hand.[16]

Similar cases were reported in the early 1900s and suggest that the right hemisphere controls singing.

Other evidence consistent with this idea comes from clinical reports that damage to the right half of the brain may result in the loss of musical ability, leaving speech unimpaired. This disorder, known as *amusia,* was most frequently reported in professional musicians who suffered from stroke or other brain damage. By the 1930s, the medical literature contained many case histories of people who suffered impairments in various aspects of musical ability after damage to the right hemisphere. Similar reports following damage to the left hemisphere were rarer, again suggesting that the right hemisphere is in some way critically involved in music.[17]

...

Why "Discovery" of the Right Brain Took So Long

All this evidence shows that the view of the right hemisphere as the minor or passive hemisphere is inappropriate. Why did it take most scientists 70 years after Broca's findings concerning the left hemisphere to recognize that the right hemisphere controls important functions? There may be several reasons for this time lag.

First, it seemed that the right hemisphere was able to withstand greater damage without producing any obvious impairments. Small lesions in particular areas of the left hemisphere drastically affected speech abilities, but comparable damage in the right hemisphere did not appear to cause any serious dysfunction. This disparity was originally interpreted as a sign of the less important role played by the right hemisphere in human behavior. It has been suggested more recently, however, that this difference simply reflects the way processes are organized in the right hemisphere: Specific processes are distributed over larger regions of brain tissue in the right half of the brain than in the left half.[18]

The most likely reason for the slow recognition of the importance of the right hemisphere, however, is that disabilities caused by lesions in the right hemisphere were not so easy to analyze and fit into the traditional ideas about brain function. Most damage to the right hemisphere did not abolish any obvious human abilities in an all-or-none fashion; instead, it disturbed behavior in fairly subtle ways. Some of the problems occurring with right-brain damage were not so easy to label as the problems associated with left-hemisphere injury. They often went unnoticed or were masked by more obvious physical disabilities, such as those found in most stroke victims.

It is important to keep in mind that the most debilitating effect of a stroke is the paralysis it often causes. The paralysis tends to be the patient's chief complaint or problem. Brain damage that arises from traumas such as accidents or gunshot wounds is also accompanied by complications that make it difficult to separate out subtle intellectual impairments from a host of other problems.

Despite its camouflaged role, the right hemisphere does play a vital part in human behavior. It is now clear that both hemispheres contribute to complex mental activity while differing in their function and organization. The idea that each hemisphere is specialized for different functions is known as complementary specialization.

·········

HANDEDNESS AND THE HEMISPHERES

It is frequently the case in science that ideas are challenged by new evidence just as they have gained widespread acceptance. We have already seen how an extreme view of cerebral dominance was called into question by new findings concerning the role of the right hemisphere. In the same way, Broca's rule linking aphasia with damage to the hemisphere opposite the preferred hand was shown to be an oversimplification soon after Broca proposed it.

The rule accounted nicely for the relationship between damage to the left hemisphere and aphasia in right-handers. But left-handers appeared to come in two varieties: those with speech in the hemisphere opposite their preferred hand (as predicted by Broca) and those with speech in the left hemisphere. The existence of the latter group was discovered through observations of left-handed patients who become aphasic following damage to the left hemisphere. These patients, often referred to as having *crossed aphasia,* show rather dramatically that left-handedness is not necessarily the simple converse of right-handedness.[19]

The relationship of handedness to hemispheric asymmetry of function remains one of the most important questions to be resolved in the study of brain organization. We shall return to it several times in later chapters.

·········

FURTHER INSIGHTS FROM THE CLINIC

To complete our brief account of the contributions of clinical data to the understanding of hemispheric asymmetry of function, we should mention two highly specialized neurosurgical procedures developed in the 1930s and 1940s. Both were designed to help the neurosurgeon determine which hemisphere was controlling speech and language function in an individual about to undergo brain surgery for epilepsy. These procedures have also contributed significantly to our knowledge of hemispheric asymmetry of function in general.

···

Direct Electrical Stimulation of the Hemispheres

Epilepsy, a disorder involving abnormal electrical activity generated within the brain, produces reactions that may range from short blackouts lasting a second or two to full-blown grand mal seizures. During an epileptic attack, the abnormal electrical activity often originates from a specific part of the brain and then spreads to other regions.

In the early 1930s, Wilder Penfield and his associates at the Montreal Neurological Institute pioneered the use of surgery to remove the area of the brain where the abnormal activity begins, as a treatment for epilepsy in patients who did not respond well to drug therapy. Although the procedure proved to be successful in many instances, surgeons were reluctant to undertake cases requiring the removal of tissue that was close to the parts of the brain controlling speech and language. They wished to avoid these regions to reduce the likelihood that the surgery would merely substitute one debilitating disorder (aphasia) for another (epilepsy). Penfield's own words aptly describe the situation facing him and his colleagues:

> Twenty-five years ago we were embarking on the treatment of focal epilepsy by radical surgical excision of abnormal areas of brain. In the beginning it was our practice to refuse radical operation upon the dominant hemisphere unless a lesion lay anteriorly in the frontal lobe or posteriorly in the occipital lobe. Like other neurosurgeons, we feared that removal of cortex in other parts of this hemisphere would produce aphasia. [The] aphasia literature gave no clear guide as to just what might and what might not be removed with impunity.[20]

Clearly, what was required was a method for determining with precision the location of the centers controlling speech and language in a given patient. To meet this need, Penfield and his colleagues developed a procedure that involved mapping these areas by using direct electrical stimulation of the brain at the time of surgery.

Direct electrical stimulation of exposed brain tissue was not in itself a new procedure. Preliminary work in the early 1900s had shown that, because the brain itself does not contain pain receptors, it is possible for a patient to remain fully conscious while a neurosurgeon removes a flap of skull under local anesthesia and applies small electrical currents directly to the brain surface. The electrode used for the procedure could be moved to stimulate different regions of the brain. Such studies had shown that electrical stimulation of specific parts of the brain caused patients to see, hear, smell, or feel in an elementary way. Stimulation of other regions caused involuntary motor responses, such as the movement of an arm or a leg. The major contribution made by the Montreal group was the use of direct electrical stimulation as a tool for determining the location of the centers controlling speech and language in a given individual.*

---

* *Their work also had important implications for the way in which memories are stored in the brain, a topic that we discuss in Chapter 7. The interested reader is directed to* Speech and Brain Mechanisms, *by W. Penfield and L. Roberts, a fascinating, well-written account of three decades of research on brain stimulation at the Montreal Neurological Institute.*

During a typical procedure using direct electrical stimulation to map speech areas, the patient and surgeon are separated by a tent constructed of surgical drapes. A third person, acting as an observer, sits with the patient under the tent. During the time an electrical current is being applied to the regions of the brain normally employed for speech, the patient is unable to speak. The interference is known as aphasic arrest.[21]

The critical areas are determined by having the observer show the patient a series of pictures and asking the patient to identify each one. As the neurosurgeon moves the stimulating electrode over the surface of the brain to locate areas that produce interference with naming, small sterile squares of paper are dropped on the brain at the point of application of the electrode to provide a record of the areas stimulated. Throughout the procedure, lasting about 15 minutes, the patient is fully conscious but unaware of when and where the electrode will be placed. Figure 1.5 maps the points on the left hemisphere where stimulation has resulted in speech disturbance.

Aphasic arrest following the stimulation of a particular part of the brain is a sure sign that the region is part of the speech area of the language-specialized hemisphere. Penfield noted that aphasic arrest never follows from the stimulation of sites within the non-language-specialized half of the brain.

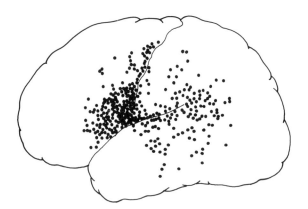

FIGURE 1.5   Points along the surface of the left hemisphere where electrical stimulation resulted in interference with speech. The interference included total speech arrest, hesitation, slurring, repetition of words, and inability to name. [From Penfield and Roberts, *Speech and Brain Mechanisms*, Fig. VII-3, p. 122. (Princeton, N.J.: Princeton University Press, 1959). Reprinted by permission of Princeton University Press.]

Several hundred patients have undergone direct electrical stimulation of the brain at the Montreal Neurological Institute and other institutions. Over the last 15 years, neurologist George Ojemann has conducted an extensive series of studies based on Penfield's pioneering technique. Together with earlier data, this recent work on direct electrical stimulation of the brain has proved to be of great theoretical and clinical value in localizing function within a hemisphere.[22]

...

The Wada Test: Anesthetizing a Hemisphere

Another test—known as the Wada test after its inventor, Juhn Wada—has been very valuable in localizing functions across hemispheres. In the Wada test, the neurosurgeon temporarily anesthetizes one hemisphere at a time on separate days before surgery so that it can be determined which side of the brain normally controls the ability to speak.[23] The first step in the Wada test is the insertion of a small tube, or catheter, into the carotid artery on one side of the patient's neck. The catheter permits the neurosurgeon to inject the drug sodium amobarbital into that artery at a later time. The carotid artery on each side brings blood to the hemisphere on the same side as the artery. Thus, sodium amobarbital injected into the right artery is carried to the right hemisphere. The drug is a barbiturate, chemically similar to the ingredients used in sleeping pills. However, because of the way it is administered in the Wada test, it puts only one-half of the brain to sleep at a time.

Moments before the drug is injected, the fully conscious patient lies flat on his or her back and is asked to count repeatedly from 1 to 20. The patient is also asked to keep both arms raised in the air while counting. Without prior warning, the drug is then slowly injected through the tube into the carotid artery. Within seconds of the injection, dramatic results occur.

First, the arm opposite the side of the injection falls limp. Because each half of the brain controls the opposite side of the body, the falling arm tells the neurosurgeon that the drug has reached the proper hemisphere and has taken effect. Second, the patient generally stops counting, either for a few seconds or for the duration of the drug's effect, depending on which hemisphere is affected. If the drug is injected on the same side as the hemisphere controlling speech, the patient remains speechless for 2 to 5 minutes, depending on the dose administered. If it is injected on the other side, the patient generally resumes counting within a few seconds and can answer questions with little difficulty while the drug is still inactivating the other half of the brain.[24]

Sodium amobarbital work has been the basis for the most commonly cited data about the relationship between handedness and brain organization. In the largest study of this type, reported in 1977, over 95 percent of all right-handers without any history of early brain damage had speech and language controlled by the left hemisphere; the remainder had speech controlled by the right hemisphere. Contrary to Broca's rule, a majority of left-handers also showed left-hemisphere speech; however, the percentage (about 70 percent) was smaller in left-handers than in right-handers. Roughly 15 percent of left-handers had speech in the right hemisphere, and 15 percent or so showed evidence of speech control in both hemispheres (bilateral speech control).[25] More recent evidence from studies using the amobarbital technique, however, suggested that the incidence of pure right-hemisphere speech may actually be much lower than previously reported in patients with no history of early damage.[26] What was believed to be right-hemisphere speech was, in reality, bilateral speech representation in many such cases.

The same 1977 study reported use of the Wada technique in patients who were known to have had some damage to the left hemisphere early in life. These patients showed a much higher incidence of right-hemisphere or bilateral speech: 70 percent of the left-handers and 19 percent of the right-handers fell into one or the other of these categories. This evidence points to the adaptability of the brain and to the limited value of handedness per se as an index of brain organization, particularly in left-handers.

·········

INFERRING BRAIN FUNCTION
FROM BRAIN DAMAGE:
The rise of cognitive neuropsychology

The clinical observations and neurological procedures we have just discussed formed the foundation of modern interest in hemispheric asymmetries. In the chapters that follow, we shall explore how investigators have built upon and extended these observations and techniques in many different and fascinating ways to give us our current understanding of the two hemispheres and their functions. Along with new findings and developments have also come new ways of thinking about the relationships between the brain and behavior. In this section we shall discuss the changes in approach and conceptualization that have taken place over time.

Over 100 years' worth of observations of neurological patients have firmly established the field of neuropsychology—the investigation of the disorders of perception, memory, language, thought, emotion, and action in patients suffering from neurological disease or injury. Broca's assertion that the seat of language is located in the posterior region of the left frontal lobe has been seen by many as a critical point in the establishment of neuropsychology. Broca's claim had two key parts: that language could be disrupted independently of other cognitive processes and that language could be localized to a specific region of the brain. Both were revolutionary in their implications and generated decades of research relating damage and disease in various parts of the brain to their consequences.

A model of the recognition and production of spoken and written words proposed in 1885 by neurologist L. Lichtheim nicely illustrates the early neuropsychological approach.[27] Based on observations of a number of patients with brain injury, Lichtheim's model has five different "centers" that are interlinked. Figure 1.6 shows the diagram that was derived from that model and used to explain several kinds of language disorders. For example, a person with a problem articulating words, but no other language impairment, was believed to have damage to center M; a patient who had difficulty repeating spoken words, but who could both understand and produce them, was seen as having an impairment to the connection between A and M.

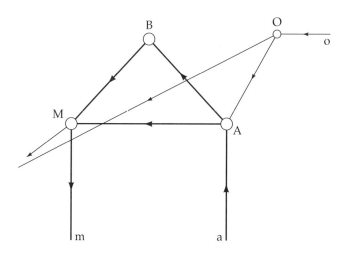

FIGURE 1.6   Lichtheim's model of word recognition and production.

This approach to neuropsychology, often referred to as diagram-making, enjoyed popularity into the early part of the twentieth century. As additional data were collected, however, diagram-making fell into disfavor because the actual observations of individual patients offered as support for the diagram models were often disappointingly weak and unconvincing. The approach was also criticized because anatomical data did not support the precise localization of centers controlling different functions that were postulated.

Even though some investigators continued to work within Lichtheim's diagram-maker tradition, by the 1930s a different approach to neuropsychology gained prominence. This new approach questioned the value of analyzing and reporting on single cases, as the the diagram-makers had done, and substituted a group approach to data analysis. Patients were assigned to a group, based on general information about the site of brain injury (e.g., left or right temporal lobe), and the performance of the groups was then compared in a series of standardized, quantifiable tests to see whether the groups showed different patterns of deficits. The use of control groups of normal subjects matched for important variables (age, sex, and education, for example) also became an important part of neuropsychological investigations.

Although sound in principle, the group study also has problems that limit its usefulness. Because the members of each group can be expected to show variation in severity of impairment, preinjury levels of performance, and so on, large numbers of subjects are required to obtain differences between groups that are statistically significant. Thus, it could (and did) take ten years of collecting data to complete some studies. Furthermore, interesting, and potentially very important, differences between subjects get "washed out" or lost in the analysis. The group study is based on averaging results across large numbers of people, and differences between individuals are obscured.

The mid-1960s saw the development of yet another approach to neuropsychology that would dramatically transform the field. The late neurologist Norman Geschwind, whose work plays a prominent role throughout many of the chapters that follow, is often credited with being instrumental in starting that transformation.[28] His own research led Geschwind to reconsider and appreciate the value of the diagram-makers and the single case study approach, and he called on his fellow investigators to reconsider as well.[29] At the same time, the discipline of cognitive psychology, which focuses on theories and models of normal cognitive function, began to firmly establish itself. The approaches of cognitive psychology were warmly embraced by Geschwind and other neurologists and neuropsychologists seeking to understand higher mental function both in the normal brain and in the diseased or injured brain. The union of cognitive psychology and the renewed interest in the single case study approach to neuropsychology established the discipline now known as cognitive neuropsychology.

···

Cognitive Neuropsychology

Cognitive neuropsychology studies the underlying mechanisms of the psychological processes that are the basis of our mental life—thinking, reading, speaking, recognizing, remembering—through the effects of brain injury. Its first aim is to relate the patterns of cognitive performance in brain-injured patients to psychological operations that are necessary for normal cognitive function; the second is to actually draw conclusions about normal cognitive processes from observations of the effects of brain injury.[30] Thus, cognitive neuropsychologists not only attempt to explain how brain injury disrupts normal function but also seek to increase our understanding of the way the normal brain and mind are organized by studying deficits that occur following brain injury.

The distinction between a traditional neuropsychological approach and that of the newer field of cognitive neuropsychology is nicely made when considering a patient who, following brain injury, could no longer remember, or "find," many words that had long been part of his vocabulary. This condition is known as anomia. Is it better to say "He is anomic because of damage to his left hemisphere," asks neuropsychologist Andrew Ellis, or "He is anomic because of damage to the psychological processes which mediate spoken word finding?"[31] We shall present both approaches. Our interest in the left and right hemisphere implies attention to "where," whereas our overall concern with function and process will lead us to deeper issues of "how" and "why."

···

The Logic of Associations and Dissociations

Central to the logic of relating normal functioning to the effects of brain injury is the concept of dissociations. A dissociation occurs when a patient performs very poorly on a task (e.g., reading) and normally or at a much higher level on another task (e.g., recognizing faces). We could argue that different cognitive processes are involved in each case. However, another explanation could be equally plausible. Perhaps the same cognitive processes are involved in both tasks, but reading is more difficult than face recognition. If this were the case, we would be observing differences in performance due to level of difficulty and not differences in the cognitive processes involved.

This logical problem can be addressed if we can identify patients who show the reverse patterns of symptoms, for example, greater impairment in face recognition and normal performance in reading. This situation, known as a double dissociation, makes a much stronger case for the existence of separate processes involved in the tasks in question.

In yet another situation, impairment in one task may be associated with impairment in other tasks. One plausible interpretation of this kind of observation is that all the tasks share a common process that is disrupted by brain damage. However, it is also possible that different sets of processes are involved, one for each task, and that these processes are mediated by areas in the brain close enough to be affected by one lesion. Such an association would be of neurological importance but of less interest from the perspective of a cognitive neuropsychologist.

...

The Concept of Modularity

The caveats about drawing conclusions from associations and dissociations follow from a view of mind-brain organization in which there are large numbers of semi-independent cognitive processes (or modules) that can be impaired independently. Mental life, according to the modularity hypothesis, is the result of the coordinated activity of many different modules, each of which engages its own form of processing independently of the activity in others.

The work of the late David Marr, who used computers to simulate complex human abilities, led him to propose that complex systems, be they brain or machines, evolve toward modular organization because of the potential for improvement and ease of detecting and correcting errors. In support of this idea he stated:

> Any large computation should be split up and implemented as a collection of small sub-parts that are as nearly independent of one another as the overall task allows. If a process is not designed in this way, a small change in one place will have consequences in many other places. This means that the process as a whole becomes extremely difficult to debug or to improve, whether by a human designer or in the course of natural evolution, because a small change to improve one part has to be accompanied by many simultaneous compensating changes elsewhere.[32]

Modularity is one of the key assumptions underlying cognitive neuropsychology, although it cannot be directly proved or disproved. Several other assumptions are also implicit in the approach taken by cognitive neuropsychologists, and we shall discuss these in greater detail in Chapter 6. For the moment it is sufficient to understand that these assumptions form the basis for the belief that a careful analysis of the pattern of intact and impaired performances and the pattern of errors shown by a patient after brain injury should lead to valid conclusions about the nature and normal function of the processing components. In other words, the patient's pattern of performances will provide a guide to the nature of the underlying disruption. This in turn will refine our understanding of normal cerebral organization.

There are, however, obstacles to the interpretation of the pattern of symptoms shown by a patient. These include individual variation in performance, the effects of the brain compensating for the injury, and the fact that most injuries cause fairly widespread damage and probably affect multiple processes, or modules. These confounding factors have been acknowledged for many years as problems for neuropsychology and for all attempts at inferring brain function from brain damage.

The basic problem is that there is no simple way to relate the function of a piece of destroyed brain tissue to the disabilities a patient seems to incur as a result of the damage. The oldest idea was to say simply that whatever a patient could not do was normally controlled by the area of the brain that was damaged. If a person had a lesion and could not see, for example, then the damaged area was said to control vision. If someone had a lesion in a different region and could not understand spoken language, then the area involved was said to be responsible for speech comprehension.

That approach has turned out to be much too simplistic. For one thing, most of the processes neatly labeled as visual perception, speech production, voluntary movement, or memory are really the result of many complex cerebral interactions. Whether they are diffusely spread over large areas of the brain or are limited to particular regions appears to be determined by which function we are studying, how precisely we are defining it, and how successfully we are able to limit our tests to what we assume they are testing. Just about any fairly limited damage to the brain is likely to interfere with a step or phase of some larger process (although not the entire process). It is also likely to interfere with a step or phase of more than one process. It is not unusual to see damage to a small area of the brain result in deficits in a number of different functions.

Another major problem in deducing brain function from clinical data is the fact that the brain tends to adjust its operations as best it can in the presence of damage. We cannot assume that the remaining intact areas of a damaged brain are operating as they would in a normal brain. It is not as though a piece is missing but everything else is working as it was before. In most cases of brain damage, there is some recovery of function over time—sometimes fairly dramatic recovery. The recovery can involve changes in the undamaged areas and is a tribute to the adaptability of the brain. This plasticity is a fascinating and obviously very useful feature, but it complicates the efforts of those who are trying to deduce brain function from clinical data.

These problems have not been eliminated by the assumptions of modern cognitive neuropsychology but have been placed in a slightly different perspective. Adjustments or compensation by the brain to injury is acknowledged as an important factor but is viewed as occurring strictly due to changes in the operations of undamaged modules, not to the creation of new modules. This notion allows investigators to assume that what appears to be missing at first, post injury, is in fact attributable to the functions of impaired modules and that changes postinjury are due to reorganization of other modules.

The knowledge we gain about the role of particular brain regions from the effects of brain damage is extremely valuable but tentative and most useful in combination with knowledge of brain function obtained in other ways. Other approaches are necessary both to corroborate brain-damage data and to add whatever knowledge can be gleaned from techniques that do not depend on great intrusions into normal functioning. We shall examine some of these approaches, including the use of neuroimaging—techniques to visualize both the structure and certain aspects of the function of the brain—in the following chapters. We shall return to what has been discovered by neuropsychological studies of brain damage in Chapters 6 and 7. Together these approaches produce converging lines of evidence about the workings of the left brain, the right brain, and the two together.

TWO

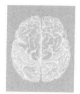

THE HUMAN SPLIT BRAIN:
Surgical Separation
of the Hemispheres

In 1940 a scientific report appeared that described the spread of epileptic discharge from one hemisphere to the other in the brains of monkeys.[1] The author concluded that the spread occurred largely or entirely by way of the corpus callosum, the largest of several commissures—bands of nerve fiber connecting regions of the left brain with similar areas of the right brain. Other investigators had already observed that damage to the corpus callosum from a tumor or other problem sometimes reduced the incidence of seizures in human epileptics.[2] Together, these findings paved the way for a new treatment for patients with epilepsy that could not be controlled in other ways: the split-brain operation.

In split-brain surgery—or commissurotomy—some of the fibers that connect the two cerebral hemispheres are cut. The first such operations to relieve epilepsy were performed in the early 1940s on about two dozen patients. These patients gave scientists an opportunity to study systematically the role of the corpus callosum in humans.

The role of the corpus callosum was a mystery to early researchers, who expected to find functions commensurate with its large size and strategic location within the brain. Animal research, however, showed that the consequences of split-brain surgery on a healthy organism are minimal. The behavior of a split-brain monkey, for example, appeared indistinguishable from that monkey's behavior before the operation. The apparent absence of any noticeable changes following commissurotomy led some scientists to suggest facetiously that the corpus callosum's only function was to hold the halves of the brain together and keep them from sagging.

Speculation about the consequences of split-brain surgery goes back to the nineteenth century and the writings of Gustav Fechner, considered by many to be the father of experimental psychology. Fechner believed that consciousness was an attribute of the cerebral hemispheres and that continuity of the brain was an essential condition for unity of consciousness. If it were possible to divide the brain through the middle, he speculated, something like the duplication of a human being would result. "The two cerebral hemispheres," he wrote, "while beginning with the same moods, predispositions, knowledge, and memories, indeed the same consciousness generally, will thereafter develop differently according to the external relations into which each will enter."[3] Fechner, however, considered this "thought experiment" involving separation of the hemispheres impossible to achieve in reality.

Fechner's views concerning the nature of consciousness did not go unchallenged. William McDougall, a founder of the British Psychological Society, argued strongly against the position that unity of consciousness depends on the continuity of the nervous system. To make his point, McDougall volunteered to have his corpus callosum cut if he ever got an incurable disease. He apparently wanted to show that his personality would not be split and that his consciousness would remain unitary.

McDougall never got the opportunity to put his ideas to the test, but the surgery Fechner thought an impossibility took place for the first time almost a century later. The issues these men raised have been among those explored by scientists seeking a fuller understanding of the corpus callosum through the study of split-brain patients.

·········

CUTTING 200 MILLION NERVE FIBERS:
A search for consequences

...

The First Split-Brain Operations on Humans

William Van Wagenen, a neurosurgeon from Rochester, New York, performed the first split-brain operations on humans in the early 1940s. Postsurgical testing by Andrew Akelaitis showed surprisingly little evidence of deficits in perceptual and motor abilities.[4] The operation seemed to have had no effect on everyday behavior. Unfortunately, success in relieving seizures seemed to vary greatly from patient to patient, and some patients showed little or no improvement after commissurotomy.

In retrospect, this variability can be attributed to two factors: (1) individual differences in the nature of the epilepsy in the patients and (2) variations in the actual surgical procedures used with each patient. Figure 2.1 shows the corpus callosum and the adjacent smaller commissures. Van Wagenen's operations varied considerably but usually included sectioning of the forward (anterior) half of the corpus callosum. In two patients he also sectioned a separate fiber band known as the anterior commissure.

At the time, the importance of these factors was not known, and Van Wagenen soon discontinued the commissurotomy procedure in cases of intractable epilepsy because it was not producing the dramatic results he had hoped for. Despite these discouraging findings, other investigators continued to study the functions of the corpus callosum in animals. A decade later, in the early 1950s, Ronald Myers and Roger Sperry made some remarkable discoveries that marked a turning point in efforts to study this enigmatic structure.

Myers and Sperry showed that visual information presented to one hemisphere in a cat with a sectioned corpus callosum was not available to the other hemisphere.[5] In most higher animals, the visual system is arranged so that each eye normally projects to both hemispheres. But by cutting into the optic-nerve crossing—the optic chiasm—experimenters can limit the sites where each eye sends its information. When this cut is made, the remaining fibers in the optic nerve transmit information to the hemisphere on the same side: Visual input to the left eye is sent only to the left hemisphere, and input to the right eye projects only to the right hemisphere.

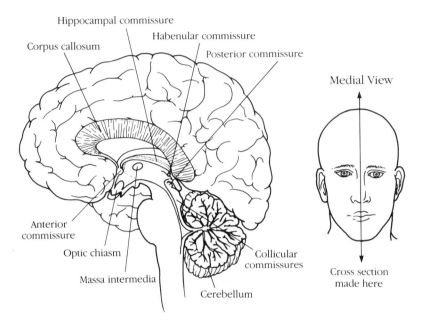

FIGURE 2.1   Major interhemispheric commissures. This is a sectional view of the right half of the brain as seen from the midline. [From Sperry, "The Great Cerebral Commissure," *Scientific American*, 1964. All rights reserved.]

Myers performed this operation on cats and subsequently taught each animal a visual discrimination task while it had one eye covered. A discrimination task involves, for example, pressing a lever when the animal sees a circle but not pressing the lever when it sees a square. Even when this training is done with one eye covered, a normal cat can later perform the task using either eye. Myers found that cats with sectioned optic chiasms were also able to perform the task using either eye when tested after the one-eyed training.

When Myers cut both the corpus callosum and the optic chiasm, however, the results were dramatically different. The cat trained with one eye open and one eye patched would learn to do a task well; but when the patch was switched to the other eye, the cat was totally unable to do the task. In fact, it had to be taught over again, taking just as long to learn the task as it had the first time. Myers and Sperry concluded that cutting the corpus callosum prevented the information going into one hemisphere from reaching the other hemisphere. They had, in effect, trained only one-half of a brain. Figure 2.2 schematically illustrates the different conditions of their experiment.

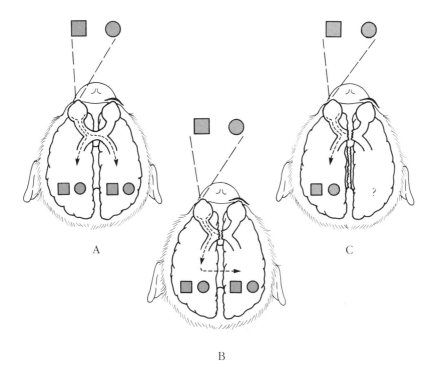

FIGURE 2.2   Split-brain experiment with cats. In a control situation, both eyes and both hemispheres see the stimuli. Experimental conditions alter this in the following ways: A. When one eye is patched, the other eye continues to send information to both hemispheres. B. When one eye is patched and the optic chiasm is cut, the visual information is transmitted to both hemispheres by way of the corpus callosum. C. When one eye is patched and both the optic chiasm and corpus callosum are cut, only one hemisphere receives visual information.

These findings, as well as later studies, led two neurosurgeons working near the California Institute of Technology, in Pasadena, California, to reconsider the use of split-brain surgery as a treatment for intractable epilepsy in human beings. The neurosurgeons, Philip Vogel and Joseph Bogen, reasoned that some of the earlier work with human patients had failed because the disconnection between the cerebral hemispheres was not complete. On the basis of this logic, coupled with new animal data showing no ill effects from the surgery, Bogen and Vogel performed a complete commissurotomy on the first of what was to be a new series (the California series) of patients suffering from intractable epilepsy.

Bogen and Vogel's reasoning proved to be correct. In some of the cases, the medical benefits of the surgery even appeared to exceed expectations. In striking contrast to its consequences for seizure activity, the operation appeared to leave patients unchanged in personality, intelligence, and behavior in general, just as had been the case with Van Wagenen's patients. More extensive and ingenious testing conducted in Roger Sperry's California Institute of Technology laboratory, however, soon revealed a more complex story, for which Sperry was awarded the 1981 Nobel Prize in Physiology or Medicine.

...

Testing for the Effects of Disconnecting Left from Right

Split-brain patient N.G., a California housewife, sits in front of a screen with a small black dot in the center. She is asked to look directly at the dot. When the experimenter is sure she is doing so, a picture of a cup is flashed briefly to the right of the dot. N.G. reports that she has seen a cup. Again, she is asked to fix her gaze on the dot. This time, a picture of a spoon is flashed to the left of the dot. She is asked what she saw. She replies, "No, nothing." She is then asked to reach under the screen with her left hand and to select, by touch only, from among several items the one that is the same as the one she has just seen. Her left hand palpates each object and then holds up the spoon. When asked what she is holding, she says, "Pencil."

Once again the patient is asked to fixate on the dot on the screen. A picture of a nude woman is flashed to the left of the dot. N.G.'s face blushes a little, and she begins to giggle. She is asked what she saw. She says, "Nothing, just a flash of light," and giggles again, covering her mouth with her hand. "Why are you laughing, then?" the investigator inquires. "Oh, doctor, you have some machine!" she replies.

The procedure just described is frequently used in studies with split-brain patients, and the testing arrangement is illustrated in Figure 2.3. The patient sits in front of a tachistoscope, a device that allows the investigator to control precisely the duration for which a picture or pattern is presented on a screen. The presentations are kept brief, about one- or two-tenths of a second (100 to 200 milliseconds), so that the patient does not have time to move his or her eyes away from the fixation point while the picture is still on the screen.* This procedure is

---

* *The rapid eye movements that occur when gaze is shifted from one point to another are known as saccadic eye movements or saccades. Although, once started, saccades are extremely rapid, they take about 200 milliseconds to initiate with the eye at rest. If a stimulus is presented for less than 200 milliseconds, then the stimulus is no longer present by the time an eye movement can occur.*

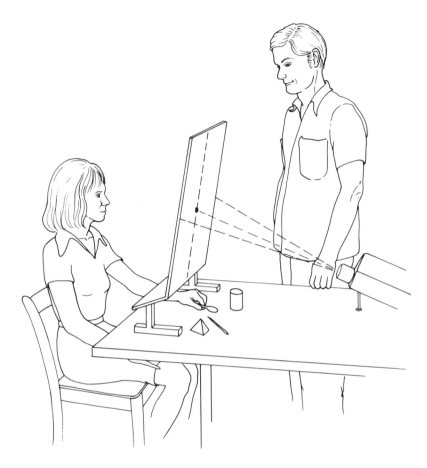

FIGURE 2.3   Basic testing arrangement used to lateralize visual and tactile information and allow tactile responses.

necessary to ensure that visual information is presented initially to only one hemisphere. Stimuli presented to only one hemisphere are said to be lateralized.

The design of the human nervous system is such that each cerebral hemisphere receives information primarily from the opposite half of the body. This contralateral rule applies to vision and hearing as well as to body movement and touch (somatosensory) sensation, although the situation in vision and hearing is more complex.

In vision, the contralateral rule applies to the right and left sides of one's field of view (visual field) rather than to the right and left eyes per se. When both eyes are fixating on a single point, stimuli to the right of the point of fixation are registered in the left half of the brain, while the right half of the brain processes everything occurring to the left of the fixation point. This split and crossover of visual information results from the manner in which the nerve fibers from corresponding regions of both eyes are divided between the cerebral hemispheres. Figure 2.4 shows both the optics and the neural wiring involved.

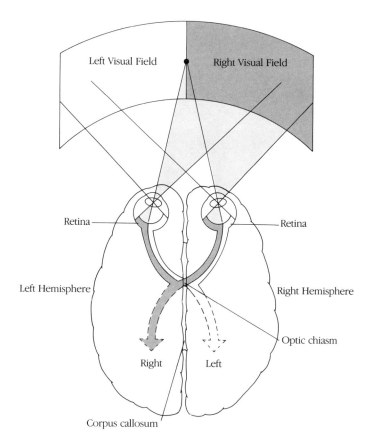

FIGURE 2.4   Visual pathways to the hemispheres. When fixating on a point, each eye sees both visual fields but sends information about the right visual field only to the left hemisphere and information about the left visual field only to the right hemisphere. This crossover and split is a result of the manner in which the nerve fibers leading from the retina divide at the back of each eye. The visual areas of the left and right hemisphere normally communicate through the corpus callosum. If the callosum is cut and the eyes and head are kept from moving, each hemisphere can see only half of the visual world.

In animal studies, as we have seen, visual information can be directed to one hemisphere by cutting the optic chiasm so that the remaining fibers in the optic nerve are those transmitting information to the hemisphere on the same side as the eye. This sectioning technique allows experimenters to present a stimulus to either hemisphere alone by simply presenting the stimulus to the appropriate eye. The procedure is used only with animals, however, because cutting the chiasm substantially reduces peripheral vision, eliminates binocular depth perception, and plays no part in the rationale for the split-brain operation on humans. For these reasons, investigators wishing to transmit visual information to one hemisphere at a time in a human split-brain patient must do so through a combination of controlling the patient's fixation and presenting information to one side of space.

With this information as background, let us return to an analysis of the tests administered to patient N.G. In those tests, the patient saw the left half of the screen (everything to the left of the fixation point) with the right side of her brain and everything to the right with her left hemisphere. The split in her brain prevented the normal interchange of information between the two sides that would have occurred before her surgery. In effect, each side of her brain was blind to what the other side was seeing, a state of affairs dramatically brought out by the knowledge that only one hemisphere controls speech.

As a consequence, the patient reported perfectly well any stimuli falling in the right visual field (projecting to the verbal left hemisphere), although she was unable to tell anything about what was flashed in her left visual field (sent to the mute right hemisphere). The fact that she "saw" stimuli in the left visual field is amply demonstrated by the ability of her left hand (basically controlled by the right brain) to select the spoon from among several objects that were hidden from her view. It is also demonstrated by her emotional reaction to the nude picture, despite her claim not to have seen anything.[6]

The patient's response to the nude picture is particularly interesting. She seemed puzzled by her own reactions to what had appeared. Her right hemisphere saw the picture and processed it sufficiently to evoke a general, nonverbal reaction—the giggling and the blushing. The left hemisphere, meanwhile, did not "know" what the right had seen, although its comment about "some machine" seems to be a sign that it was aware of the bodily reactions induced by the right hemisphere. It is very common for the verbal left hemisphere to try to make sense of what has occurred in testing situations where information is presented to the right hemisphere. As a result, the left brain sometimes comes out with erroneous and often elaborate rationalizations based on partial cues.

·········

EVERYDAY BEHAVIOR
AFTER SPLIT-BRAIN SURGERY

It is natural to wonder what disconnection effects can be observed in the everyday behavior of split-brain patients. Some instances of bizarre behavior have been described by both patients and onlookers and are frequently mentioned in popular articles on split-brain research. One patient, for example, described the time he found his left hand struggling against his right when he tried to put his pants on in the morning: One hand was pulling them up while the other hand was pulling them down. In another incident, the same patient was angry and forcibly reached for his wife with his left hand while his right hand grabbed the left in an attempt to stop it.[7]

The frequency with which such stories are mentioned would lead one to believe that they are commonplace events. In fact, the frequency of such events is low in most patients. However, there are exceptions. One example is P.O.V., a female patient operated on by neurosurgeon Mark Rayport of the Medical College of Ohio. The patient reported frequent dramatic signs of interhemispheric competition for at least three years after surgery. "I open the closet door. I know what I want to wear. As I reach for something with my right hand, my left comes up and takes something different. I can't put it down if it's in my left hand. I have to call my daughter."[8]

Cases such as these support the concept that the cerebral commissures transmit information that is inhibitory in nature. In other words, activity in one hemisphere leads to callosal transmissions that serve to moderate, decrease, or stop certain activities in the other.

Research with animals indicated that the cerebral commissures pass both excitatory and inhibitory information.[9] Colwin Trevarthen reported that split-brain baboons at times reached for an object with both forelimbs at the same time, presumably because no inhibitory processes were available to establish unilateral control over the action.[10] Other work demonstrated that monkeys whose corpus callosum was cut reached to grasp presumably hallucinated objects when the occipital region of one hemisphere was electrically stimulated.[11] This action did not occur in animals with intact commissures, a result suggesting that in normal animals the unstimulated hemisphere "disconfirms" the hallucination through inhibitory information passed via the callosum.

It seems likely that corpus callosum-mediated inhibition is an important process in maximizing efficiency in behavioral performance and perhaps even in producing new kinds of functions. It is very apparent, however, that these functions are quickly masked by compensatory mechanisms in most split-brain patients. In fact, in a large majority of cases the two sides of the body appear to continue to work in a coordinated fashion. Perhaps the rarity of patients with persistent disconnection effects indicates that more than callosal damage is necessary to prevent adjustment to the commissurotomy.

A battery of sophisticated tests specifically designed to detect unusual behaviors is generally needed to identify a commissurotomy patient. However, there are reports of subtle changes in behavior or ability after surgery. Although some of the reported changes have not held up when carefully studied, others do appear to be verifiable consequences of the operation.

...

Subtle Deficits Following Surgery

Several patients have reported great difficulty in learning to associate names with faces after surgery. Verification of this problem came from a study in which subjects had to learn first names for each of three pictures of young men.[12] This procedure was only incidental to the main purpose of the study, but it proved to be a major stumbling block for the subjects. The investigators reported that subjects eventually learned the name-face associations by isolating some unique feature in each picture (for example, "Dick has glasses") rather than by associating the name with the face as a whole. This finding suggests that the deficit in the ability to associate names and faces may be due to a disconnection of the verbal naming functions of the left side of the brain from the facial-recognition abilities of the right side.

Deficits in the ability to solve geometric problems have been anecdotally linked to the sectioning of the corpus callosum. Patient L.B., a high school student with an IQ considerably above average, was transferred out of geometry into a class in general math after he experienced inordinate difficulty with the course. Another report told of a college student who had exceptional difficulty with geometry despite average grades in other courses. Studies with split-brain patients to determine the ability of each hemisphere to match two- and three-dimensional forms on the basis of common geometric features showed that the right hemisphere was markedly superior, especially on the most difficult matches.[13] Thus, as in the preceding example, the patient's deficits may be the result of the disconnection of the speaking left hemisphere from the right-hemisphere regions specialized for such tasks.

Another complaint of some split-brain patients is that they no longer dream. Because dreaming is primarily a visual-imaging process, investigators have speculated that it might be the responsibility of the right half of the brain. The operation may disconnect this aspect of the patient's mental life from the speaking left hemisphere and thus result in verbal reports that the patient does not dream.

This idea, however, has not been confirmed by further research. Split-brain patients were monitored for brain-wave activity while sleeping and were awakened whenever the recordings indicated that they were dreaming. When asked to describe the dreams they had just been having, the patients provided the experimenters with descriptions of their dreams, a result contradicting the prediction that they would be unable to do so.[14]

Other anecdotal evidence documents poorer memory after surgery. Recent work suggests a physiological basis for these observations. Some patients, specifically those with damage to the hippocampal commissures*or other extracallosal structures, display memory deficits, whereas others do not.[15] In another study involving pre- and post-surgical memory tests, patients with commissurotomies that included the posterior region of the callosum showed memory impairments, with recall more affected that recognition. Patients with partial callosal sections that excluded the posterior region did not show these deficits.[16] The investigators concluded that these results were consistent with the earlier work, since the hippocampal commissure is usually damaged during posterior sectioning, but not during anterior sectioning, of the corpus callosum. Much more work needs to be done, however, to clarify the nature of the deficit and the neuroanatomical structures involved.

It is not clear why a few patients seem to show persistent patterns of deficit after commissurotomy, whereas the majority of patients do not. Important differences among patients in their preoperative condition and surgical treatment probably exist, although we do not yet know what they are. There are some consequences of commissurotomy, however, that are dramatic and quite consistent across patients but are short lived.

---

* The hippocampus is a subcortical structure that is divided into two parts connected by a band of fibers. It is believed to play an important role in memory and is discussed in Chapter 7.

...

Acute Disconnection Syndrome

Commissurotomy patients are often mute for a time after surgery. Sometimes they have difficulty controlling the left side of the body, which may even be paralyzed at first. As the patient recovers use of the left hand, competitive movements between the left and the right hands sometimes occur. This syndrome, known as the acute disconnection syndrome, usually passes quickly. It is probably due to the surgical division of the commissures and to general trauma resulting from the compression of the right hemisphere required to provide access to the nerve tracts between the hemispheres.

After recovering from the initial shock of major brain surgery, most patients report a feeling of improved well-being. Less than two days after surgery, one young patient was well enough to quip that he had a "splitting headache." Within a few weeks, the symptoms of the acute disconnection syndrome subside, making it necessary to use carefully contrived laboratory tests to reveal the effects of the operation.

....

CROSS CUING

As more split-brain patients were studied, certain inconsistencies in the findings began to appear with greater frequency. Patients previously unable to verbally identify objects held out of sight in the left hand began to name some items. Some pictures flashed in the left visual field (to the right hemisphere) were also correctly identified verbally. One interpretation of these results was that, over time, the right hemispheres of the patients acquired the ability to produce speech. Another was that information was being transmitted between the hemispheres by way of pathways other than those that had been cut.

Although these were interesting and exciting possibilities, Michael Gazzaniga and Steven Hillyard proposed a much simpler explanation for their findings.[17] They coined the term *cross cuing* to refer to patients' attempts to use whatever cues are available to make information accessible to both hemispheres. Cross cuing is most obvious in the case where a patient is given an object to hold and to identify only with his or her left hand; the object is out of sight and thus disconnected from the verbal left hemisphere. When, for example, a comb or a toothbrush is placed in the patient's left hand, the patient will often stroke the brush or the surface of the comb, and then immediately identify the object—because the left hemisphere hears the tell-tale sounds.

Cross cuing provides a way for one hemisphere to provide the other with information about what it is experiencing and can be quite subtle. A good example of this is the patient who was able to indicate verbally whether a 0 or a 1 had been flashed to either hemisphere. The same patient was unable to verbally identify pictures of objects flashed to the right hemisphere, a test suggesting that he lacked the ability to speak from the right hemisphere. Instead, the investigators proposed that cross cuing was involved; they hypothesized that the left hemisphere would begin counting "subvocally" after a presentation to the left visual field and that these signals were picked up by the right hemisphere. When the correct number was reached, the right hemisphere would signal the left to stop and report that digit out loud.

To test this idea, the patient was presented with an expanded version of the task: The digits 2, 3, 5, and 8 were added without his knowledge. At first the subject was very surprised when a new number was presented. With a little practice, however, he was able to give the correct answer for all the numbers presented to the right hemisphere, but with some hesitation when the number was high. In contrast, responses to the same digits presented in the right visual field (to the left hemisphere) were quite prompt.

These findings supported the idea that the left hemisphere began counting subvocally after a digit was presented to the right hemisphere. The larger the number of potential digits, the longer the list of numbers the left hemisphere had to go through before reaching the correct one.

Cross cuing generally is not a conscious attempt by the patient to trick the investigator. Instead, it is a natural tendency by an organism to use whatever information it has to make sense of what is going on. This tendency, in fact, contributes further insight into why the common, everyday behavior of split-brain patients seems so unaffected by the surgery.

·········

LANGUAGE AND THE HEMISPHERES

Split-brain research has dramatically confirmed that, in most persons, control of speech is localized to the left hemisphere. But what about other language abilities? How well can the right hemisphere understand language, either written or spoken? The earliest split-brain studies to consider these questions flashed printed words to either the left or the right hemisphere. However, the brief presentation time necessary to ensure that the stimuli reached only one hemisphere placed severe limitations on the kinds of words that could be used. This problem was eliminated with the development of a new method of restricting visual stimuli to one hemisphere. Developed by Eran Zaidel, who worked extensively with two of the patients in the original California series, it utilizes a device known as the Z lens, which is illustrated in Figure 2.5.[18] The Z lens is a contact lens that permits the patient to move his or her eyes freely without a time limit when examining something, but at the same time ensures that only one hemisphere of the patient's brain receives the visual information.

Zaidel's strategy was to test the comprehension abilities of each hemisphere by using a variety of stimuli that had been used previously both with children and with aphasic patients. The goal was to obtain data that would allow him to compare the abilities of the right hemispheres of split-brain patients with the right-hemisphere abilities of the two other groups, for which norms were already available.

In the auditory vocabulary test, two split-brain patients heard a single word spoken by the experimenter and then viewed a display of three pictures through the Z lens. Each patient's task was to select the picture that corresponded with the word. Because the pathways of the auditory system are arranged so that each ear sends information to both hemispheres, under ordinary conditions it is not possible to tell whether one or both hemispheres have understood a spoken message. The Z lens, however, allowed Zaidel to lateralize the response alternatives to one hemisphere so that he could determine how well each half of the brain matched a spoken word to its written counterpart.

The same procedure was used with the token test, in which the subject was asked to arrange plastic shapes of different colors and sizes according to verbal instructions, such as "Put the yellow square under the green circle." Again, instructions were delivered orally while the objects to be arranged were viewed through the Z lens. The token test is commonly used as a test of damage to left-hemisphere language zones, because it is sensitive to impairments not picked up by other aphasia tests.

Zaidel's work revealed a surprising degree and array of comprehension abilities in the right hemisphere.[19] The pattern of results was complex, however, and it was not possible for Zaidel to make a simple summary statement about the right hemisphere's linguistic "age" or "health." On the vocabulary tests, the right hemisphere generally performed at least as well as a normal ten-year-old; whereas on the token test, it experienced difficulties characteristic of aphasic impairments.

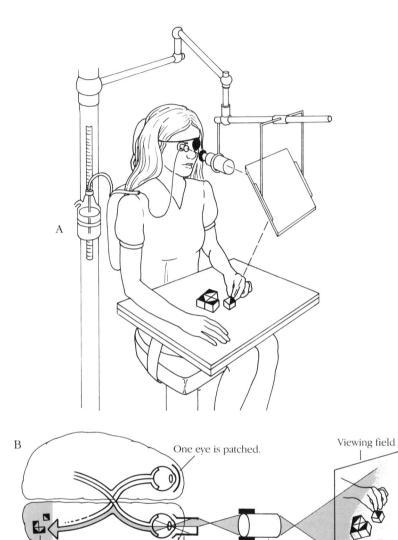

The image projects to only one hemisphere even though the subject can scan the entire viewing field.

Z lens allows the image to fall on only one half of the retina.

Telescope reduces the viewing field to the small image projected onto the surface of the contact lens.

One eye is patched.

Viewing field

FIGURE 2.5   The Z lens. A. The Z lens setup keeps the patient's field of view lateralized to one hemisphere. B. One eye is patched, and the image is projected to only one-half of the retina of the other eye. [Part A adapted from Zaidel, "Language Comprehension in the Right Hemisphere Following Cerebral Commissurotomy," in *Language Acquisition and Language Breakdown: Parallels and Divergencies,* ed., A Caramazza and E. Zurif, Fig. 12.2, p. 233, (Baltimore, Md.: The Johns Hopkins University Press, 1978).]

The language asymmetries we have reviewed so far are those found in typical split-brain patients—if it is appropriate to talk of "typical" patients, in view of their varied neurological history. The question of whether findings from these patients reflect the division of functions between hemispheres in the normal brain is highlighted when we consider how neurological histories can produce dramatic departures from this picture.

...

The Right-Hemisphere Language Controversy

On the basis of his review of research dealing with the role of the right hemisphere in language, Michael Gazzaniga argued that the normal right hemisphere is nonlinguistic.[20] Signs of linguistic ability in the right hemisphere of split-brain patients are attributable, he claimed, to early left-hemisphere damage resulting in reorganization of language functions to the right hemisphere. Gazzaniga noted that only 3 of the 28 patients operated on by the late Donald Wilson of the Dartmouth Medical School, showed evidence of right-hemisphere language to some degree; in each of these cases, signs of early left-hemisphere injury were present. He further noted that only two patients from the California series, L.B. and N.G., showed evidence of right-hemisphere language, that these were the same patients extensively studied by Zaidel using the Z lens, and that both are suspected of having left-hemisphere injury.

Zaidel disagreed with Gazzaniga's conclusions.[21] He claimed that six, not two, California split-brain patients showed evidence of right-hemisphere language and that there is little reason to believe that L.B. and N.G. had the kind of left-hemisphere lesion that would result in right-hemisphere takeover of language function. He further pointed to clinical data suggesting a role for the right hemisphere in language, citing right-hemisphere recovery of some language functions in aphasia and the fact that selective language deficits do occur following right-hemisphere lesions in right-handers. He suggested that differences among aphasic patients in the degree to which the right hemisphere takes over language functions result from variability in the amount of interference to the right hemisphere caused by different kinds of left-hemisphere lesions. He also noted that there may be inherent variability among right-handers in the language functions of the right hemisphere.*

---

* See Chapter 6 for a more extensive discussion of the role of the right hemisphere in language and in recovery from aphasia.

In a recent review of language functions following commissurotomy and hemispherectomy (removal of one-half the brain), Zaidel presented additional data to strengthen the case for the existence of right-hemisphere language. He acknowledged, however, that much is still unknown about language abilities in the disconnected hemispheres.[22] It is clear that existing data are not sufficient to clarify the very important question of the nature and extent of right-hemisphere involvement in language in the normal brain. The issue is one of considerable theoretical as well as practical significance, however, and is currently the focus of a great deal of research.

...

Some Cautions About Interpreting Data

The preceding controversy points to the need for caution in extending any research finding with split-brain subjects to normal subjects. Both the factors that produced the epilepsy in the first place and the epilepsy itself may have produced changes in the brains of split-brain patients, making their brains fundamentally different from those of normal subjects. Norman Geschwind noted that some commissurotomy patients probably suffered epilepsy as a result of brain lesions occurring in utero. Such prenatal lesions have been shown to result in significant reorganizations of the brain that differ from those occurring after birth. Geschwind also pointed out that long-standing epilepsy may itself produce major changes in brain organization. Perhaps the epilepsy has modified the use of brain pathways, thereby making the patients different from the unaffected adult population.

Summarizing his views on this issue, Geschwind observed that "many of the arguments in the literature between different investigators as to the effects of callosal section probably do not reflect a real difference in the adequacy of the data, but simply arise because the investigators have been studying patients in whom the patterns of brain development and connections are simply not equivalent."[23] Some researchers would dismiss split-brain research because of the problems in interpreting results. A better approach, we think, is to continue to learn what we can about the brain from the study of split-brain patients, remembering that such research will be but one of many sources of evidence about hemispheric asymmetries.

·········

VISUOSPATIAL FUNCTIONS
IN THE HEMISPHERES

On the basis of split-brain studies, the most general statement that can be made about right-hemisphere specializations is that they are nonlinguistic functions that seem to involve complex visual and spatial processes.

The perception of part–whole relations, for example, seems to be superior in the right hemisphere. In one task, patients viewed line drawings of the separated pieces of geometric shapes that had been cut up. The task was to decide which of three solid alternatives felt with one hand, but not seen, was represented by the fragmented figure. The left hand was far superior on this task; the right hand showed chance performance in six of seven patients. In another study, arcs (sections of circles) were presented to either the left or the right visual field of commissurotomy patients. After each presentation, they were asked to choose which circle from a set of different-sized circles would be formed by the arcs they saw. The patients performed much better when their judgments were based on arcs presented to the left visual field (right hemisphere).[24]

One of the most dramatic demonstrations of right-hemisphere superiority in visuospatial tasks was recorded on film by Gazzaniga and Sperry while they were testing W.J., the first patient of the California series. W.J. was presented with several cubes, each containing two red sides, two white sides, and two half-red and half-white sides divided along the diagonal. His task was to arrange these blocks to form squares with patterns identical to those shown on a series of cards. Figure 2.6 illustrates the task.

The beginning of the film shows W.J. readily assembling the blocks with his left hand to form a particular pattern. When he tries to form a pattern with his right hand, however, he experiences great difficulty. Slowly and with considerable indecision, the right hand arranges the blocks. At one point, the left hand moves into the picture and begins to assemble the blocks in the correct pattern. It is gently but firmly removed from the table by the investigator, while the right hand continues to fumble, unaided by the more skillful left.

Other evidence pointing to right-hemisphere superiority in visuospatial ability comes from differences in the abilities of the two hands of

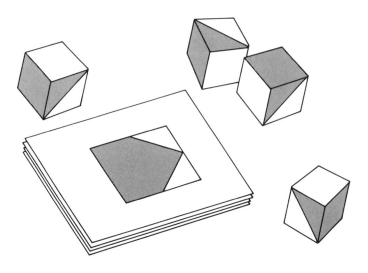

FIGURE 2.6   A block-design task. The subject is asked to arrange the colored blocks to match the pattern shown on a card.

the split-brain patient to draw a figure of a cube. Invariably, the left hand produces a better drawing. Examples are shown in Figure 2.7.

What is the basis for the right hemisphere's superior abilities in these visuospatial tasks? Two possibilities suggested themselves to investigators. First, the right hemisphere could be dominant for the expression of visual understanding, just as the left hemisphere is dominant for the expression of language understanding, although both halves of the brain might be equally skilled in perceiving spatial relationships. This view emphasizes an asymmetry in the ability to perform the complex motor acts required by the tasks. An alternative interpretation holds that there are true differences in perceptual abilities between hemispheres.

Laura Franco and Roger Sperry tested each hand of right-handed commissurotomy patients and normal control subjects on matching unseen objects by touch with geometric shapes presented in free vision. They found that the left hands of the split-brain subjects performed consistently better than did the right hands. Furthermore, this left-hand (right-hemisphere) superiority increased as the shapes became less geometric and more free form. When the sets of objects to be matched consisted only of free-form contours, the right hand (left hemisphere) performed barely above choice level. Normal subjects did equally well with either hand on these tasks.[25]

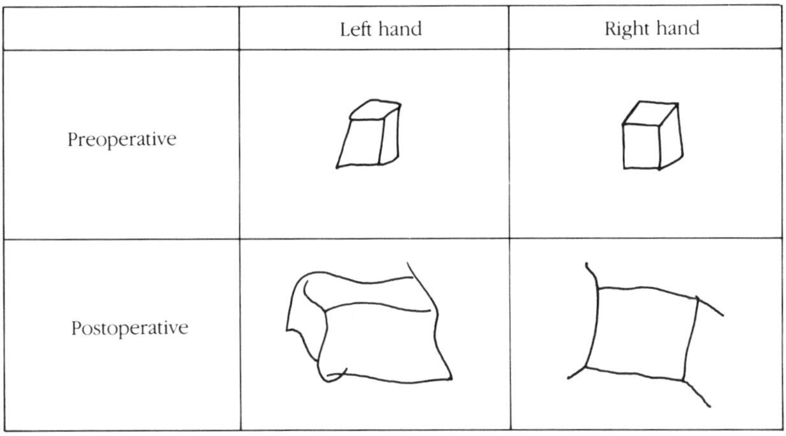

	Left hand	Right hand
Preoperative		
Postoperative		

FIGURE 2.7   Cube drawings before and after commissurotomy. Preoperatively, the patient could draw a cube with either hand. Postoperatively, the right hand performed poorly. The patient was righthanded. [From Gazzaniga and LeDoux, *The Integrated Mind*, Fig. 18, p. 52 (New York: Plenum Press, 1978).]

One can argue that left-hemisphere difficulty increased as the objects became less describable verbally or, perhaps, less structurally constrained. In either case, the results showed that matching such objects by touch and visual perception requires the involvement of the right hemisphere, for it seems that simply disconnecting the two half-brains results in a severe breakdown in the performance of the preferred right hand. What seems most important in solving the matching tasks is not the tactile manipulation and sensations from the fingers of the hand but "knowing what kind of shaped object to feel for . . . this in turn requires being able to subjectively visualize what the seen figure would look like if folded up."[26] Thus, the right-hemisphere superiority is not just in spatially related hand activities but also in visual mental manipulations. We shall discuss some further implications of this issue in Chapter 12.

·········

IMAGERY

The subject of visual mental imagery has enjoyed a recent surge of attention as investigators have sought to understand how visual imagery is generated and what parts of the brain are involved in it. Although the visual, nonverbal nature of imagery initially suggests greater involvement of the right hemisphere, some investigators have reported evidence of a special role for the left hemisphere.[27]

Split-brain patients appear to be close to ideal subjects in which to study visual imagery. With this in mind, Martha Farah and her colleagues presented J.W., a male patient who is part of the Wilson series, with uppercase letters in the left or right visual field and asked him to indicate whether their lowercase counterparts were tall or short by pushing one of two buttons. For example, lowercase versions of B, D, and F are tall, whereas lowercase versions of A, C, and E are short. J.W.'s task was to image the lowercase form of the letters as each was presented and to respond appropriately. J.W. did well when the stimuli were presented in the right visual field (left hemisphere), but he could not make these judgments above chance level when the stimuli were presented in the left visual field (right hemisphere).[28]

This finding was consistent with Farah's earlier analysis of single case studies of brain-damaged patients displaying loss of visual imagery; all were seen as pointing to left-hemisphere specialization for image generation.[29] Stephen Kosslyn has taken this analysis further and suggested that the left hemisphere is specialized at generating fully detailed, multipart images, whereas the right hemisphere generates "skeletal" images.[30] This conclusion was supported by work with split-brain patient J.W. Tasks involving decisions about parts of imaged objects could not be handled by his right hemisphere, although tasks involving the overall shape of objects were successfully performed.

Justine Sergent, however, has challenged the validity of the claim for left- hemisphere specialization for imagery.[31] Her arguments are based on her own work with additional split-brain patients, her review of other findings, and her critical reanalysis of the evidence from single case studies. She concluded, "As far as can be inferred from the existing evidence, neither hemisphere has an exclusive competence at generating visual images and, at present, a conservative interpretation of the findings points to a simultaneous involvement of the two hemispheres in this process."[32]

It is clear that much remains to be learned about the brain mechanisms involved in various aspects of visual imagery; at the present time, however, a convincing case has yet to be made for lateralization to one hemisphere, either left or right.

·········

PARTIAL COMMISSUROTOMY

Since the split-brain operations of the early 1960s, several neurosurgeons have attempted to control intractable epilepsy with a procedure less radical than the severing of all the forebrain commissures. The idea was to limit the surgery to the areas of the corpus callosum and anterior commissure most likely to transmit epileptic discharges in any particular patient. If the source of the epileptic discharges could be localized to some specific region of the brain, they reasoned, then cutting only those fibers connecting that area with the opposite hemisphere should help control the epilepsy.

Evidence gathered from patients who have undergone partial commissurotomy (where only selected portions of the corpus callosum are cut) has suggested that there is a high degree of specificity of function within the cerebral commissures of humans. Parts of the front region of the corpus callosum are responsible for somatosensory—or touch—transfer. The rear third of the corpus callosum, the splenium, transfers visual information.

A patient with the front half of the callosum cut is not able to tell what he has in the left hand but is able to verbally identify an image flashed in the left visual field. The tactile information is not accessible to the verbal left hemisphere, whereas the visual information gets across. A patient with only the splenium cut shows the reverse pattern of information transfer.[33]

·········

INFORMATION PROCESSING IN THE
TWO HEMISPHERES

As research into the specialized functions of the two hemispheres continued, the pattern of results suggested a new way to conceptualize hemispheric differences. Instead of a breakdown based on the type of tasks (for example, verbal or spatial) best performed by each hemisphere, a dichotomy based on different ways of dealing with information in general seemed to emerge.

According to this analysis, the left hemisphere is specialized for language functions, but these specializations are a consequence of the left hemisphere's superior analytic skills, of which language is one manifestation. Similarly, the right hemisphere's superior visuospatial performance is derived from its synthetic, holistic manner of dealing with information. Much of the work that led to this reanalysis of hemispheric differences was conducted by Jerre Levy and her colleagues working with the California series of patients.

One of the first suggestions that the two hemispheres have different information-processing styles came from a study in which split-brain patients were asked to match small wooden blocks held in the left or the right hand with the appropriate two-dimensional representation selected from drawings of blocks shown in "opened-up" form. Overall, the left hand was considerably better than the right at this task, but the most interesting finding was that the two hemispheres appeared to use different strategies in approaching the problem.

An analysis of errors showed that the patterns the right hand (left hemisphere) found easier to deal with were the patterns that were easy to describe in words but difficult to discriminate visually. For the left hand (right hemisphere), the reverse was true. Thus, the left hemisphere appeared to make its matches on the basis of verbal descriptions of the properties of the blocks and the two-dimensional patterns. It seemed unable to fold up the two-dimensional representation mentally so that a match could be made on the basis of overall appearance.[34]

Other work has shown that the two hemispheres differ in the kinds of information they pick up from visual stimuli. We shall discuss these studies at greater length later in this chapter. For now, we need only point out that pictures that can be matched either by their functions (such as a cake on a plate matched with a spoon and a fork) or, by their appearances (such as a cake on a plate matched with a hat with a brim) are handled differently by the two hemispheres. See Figure 2.8 for examples of the stimuli. When given ambiguous instructions—simply to match similar stimuli—the left hemisphere of the split-brain patient matches by function and the right hemisphere matches by appearance.

Levy concluded that the left hemisphere's strategy in dealing with incoming information is best characterized as analytic, whereas the right hemisphere appears to process information in a holistic manner.[35] There are other ways to interpret the differences we have just considered, but the analytic-holistic distinction has been the most influential in moving thinking about hemispheric differences away from the verbal-nonverbal dichotomy. The latter is clearly too simplistic to explain all the results found with brain-damaged, split-brain, and (as we shall see in the next chapter) normal subjects.

·········

VISUAL COMPLETION

Patient N.G. sits in front of a screen. Once again, she is asked to gaze at a spot marked in the middle. A strange picture appears briefly on the

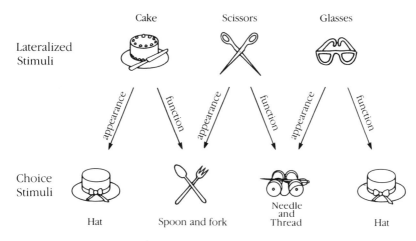

FIGURE 2.8   Function and appearance matches by split-brain patients. The stimuli in the top row are visually presented to one hemisphere at a time. The patient is instructed to pick the best "match" from the choice stimuli. When the left hemisphere sees the stimuli, it tends to match by function. When the right hemisphere sees the stimuli, it tends to match by appearance. [Adapted from Levy and Trevarthen, "Metacontrol of Hemispheric Function in Human Split Brain Patients," Fig. 1, p. 302, *Journal of Experimental Psychology*, 2, 1976, (American Psychological Association), Reprinted by permission.]

screen. It is a split face made up of the left half of one face and the right half of another, joined down the middle. On the right is half of the face she has been taught to identify as "Dick"; on the left, the face belonging to "Tom." A split stimulus such as this is known as a chimeric figure. It is named after Chimera, a mythical monster made up of parts of different animals. N.G. is asked to report what she saw. She says she saw "Dick." When questioned further, she denies that there was anything odd about the picture. Later, the same composite picture is flashed on the screen. This time she is asked not to say anything. Instead, she is shown several faces in full view and is asked to point with either hand to the one she saw. This time she points to the picture of "Tom."

This experiment, illustrated by a similar task in Figure 2.9, again shows that each half of the brain is blind to what the other side is seeing. What is particularly striking is that in this split-face study, each half of the brain seems to see a normal, symmetrical face, despite the unusual composition of the stimulus. In addition, the patient's report of what she sees changes with the nature of the response she is asked to make. The patient shows no sign of conflict when this occurs.

Completion, the tendency for split-brain patients to see as whole what are really partial figures falling at the visual midline, was first noted when patients showed the ability to identify accurately a square

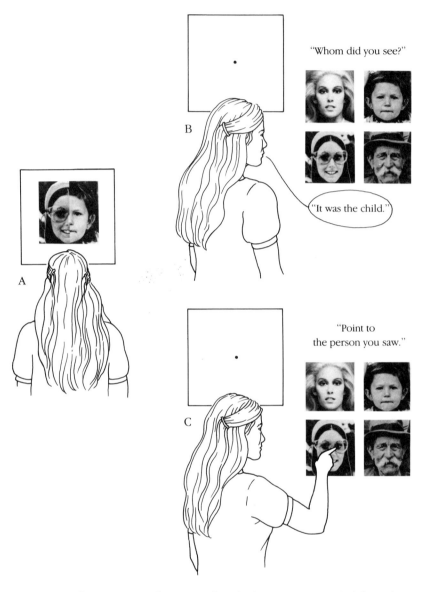

FIGURE 2.9   Chimeric-stimuli tests with split-brain patients. A. The subject is told she will see a picture. She is asked to fixate on the center of the screen; a composite picture is flashed. The subject is asked to identify the picture, either verbally (B) or by pointing with one hand or the other (C). Split-brain patients seem unaware that the chimeric stimulus is incomplete or conflicting. When asked to vocalize the answer, they choose the picture from which the right-field half of the composite was made. When asked to point, they choose the picture from which the left-field half was made. [Adapted from Levy, Trevarthen, and Sperry, "Perception of Bilateral Chimeric Figures Following Hemispheric Disconnection," Fig. 4, p. 68, *Brain* 95 (1972).]

flashed briefly in the center of the visual field. Because the left half of the square is projected to the right hemisphere and the right half to the left hemisphere, the fact that the patients reported seeing a normal square meant that the left hemisphere had "completed" the partial figure presented to it. The right hemisphere also perceived a normal square, for the left hand would draw a complete figure when a patient was asked to sketch what he or she saw with that hand.[36] Later studies have shown that chimeric figures such as the composite pictures presented to patient N.G. also give rise to visual completion.

The completion phenomenon is also seen in some patients who have unilateral damage to the visual regions of the brain. It is not well understood in either case, but it is clearly one of the reasons split-brain patients report that the world appears normal. In conjunction with eye movements that bring information to both hemispheres, completion helps bring to visual experience a unity that extends across the visual field.

·········

METACONTROL:
Who is in charge here, anyway?

Jerre Levy and Colwyn Trevarthen constructed chimeric figures from drawings of common objects and asked subjects to point to a similar picture from an array viewed in free vision.[37] Objects could be matched on the basis of either their function or their appearance. (Examples are shown in Figure 2.8.) Function and appearance matches for stimuli to both the left and right hemispheres were included among the choices on each trial, allowing the investigators to see whether each hemisphere had a preferred "mode" for making matches. Levy and Trevarthen hypothesized that function matches would be best performed by the left hemisphere and appearance matches would be the specialty of the right.

This prediction was supported by the data from one patient who was given the ambiguous instruction to match "similar" objects. Responses to left-hemisphere stimuli were overwhelmingly based on function, whereas responses to right-hemisphere stimuli were based on appearance. The investigators then specifically instructed the same subject and other patients to perform matches on the basis of only function or appearance. In general, function instructions elicited function matches to left-hemisphere stimuli, and appearance instructions elicited appearance matches to right-hemisphere items.

A large number of responses, however, deviated from the expected pattern. In some cases, the appearance instruction resulted in a response to the right-hemisphere stimulus, but the subject made a function match. Similarly, function instruction sometimes resulted in a response to the left-hemisphere stimulus that was based on appearance. In these cases, the hemisphere appropriate to the instructions responded, but in an "inappropriate" way. The reverse also occurred: The hemisphere inappropriate in terms of the instruction sometimes controlled the response, using the "appropriate" processing strategy. For example, the right hemisphere might respond under the function instruction, making its decision on the basis of function, or the left hemisphere might respond under the appearance instruction, with the response based on appearance.

These results showed that a given hemisphere does not always do the tasks for which it is thought superior, nor in performing a task does it always process information in the manner expected of it. This surprising result led Levy to speculate that "hemispheric activation does not depend on a hemisphere's real aptitude or even on its actual processing strategy on a given occasion, but rather on what it thinks it can do."[38]

The "thinking" that Levy referred to is actually part of an interaction between higher cortical processes and brain-stem "arousal" that she refers to as "metacontrol." In Levy's view, each hemisphere processes a given set of instructions; based on these evaluations, signals are sent to the brain stem, biasing control to either the left or right hemisphere. Thus, the control of hemispheric dominance, that is, which side is "in charge," is mediated by a system that is highly sensitive to task instructions but is distinct from that determining the actual processing by a hemisphere once it is in charge.[39] According to Levy, dissociations occur precisely because the underlying mechanisms governing hemispheric arousal are different from those involved in the task processing.

·········

SEPARATED AWARENESS AND UNIFYING MECHANISMS

Under certain conditions, each hemisphere of a split-brain patient appears to function as an independent processor, producing results reminiscent of the behavior of two separate individuals. As Sperry has observed:

Each hemisphere . . . has its own . . . private sensations, perceptions, thought, and ideas all of which are cut off from the corresponding experiences in the opposite hemisphere. Each left and right hemisphere has its own private chain of memories and learning experiences that are inaccessible to recall by the other hemisphere. In many respects each disconnected hemisphere appears to have a separate "mind of its own."[40]

Yet, casual observers do not notice anything unusual about most split-brain patients shortly after commissurotomy. In fact, a patient who recovered from the operation without complications could probably go through a routine medical checkup a year or two later without giving away his surgical history to anyone not already acquainted with it. Speech, language comprehension, personality, and motor coordination are remarkably preserved in patients without a corpus callosum and other commissures.

What keeps the two separate hemispheres acting as a unit during the everyday activities of these patients? A variety of unifying mechanisms, some of which we have already considered, seem to compensate for the absence of the cerebral commissures. Conjugate eye movements, as well as the fact that each eye projects to both hemispheres, play an important role in establishing unity of the visual world. The eye movements initiated by one hemisphere to bring an object into direct view serve to make that information available to the other hemisphere as well. Much of the conflict that would result from having the two hemispheres view different halves of the visual field is thus avoided.

Information from the touch modality provides another means by which each hemisphere is made aware of stimulation from both sides of the body. Up to now we have considered only the crossed, or contralateral, nerve fibers that allow each hemisphere to control the hand opposite to it. However, a much smaller number of same-side, ipsilateral, fibers allow each hemisphere to exert some limited control over the hand on the same side of the body. Ipsilateral sensory information is generally incomplete and inadequate to enable a patient to verbally identify an object held in the left hand; however, the ipsilateral pathways do provide partial information.

Yet another way information is made available to both hemispheres is by commissures located in the lower regions of the brain. The human split-brain operation severs only the nerve bundles connecting the cortical levels of the brain. These are the major fibers connecting the hemispheres, but other, smaller commissures remain intact. These other commissures connect paired structures that are part of the midbrain. They are shown in Figure 2.10.

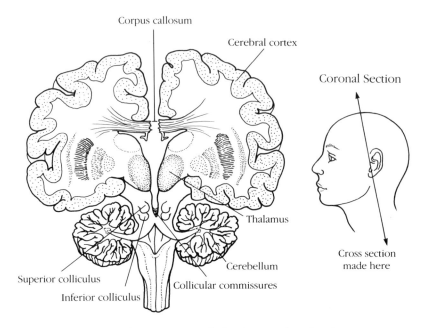

FIGURE 2.10   Extent of separation of the brain after forebrain commissurotomy. The structures of the midbrain remain connected by the collicular commissures. [From Sperry, "The Great Cerebral Commissure," *Scientific American*, 1964. All rights reserved.]

One such structure, the superior colliculus, is involved in the location of objects and the tracking of their movements. The colliculus is believed to process the "where" aspects of the visual world, as opposed to the "what," or finely detailed, aspects of vision. The left and right superior colliculi communicate through the commissures connecting them, so each hemisphere is provided with information about the location of objects regardless of where the objects fall in the visual field. Such crude location information could explain the phenomenon of visual completion mentioned earlier.

...

Evidence for Information Sharing Between
the Disconnected Hemispheres

Data from a more recent series of studies with split-brain patients suggested that both hemispheres have access to selected aspects of a stimulus presented to one hemisphere alone. The stimulus used in a study of visual attention consisted of a three-by-three grid located either to the left or to the right of the subject's point of fixation.[41] On each trial, a target digit was presented briefly in one of the nine cells; the subject's task was to indicate whether the target was odd or even. On within-field trials, before the onset of the target, an X (spatial cue) appeared either briefly in one of the nine cells or was superimposed on the fixation point. When it appeared in one of the nine cells, it occurred either in the cell corresponding to the position of the target digit to follow or in a different cell. On between-fields trials, two grids appeared, one in each field, with the X appearing in a cell in one field and the target presented subsequently in a cell in the other field. Figure 2.11 illustrates this task.

Earlier work in neurologically normal subjects showed that reaction time is faster when the spatial cue indicates the target's subsequent location and longer when the spatial cue directs the subject's attention to an incorrect location. Would this effect be found in split-brain patients when the task required access to information from both hemispheres (between fields)? The results were quite clear: For each of the two split-brain subjects tested, reaction time decreased when the subject had prior information about the target's spatial location in both the between-fields and within-field conditions and increased when an invalid cue was presented. Another experiment showed that specific information about the location of a stimulus presented in one visual field is not available to the other hemisphere.

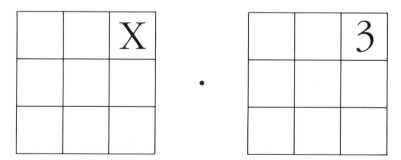

FIGURE 2.11   Example of stimuli for a trial in the between-fields condition. For the first part of each trial, two empty grids were presented on either side of a fixation dot. Next, the spatial cue (X) appeared for 150 milliseconds in one of the grid cells. After a 1.5-second interval in which only the empty grids were shown, the target digit was presented in the opposite grid either in the same relative position as the cue or in a different position. This figure illustrates a valid cue (same position) trial.

The investigators suggested that these data provide evidence for distinguishing between stimulus information needed for explicit identification of spatial location and stimulus information needed to direct visual attention. They argued that different neural pathways are involved in these two functions and that commissurotomy does not disrupt the access of either hemisphere to information needed to direct visual attention.

Justine Sergent has presented additional evidence for hemispheric sharing of some aspects of information in selected patients from the California series.[42] In one task, subjects were unable to make same-different judgments between two digits projected simultaneously, one to each hemisphere. When the task instructions were modified, however, so that subjects had to indicate whether one digit was higher than the other, performance improved dramatically. In another task, subjects were unable to describe the features of faces projected to the right but were able to accurately respond to a series of focused questions about the faces, for example, young/old or man/woman. Sergent interpreted these findings as reflecting the role of subcortical structures in the sharing of semantic information, or meaning. Thus, she argued, subcortical structures contribute to keeping the two hemispheres informed of their respective "informational contents," but the shared information is not highly specific.

Subsequent work by other investigators with Donald Wilson's patients, however, failed to replicate these findings.[43] The basis for this discrepancy remains to be clarified, and along with it, the role of subcortical structures in the interhemispheric sharing of information.

·········

WHAT DO THE CEREBRAL COMMISSURES REALLY DO?

We started this chapter with an account of the mystery surrounding the function of the corpus callosum. Are we now any nearer to understanding it? A simple answer would be to say, "Yes, we know that the cerebral commissures transfer information obtained by one hemisphere over to the other hemisphere." Although this is true, it is not a particularly revealing or complete answer. At the very least, we want to know the nature of the information that is transferred and how it is used by the hemispheres.

...

A Model of Brain Asymmetry

It has been postulated that in the course of evolution the functions of the left and right hemispheres began to diverge. Areas in the left hemisphere became more adept at generating rapidly changing motor patterns, such as those involved in fine control of the hands and the vocal tract. They also became more skilled at processing the rapidly changing auditory patterns produced by the vocal tract during speech.

Further speculation has led to the idea that the left hemisphere is skilled at sequential processing in general and, therefore, is the more analytic of the two hemispheres. This analytic mode of information processing is thought to apply to all incoming information, not just to speech. Visual information, for example, would be treated in an analytic manner by being broken up and reorganized in terms of features.

Areas of the right hemisphere, by contrast, became more adept at simultaneously processing the type of information required to perceive spatial patterns and relationships. Some investigators have claimed that the right hemisphere's specialties are an outgrowth and elaboration of the processes considered basic to vision and visual memory. Further speculation has led to the idea that the right hemisphere is the more holistic and synthetic of the two in handling all kinds of information.

Although some of these labels describing the functions of the left and right hemispheres are vague and await further work to clarify them, it is clear that differences along these lines do exist. Some investigators have argued that a basic incompatibility between the mechanisms generating these processing styles accounts for their evolutionary development in different hemispheres.

A question that immediately comes to mind is how the two hemispheres share control of behavior in everyday situations. The first possibility investigators have considered is that one hemisphere, usually the left, dominates the control of behavior. The original concept of cerebral dominance was based on this idea. It gained support from early findings with split-brain patients showing that the left hemisphere assumed control of responding in situations where there were simultaneous and different inputs to the two hemispheres. What was overlooked was the fact that these tests generally involved linguistic stimuli (words, for example) and often required a verbal response. Given these conditions, it is not at all surprising to find the language-rich hemisphere "dominating."

An alternative idea—that there is a constant vying for control between the hemispheres—is an outgrowth of subsequent work with split-brain patients. As a wider variety of tasks was employed, including some that could be performed better by the right hemisphere, some interesting results emerged. In the chimeric-stimuli studies, for example, we have seen that it is not always possible to predict which hemisphere will control a response, despite instructions specifically designed to "engage" one hemisphere. Observations of this sort have led to speculation that there is a delicate balance between the hemispheres, with one or the other taking over, depending on the task and other as yet unspecified factors.

Some investigators have suggested that the corpus callosum and other commissures play an important role in achieving interhemispheric harmony in the normal brain, serving to integrate the verbal and spatial modes of thinking into unified behavior. How is this harmony achieved? Is it simply a matter of ensuring that the two hemispheres have the same information available to them, or does it also involve a more complex system of inhibition or suppression of activity in the hemispheres?

...

The Commissures as Interhemispheric Integrators

Conjectures such as these bring us back to the question of the role of the cerebral commissures. There are no definitive answers yet. At this point, the role of the callosum and other commissures can perhaps best be seen as that of a conduit through which the hemispheres exchange information and perhaps handle the problems associated with conflicts among independent processing modules. Because the commissures are simply bundles of nerve fibers, they cannot in and of themselves control anything. But they can serve as channels through which synchronization of hemispheric function occurs and duplication or competition of effort is prevented.

Perhaps this integration is accomplished by the callosum's simply serving as a sensory "window," providing a separate and complete representation of all sensory input in each hemisphere. It is more likely, however, that more complex, processed signals normally traverse the commissures, informing each hemisphere about events in the other and, to an extent, controlling their respective operations. This type of communication would allow the whole brain to supersede individual hemispheric competencies.

Early in the course of evolution and in the development of bisymmetric bodily organization, the continuous transmission of sensory information from one side to the other may have been the one essential function of interhemispheric pathways. It seems likely, however, that with the development of asymmetries in brain function, the role of these pathways became more profound.

If this is the case, why do we not see evidence of serious problems in split-brain patients? We have previously discussed at least part of the answer, including the fact that the hemispheric disconnection in these patients is never really complete. Another possibility is that the role of the commissures is most important in the early developmental period following birth. Severing them later in life may not be overly critical because hemispheric differences and interhemispheric relationships have already been established. We shall delve further into models of callosal function in Chapter 12 and shall discuss the role of the corpus callosum (and its absence) in development in Chapter 9.

········

SPECIAL INSIGHTS FROM THE STUDY OF COMMISSUROTOMY PATIENTS

Our review of data from split-brain subjects has led us to the conclusion that hemispheric specialization is not an all-or-none phenomenon but represents a continuum. Recent work with split-brain patients has revealed that each hemisphere is capable of handling many kinds of tasks but often differs from the other hemisphere in both approach and efficiency. Almost any human behavior or higher mental function, however, clearly involves more than the actual specialties of either hemisphere and utilizes what is common to both hemispheres.

In research with split-brain subjects, language continues to stand out as the most salient and profound difference between the left brain and the right brain. Some investigators have claimed that all other hemispheric differences are manifestations of the verbal asymmetry.[44] They have argued that the region of the left hemisphere that developed specialization for language would no longer be available to handle the processing of spatial information formerly controlled by either half of the brain. The right hemisphere, then, would appear to be specialized for spatial skills, even though its specialization would really be a result of the left hemisphere's deficit rather than the right hemisphere's superiority. This argument provides an interesting perspective on the problem of how lateralization developed, although it is exceedingly difficult to "prove" in the usual sense.

THREE

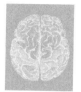

ASYMMETRIES IN THE
NORMAL BRAIN

Fortunately, most people are neurologically normal, having two un-damaged hemispheres connected by intact commissures. So what does evidence from studies of brain-damaged and split-brain patients tell us about the different roles of the two hemispheres in the rest of humanity?

The investigation of asymmetries in normal subjects has been carried out in several ways. One of the oldest and most extensively used techniques takes advantage of the natural split in human visual pathways. This split neatly divides our visual world into two fields, each of which projects to one hemisphere. By flashing material very briefly either to the left or to the right of the point on which a subject is fixating, investigators are able to lateralize inputs—that is, to present them to one hemisphere only. Because of the connections between the hemispheres, this one-sided presentation lasts only a fraction of a second, but it appears to be sufficient to allow investigators to compare the abilities of one hemisphere with those of the other.

Similarly, it has been discovered that simultaneously presenting different auditory information to each ear leads to the initial lateralization of auditory stimuli. Information presented to the left ear appears to project first to the right hemisphere, and information presented to the right ear is lateralized to the left hemisphere. This procedure, known as dichotic listening, has allowed investigators to study differences and similarities in the way the two hemispheres handle speech and other types of auditory information.

In this chapter we shall review data collected from normal subjects with whom these and other techniques have been used.

....

VISUAL-FIELD ASYMMETRIES

The investigation of visual asymmetries in normal subjects often resembles the testing situations used with split-brain patients. Visual stimuli flashed briefly in the left visual field project first to the right hemisphere; stimuli flashed in the right visual field project initially to the left hemisphere. In split-brain patients, this initial lateralization to one hemisphere or the other is maintained because the connections between the hemispheres have been cut. In a normal subject, however, the connections are intact and can transfer information between hemispheres. Nevertheless, it was found that differences could be detected in a person's performance on certain tasks, depending on whether the task was presented to the right or the left visual field.

...

Visual-Field Differences: The Result of Reading Habits or a Sign of Hemispheric Asymmetry?

In the early 1950s Mortimer Mishkin and Donald Forgays demonstrated that normal right-handed subjects were better at identifying English words briefly presented to the right of fixation than they were at identifying words flashed in the left visual field. However, when Yiddish words were presented in the same way to subjects who could read Yiddish, a slight advantage in favor of the left visual field was found. The authors concluded that acquired directional reading habits result in better processing of written English in the right visual field, whereas Yiddish, a language that uses the Hebrew alphabet and reads from right to left, is processed more accurately in the left visual field.[1]

This explanation enjoyed widespread acceptance for several years, although it did not address the question of why the advantage for the right visual field with English words was considerably greater than that for the left visual field with Yiddish words. A decade later, however, the publication of work with the California split-brain subjects suggested a reason for the lack of parallelism in the size of the visual-field differences.

Split-brain subjects, as we have seen, showed dramatic differences in their abilities to report printed English words presented in the left or the right visual field. Those differences were interpreted as a reflection of the functional differences between the hemispheres for language. Perhaps, investigators began to think, the asymmetries found in the split-brain patients contribute to the visual-field differences found in normal subjects as well. Mishkin and Forgays' findings, then, may have been due to two factors operating simultaneously: (1) The biases in favor of one visual field due to acquired reading habits in a particular language are superimposed on (2) an advantage for the right visual field resulting from differences between the left brain and the right brain.

An important test of this two-factor interpretation came from later studies investigating visual-field asymmetries with English or Yiddish words presented vertically to minimize the possible role of directional scanning. With the effects of directional scanning reduced, the two-factor interpretation predicted that the functional differences between the hemispheres should produce a right-visual-field advantage for both Yiddish and English words. Precisely this result was found.[2]

These findings, and a variety of other data that we shall consider, lend support to the idea that visual-field differences in normal subjects reflect brain asymmetries in those subjects. This conclusion is an exciting one, for it suggests that differences between the left brain and the right brain found in clinical and split-brain subjects apply to the normal brain as well and that these differences can actually be studied in normal subjects.

...

Why Does Lateralized Presentation Result in Asymmetric Performance?

Even if there are functional differences between the hemispheres in normal subjects, why are they reflected in differences in performance for the two visual fields? Despite the initial lateralization or one-sided presentation, both hemispheres have access to all incoming information. Very brief presentations to one side of the fixation point ensure that a stimulus initially is projected directly to only one-half of the brain, but the connections between the hemispheres can transmit information about the stimulus to the other side almost instantaneously. Why, then, do we find differences in performance between the visual fields?

There are two models of hemispheric asymmetry that are widely considered. The first, known as the direct access model, assumes that information will be processed by the hemisphere that first receives it, regardless of the differences in ability that may exist between the hemispheres. In this model, the first hemisphere to receive a task will be the one to handle it, although it may not be the one best equipped to do the job. The direct access model predicts an advantage in performance for information that reaches the appropriately specialized hemisphere, because processing by that hemisphere presumably would be better than processing by the other hemisphere.

The relay model, on the other hand, assumes that information is always processed by the hemisphere best equipped to deal with it. Material presented initially to the nonspecialized hemisphere, in this model, would have to reach the specialized hemisphere via the commissural fibers before processing could take place. If this transfer results in some loss of clarity of information, then an advantage should be found for stimuli reaching the specialized hemisphere directly. Some evidence for loss of information following callosal transfer is found in animal research. In monkeys, cells in one hemisphere sensitive to the shape of a stimulus respond more vigorously when a stimulus is presented in the contralateral visual field (input is sent directly to that hemisphere) than when it is presented in the ipsilateral field (information must cross over from the other side of the brain).[3]

In both the direct access and relay models, asymmetries emerge in tasks where the hemispheres do not have equal capacities to begin with. And in both, information presented directly to the hemisphere specialized for a specific function would be expected to produce better performance—that is, more accurate or faster responding than one in which information goes first to the other half. They differ, however, in their view of the participation of the nonspecialized hemisphere and in the role played by the cerebral commissures.

Perhaps the strongest evidence that visual-field asymmetries in normal subjects reflect underlying hemispheric differences is the similarity between these findings and the results of research with brain-damaged and split-brain patients. Although a right-visual-field advantage is found with normal subjects in a variety of tasks using words and letters, these normal subjects show a left-visual-field advantage for stimuli that are thought to be handled by the right hemisphere.

For example, several studies have demonstrated that normal subjects recognize faces presented in the left visual field more quickly than those presented in the right visual field.[4] Other work has shown that normal subjects more accurately remember the locations of dots presented on a card when the material is presented initially to the right hemisphere.[5] These findings provide strong support for the idea that visual-field differences reflect hemispheric differences: The right-visual-field advantage reflects left-hemisphere specialization for language functions, and the left-visual-field superiority results from right-hemisphere specialization for the processing of visuospatial stimuli.

We should point out, however, that studies using nonverbal stimuli have not produced results as consistent as those found with words or letters. Some studies using nonsense forms and geometric shapes have shown no differences for the two visual fields.[6] For the most part, however, the studies that do obtain differences between fields show the left visual field to be superior. The problem is that many studies that use stimuli believed by investigators to be processed by the right hemisphere do not find any differences between visual fields. This situation is reminiscent of the problems encountered when investigators started to look for evidence of special right-hemisphere functions in studies with brain-damaged patients. The functions of the right hemisphere proved to be much more elusive than those of the left. A similar picture has emerged in studies with neurologically normal subjects. We shall discuss these and other findings later in this chapter when we consider what has been learned about the nature of hemispheric asymmetries from visual-field and dichotic-listening studies.

·········

USING AUDITORY STIMULI
TO STUDY ASYMMETRIES

Techniques to lateralize auditory information have also been used to study hemispheric differences. Doreen Kimura, working at the Montreal Neurological Institute, noticed that under certain conditions, subjects were more accurate at identifying words presented to the right ear than they were at identifying words delivered to the left ear. Kimura was using the dichotic-listening procedure, in which subjects listen to two different spoken messages simultaneously, one message to each ear.

She wanted to compare the performances of brain-damaged subjects and normal subjects in a task involving an overload of information.

...

Dichotic Listening

The stimuli used by Kimura consisted of pairs of spoken digits, for example, "one" and "nine." The members of each pair were aligned for simultaneity of onset and were recorded on separate channels of audio tape. Subjects listened through headphones to trials consisting of three pairs of digits presented in rapid succession. After each trial, the subject was asked to recall as many of the six previously presented digits as possible, in any order.

Kimura found that patients with damage to the left temporal lobe did more poorly than patients with damage to the right temporal lobe, but regardless of where the damage was located, subjects typically reported the digits presented to the right ear more accurately. This right-ear advantage was also found in normal control subjects.[7]

The finding that patients with damage to the left hemisphere performed more poorly overall than did patients with damage to the right hemisphere was predictable. The dichotic-listening task involves the abilities to understand and to produce speech, both of which are primarily left-hemisphere functions that might be disrupted to some extent in patients with damage on the left side. The observation that the ears performed asymmetrically, however, was surprising.

A review of anatomy reveals why the asymmetry was unexpected. Unlike the retina, which sends projections contralaterally to the brain from one-half of its surface and ipsilaterally from the other half, each ear sends information from all its receptors to both hemispheres. Thus, complete information about a stimulus presented to the right ear is represented initially in both hemispheres, and vice versa. Even if speech stimuli could be processed in only one hemisphere, we would not expect to see any evidence of the asymmetry, because each ear has direct access to both hemispheres.

...

Kimura's Model of Ear Asymmetry

To explain her findings, Kimura cited evidence from animal studies suggesting that the contralateral projections from ear to brain are stronger than the ipsilateral pathways.[8] She also proposed that when two different stimuli are presented simultaneously to each ear, the difference in the strengths of the signals traversing the two pathways is exaggerated, so information sent along the ipsilateral route is suppressed. Given these assumptions, it was then possible to explain the right-ear advantage.

Under dichotic-listening conditions, the stimulus to the left ear may reach the left hemisphere in one of two ways: over the suppressed ipsilateral route or over the contralateral pathways to the right hemisphere and then across the cerebral commissures. The stimulus to the right ear, however, has a simpler task. It gains access to the left hemisphere along the contralateral route. Because it is likely to arrive at the left hemisphere for processing in better form than its left-ear counterpart, a small right-ear advantage emerges. Kimura's model is depicted in Figure 3.1.

Some support for Kimura's ideas has come from studies showing that there is basically no difference between the two ears in a subject's ability to detect or identify stimuli presented one at a time. Individual subjects may have hearing loss in one or both ears, but overall, when data are collected from large numbers of subjects, the two ears perform

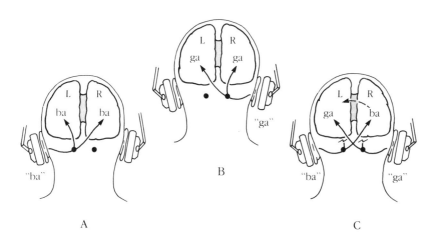

FIGURE 3.1   Kimura's model of dichotic listening in normal subjects. A. The syllable "ba" is corrrectly reported when it is presented to the left ear alone; it reaches the left and right hemispheres via ipsilateral and contralateral pathways, respectively. B. Similarly, the syllable "ga" is correctly reported when it is presented to the right ear alone. C. In dichotic presentation, ipsilateral pathways are presumed to be supressed, leaving only the contralateral pathways fully functional. The syllable "ba" is accessible to the left (speech) hemisphere only through the commissures; "ga" is usually reported more accurately. Following commissurotomy, "ba" is not accessible to the left hemisphere because the commissures are cut. The patient reports hearing only "ga."

similarly.[9] This result suggests that ordinarily, without any competition from the contralateral pathways, the ipsilateral fibers are sufficient to produce good performance.

...

Dichotic Listening in Split-Brain Subjects: Testing the Assumptions

Split-brain patients can identify words equally well in either ear, just as neurologically intact subjects do. This finding shows that the ipsilateral path from the left ear to the left hemisphere is functional under conditions of monaural presentation. If, however, speech stimuli are presented dichotically to split-brain subjects, a dramatic, highly exaggerated version of the ear asymmetry found in normal subjects occurs. The typical split-brain patient reports the right-ear items accurately, but the left-ear report is at a chance level. In fact, the patients frequently have to be coaxed into guessing about the identity of left-ear items, because they report that they hear only one stimulus.[10]

This situation with split-brain patients is consistent with Kimura's model and helps confirm it. With the corpus callosum cut, communication between the hemispheres is disrupted, but both the ipsilateral and the contralateral projections of each ear are left intact. (These pathways are subcortical and are not cut during surgery.) If, as Kimura suggested, the ipsilateral pathways are suppressed under dichotic stimulation, each ear would send its half of the information to the opposite hemisphere only over the contralateral pathway. The right hemisphere would receive input from the left ear, and the stimulus to the right ear would reach the left hemisphere. Because the right hemisphere is very limited verbally, it would not be able to talk about the word it received from the left ear. At the same time, information about the left-ear word could not transfer into the left hemisphere because the corpus callosum was cut. As a result, the left-ear items would not be identified.

...

Does Ear Asymmetry Really Reflect Hemispheric Asymmetry?

Other support for Kimura's model comes from the finding that the ear advantage reverses in subjects who have been shown to have speech controlled by the right hemisphere instead of by the left. Patients tested with sodium amobarbital to determine the hemisphere controlling speech have been given the dichotic-listening task to see whether the ear asymmetry is related to hemispheric asymmetry. Those with left-hemisphere speech centers typically show a right-ear advantage; those with right-hemisphere speech show a left-ear advantage.[11] The sodium amobarbital test, as we discussed in Chapter 1, allows a direct assessment of speech lateralization without having to infer it from the patient's handedness. Thus, in the rare cases of right-handers with right-hemisphere speech, a left-ear advantage would generally be found. These data are very important in establishing the validity of the dichotic-listening test as a measure of brain asymmetry.

The results of another study using a similar approach are even more encouraging.[12] Patients whose speech centers were previously determined by the amobarbital test were asked to monitor a sequence of dichotically presented word pairs for the occurrence of a specific target word, which appeared randomly in the series. The results were scored in terms of the number of target words correctly detected in each ear, as well as the speed with which they were detected. By incorporating both percentage correct identification and reaction time scores in the data analysis, the researchers were able to correctly classify 95 percent of the patients in terms of the hemisphere controlling their speech.

Finally, research has demonstrated that the ear asymmetry found in a given subject differs as a function of the nature of the stimuli that are presented. A left-ear advantage has been found with stimuli believed to be processed by the right hemisphere—stimuli such as musical chords and melodies.[13]

·········

WHAT HAS BEEN LEARNED FROM VISUAL AND AUDITORY ASYMMETRIES?

During the last 20 years, a great many studies used the techniques of dichotic listening and lateralized tachistoscopic presentation with normal subjects. As in the research with split-brain patients, there has been a gradual evolution of ideas about the nature of hemispheric asymmetries as new data suggest different interpretations of earlier work.

...

The Nature of Information: The Verbal–Nonverbal Distinction

Much of the early work on the left brain and the right brain in normal subjects led investigators to believe that the two hemispheres differ basically in terms of the nature of the stimuli they are best prepared to deal with. A typical visual task involved the lateralized presentation of stimuli that the subject was asked to identify. A similar procedure was employed with dichotic stimuli as well: Two items were presented simultaneously, and the subject was asked to report what was heard. Sometimes the basic task was modified so that the subject was required to recognize a specific stimulus, rather than identify each item, and sometimes the experimenter was interested primarily in how quickly a subject could respond to a stimulus instead of how accurate the response was. Often, both speed and accuracy were measured in the same study.

Stimuli were said to show a left-hemisphere advantage if performance was superior when items were presented to the right ear or in the right visual field. A right-hemisphere advantage was assumed if performance was superior when items were presented to the left ear or in the left visual field. Differences in performance between sides were quite small—frequently, just a few percentage points better in identification or a few milliseconds faster in response—but anywhere from 70 to 90 percent of the right-handed subjects tested in a typical study showed the asymmetry.

Most of the early studies showing a right-side advantage used stimuli that were language-related in a very obvious way. Tachistoscopically presented words and even single letters produced a right-visual-field advantage.[14] Dichotically presented spoken digits and words also resulted in a right ear advantage.[15] The advantage, however, was not limited to meaningful spoken utterances. Studies have shown that nonsense syllables such as "pa" and "ka" also produce a right-ear advantage and that speech played backward produces a right-ear superiority in recognition as well.[16] Taken together, the results of these studies suggest that stimuli do not have to be meaningful to produce a left-hemisphere advantage but should be language-related or verbal in some way.

The picture for the right hemisphere is more difficult to summarize. A wide variety of visual stimuli have produced left-visual-field or right-hemisphere superiorities. We have mentioned studies that used faces and dot displays as stimuli and obtained a left-visual-field advantage. The dichotic-listening studies that result in a right-hemisphere advantage are also diverse. One of the earliest demonstrated a left-ear superiority in the recognition of melodic excerpts.[17] Two different 4-second piano melodies were presented simultaneously on each trial. The subject was asked to indicate which of the four sequentially presented excerpts played immediately thereafter had been members of the pair delivered dichotically. Other studies revealed a left-ear advantage when familiar environmental noises were presented dichotically.[18] In a typical trial, the subject would be asked to identify a pair of sounds, such as a dog barking and a train whistling.

All these "right-hemisphere" stimuli share the attribute of being nonverbal, and many investigators have argued that the distinction between the functions of the two hemispheres lies along this verbal-nonverbal dimension. In this view, all language-related stimuli are dealt with primarily in the left hemisphere, and the right hemisphere is specialized for handling certain types of nonverbal stimuli. This conclusion appears to be a neat, reasonably satisfying summary of the data we have reviewed so far. However, problems that have emerged in more recent work have led researchers to seek another explanation of the fundamental differences between the left brain and the right brain.

...

Operating on the Stimulus: The Information-Processing Approach

Consider the following experiments. The subject is given a short list of letters to memorize and then briefly views a familiar object in the left or the right visual field. The subject's task is to decide whether the first letter of the name of the object is among the letters in the memorized list. Which visual field would lead to a faster response? Or suppose that the subject viewed single letters instead of pictures and had to decide whether the letter was among those that had been memorized. What could be predicted about the speed of response in this case?

It would be reasonable to expect a left-visual-field superiority in the first case and a right-visual-field superiority in the second. Pictures, after all, are nonverbal stimuli, and letters clearly fall in the verbal domain. In fact, the results obtained were the complete reverse. Picture stimuli resulted in faster performance when they were presented to the left hemisphere, and the letters were responded to more quickly when they were projected initially to the right hemisphere.[19] Why?

What seems to be more important than the nature of the stimulus is what the subject does with the stimulus. In the case of the supposedly nonverbal pictures, the subject was asked to identify each picture and recover the initial letter of its name, a clear-cut language function that is analytic in nature. The single-letter stimuli, on the other hand, were verbal in nature but in this task did not have to be approached as verbal stimuli. The subject could readily perform the task holistically by matching the mental image of the letter against the images of the set of memorized letters. Theoretically, the subject could do this without ever knowing the name of the letter presented.

This kind of explanation emphasizes the task to be performed by the subject, analytic or holistic, rather than the nature of the stimulus per se. It reflects a shift away from left- and right-hemisphere stimuli to left- and right-hemisphere modes of processing information. Along the same lines, other investigators have made a case for describing the differences in processing by the hemispheres as global (right-hemisphere advantage) versus local (left-hemisphere advantage).[20]

Another study that highlights an information-processing approach to brain asymmetry was one that took advantage of the fact that there are alternative ways for subjects to remember pairs of words. One is to rehearse the words by repeating them out loud or subvocally; a second is to form an image of the two items interacting in some way. For example, faced with the task of remembering "flag" and "chicken," subjects can repeat the words over and over again, or they can form an image of the two words, such as a chicken carrying a flag. (The use of images of this type has been shown to be a very effective memory aid.)

The researchers hypothesized that verbal and imagery strategies would involve different cerebral hemispheres. They proposed that this difference would be tapped by having subjects indicate whether a picture flashed to the left or the right visual field corresponded to one of the words previously presented. When subjects were told to remember the word pairs by subvocal rehearsal, response time was faster for probes to the right visual field; when they were asked to form images of the pairs to be remembered, response time was faster for the left visual field.[21] These findings were in keeping with the predictions.*

Still further evidence for information-processing differences between the hemispheres comes from studies using languages other than English.

---

* In Chapter 2 we discussed the problems associated with thinking of imagery as either a left-hemisphere-only or right-hemisphere-only task. The data reviewed there suggested that the precise nature of the task was critical in determining the outcome. Given the results obtained in the study under discussion, it appears that the authors were fortunate in selecting an imagery task that showed right-hemisphere specialization.

In Japanese there are two writing systems, Kana and Kanji. The Kana system is sound based: A symbol represents the sound of a syllable without any meaning, and has a one-to-one correspondence with a syllable. The Kanji system is meaning based, with each character having several alternative meanings. Kana and Kanji also differ in terms of their graphic complexity, Kanji characters generally being more complex. Examples are given in Figure 3.2.

Studies of Japanese aphasic patients have suggested some interesting differences in the way these two types of linguistic symbols are processed in the brain. Sumiko Sasanuma has shown that a sizable number of patients exhibit selective impairment of Kana processing, whereas the ability to process Kanji remains relatively well preserved or almost intact. A much smaller number of patients show selective impairment of Kanji, with Kana processing relatively unaffected.[22] Analysis of the errors made by aphasic patients suggests that different strategies are used for the two types of symbols: visual processing for Kanji, as opposed to phonologic, or sound-based, processing for Kana.[23]

These observations have led Sasanuma and colleagues to tests of the hypothesis that Kana and Kanji represent different modes of linguistic processing differentially involving the two hemispheres.[24] To test this hypothesis with neurologically normal Japanese subjects, sets of Kana and Kanji nonsense words were prepared and presented briefly one at a time in either the left or the right visual field. Results showed that subjects showed a significant right-field superiority for identification in

MEANING	KANA	KANJI
INK	インキ (INKI)	墨
UNIVERSITY	ダイガク (DAIGAKU)	大学 (GREAT LEARNING)
TOKYO	トウキョウ (TOKYO)	東京 (EAST CAPITAL)

FIGURE 3.2   The two forms of writing in Japan. Kana is syllabic, with words articulated syllable-by-syllable. Kanji is ideographic, with each character simultaneously representing a sound and a meaning.

the Kana task and a left-field (but not significant) superiority for the Kanji task. The investigators concluded that Kana and Kanji characters are processed differently in the two hemispheres; further, Kanji processing is particularly complex because both visual and verbal functions likely play a role, depending on the specific task. Whether Kanji would show a left- or a right-visual-field superiority might depend on, among other things, the strategy used by the subject and the mode of response (verbal or nonverbal).

Taken together, the findings on Kana and Kanji point to the importance of the kind of processing a subject must perform in determining hemispheric asymmetries.

...

The Representation of Information: The Role of Spatial Frequency

Justine Sergent and colleagues have emphasized the importance of the physical characteristics of the stimulus and the conditions under which it is presented in tachistoscopic tests.[25] They noted that stimulus duration, brightness, and distance from fixation, among other variables, may affect the outcome of laterality studies, independent of the nature of the stimulus or task. For example, in laterality investigations, stimuli are typically presented briefly (to eliminate the effects of eye movements) and off to the left or the right of the fixation point (to ensure projection to the contralateral hemisphere). The result is that the representation of information in the brain is qualitatively different from the representation under normal conditions. Sergent presented evidence to show that asymmetries in a given tachistoscopic task depend, at least in part, on the unequal ability of the hemispheres to operate on these degraded representations. She argued that conditions making the extraction of stimulus attributes more difficult favor the right hemisphere.

Sergent suggested that these effects are due to differential hemispheric processing of the "spatial frequency" components of a stimulus. The concept of spatial frequency can be illustrated by a simple grating of alternating black and white stripes; the spatial frequency of the grating is a function of the number of light-dark changes (bars) in the stimulus over a given spatial interval. Any complex visual stimulus can be represented as an array of many such intensity variations, some higher (more bars) and some lower (fewer bars). Incoming visual information is broken down by the brain into discrete neural signals that represent these intensity variations. This processing is believed to be done by "channels" or filters sensitive to different spatial frequencies; the output of these channels reflects the array of spatial frequencies in the stimulus.

Sergent has argued that the right hemisphere is more sensitive to low spatial frequencies and the left hemisphere more sensitive to high ones. The effects of reducing the perceptability of stimuli can be accounted for by the spatial frequency hypothesis if it is assumed that such manipulations disrupt the processing of high spatial frequencies more than low spatial frequencies.

Stephen Christman has looked at the effects of perceptual characteristics in light of the spatial frequency hypothesis by examining factors that decrease the availability of higher spatial frequencies relative to lower spatial frequencies.[26] These factors include increases in size, distance from fixation, and amount of blur, along with decreases in brightness and exposure duration. Of the 79 experiments he reviewed, 45 showed effects in which side of hemispheric advantage and perceptual characteristics were consistent with the spatial frequency hypothesis; 25 experiments showed no significant effects; and 9 showed results that were the opposite of the spatial frequency predictions. Thus, his review provides some, but not unequivocal, support for the spatial frequency predictions.

Other studies have attempted to examine the spatial frequency hypothesis more directly, through the presentation of gratings of different spatial frequencies or stimuli treated with filters to remove specific frequency ranges. Here, too, the results are suggestive but not definitive.[27] John Bradshaw suggested that the spatial frequency hypothesis may be a special case of the analytic (high frequency)—holistic (low frequency) hypothesis, at a more sensory level. He also noted that, by its very nature, the spatial frequency hypothesis can be applied only to visual stimuli and that its usefulness is limited because it does not provide a more general hypothesis to deal with all sensory modalities.[28] A major advantage of the approach is that, unlike some other dichotomies, the predictions of the spatial frequency hypothesis can be precisely specified and rigorously tested.[29]

·········

THEORETICAL ISSUES IN INTERPRETING BEHAVIORAL STUDIES

Tachistoscopic presentation and dichotic-listening studies have served as the basis for much of our current theorizing about the nature of the left brain and the right brain in normal subjects. There is a striking correspondence between many of the hemispheric differences shown in normal subjects through these techniques and the ideas gleaned from the brain-damage clinic by several generations of neurologists and neuropsychologists. Important issues about these techniques remain unresolved, however.

···

What Are the Tests Measuring?

One concern is that these behavioral tests typically underestimate the incidence of left-hemisphere speech in right-handers compared to that determined with sodium amobarbital (Wada) testing. Studies generally find that approximately 80 percent of right-handed subjects show a right-ear or right-visual-field advantage for language stimuli; sodium amobarbital testing, in contrast, indicates that more than 95 percent of right-handed individuals have left-hemisphere language. What is causing this discrepancy?

One possibility is that the tests are not a pure measure of brain asymmetry and that other factors are involved. Perhaps individual differences in the neural pathways connecting the eyes and ears to the brain play a role in the outcome of the studies.

The strategies that subjects adopt in these tasks may also contribute in a major way to performance.[30] In dichotic listening, for example, subjects can actively shift their attention to either the left-ear or the right-ear stimulus. If the left-ear items are at a disadvantage because of hemispheric asymmetry, then some subjects may choose to direct their attention to the weaker ear, thereby producing a smaller right-ear superiority than might be found otherwise. Other subjects, in contrast, may focus their attention on the clearer of the two stimuli on any trial, without trying to identify both of them. These subjects would show a larger right-ear advantage than one would expect. M. P. Bryden has made a convincing case for the importance of attentional effects in dichotic listening. Nevertheless, he concluded that, across large numbers of studies, the expected ear asymmetries emerge, particularly when left-handers and right-handers are compared.[31] Bryden has also advanced similar arguments for the study and interpretation of visual-field asymmetries.[32]

We should also note that the discrepancy between the results of Wada testing and behavioral measures of asymmetry may be due to the possibility that each is tapping a different aspect of functional asymmetry. The Wada test is used to determine the hemisphere that controls speech output. Perhaps tachistoscopic and dichotic-listening tasks, which are basically tests of perception and not production, reflect functions that are less lateralized.*

Another problem is that visual and dichotic measures of lateralization are not highly correlated with each other. If these tests are measuring the same lateralized functions, it would be reasonable to expect them to produce results that are highly related to each other. Studies that have compared asymmetries in dichotic-listening and tachistoscopic tasks in the same subjects have found some degree of relationship, but not a high one.[33] Why? Perhaps these tests are not measuring the same thing after all.

Another concern, one that has implications for the two preceding problems as well, is that repeated testing of the same subjects does not always produce the same results. A test is reliable to the extent that repeated administrations yield similar results. Some studies have found the reliability of the dichotic-listening and tachistoscopic tests to be lower than one might expect.[34] For example, some subjects who, when first tested, showed a right-ear advantage for dichotically presented speech shifted to a left-ear advantage when tested a week later. Presumably, the organization of an individual's brain is a stable characteristic and does not change over time. Signs of variability within an individual may mean that the laterality tests are tapping functions, such as the formation of strategies to be used in performing the tasks, that can shift over brief intervals of time.

...

What Do the Tests Tell Us
About the Nature of Asymmetries?

Yet another issue raised by dichotic-listening and tachistoscopic studies is whether hemispheric differences are absolute or relative. Does a difference in performance between visual fields mean that only one hemisphere is capable of performing the task? Or does it simply reflect the fact that one hemisphere is better at the task than the other? The typical study with normal subjects does not allow us to tease apart these alternatives, because performance in the "inferior" visual field may be the result of either less efficient processing by the nonspecialized hemi-

---

* The terms lateralized and lateralization are frequently used to refer to the division of functions between the hemispheres, as well as to the restriction of information to one hemisphere.

sphere (the direct access model) or processing by the specialized hemisphere after transfer of information across the commissures (the callosal relay model). In either case, we would expect the same results: a difference in performance between the two sides.

A related issue is whether the size of the asymmetry found in different subjects can tell us anything about the degree of lateralization for certain functions in particular subjects. Although a subject's strategies may play a role in determining the size of the asymmetry effects, independent of lateralization per se, is it possible that differences in the size of the asymmetry can tell us something about the extent of lateralization? Is a subject with a large right-ear advantage more lateralized than a subject with a smaller right-ear advantage? This intriguing problem has investigators looking for ways to transform scores reflecting a subject's performance into a meaningful index of lateralization.*

...

Metacontrol

In the work with split-brain patients reviewed in Chapter 2, Jerre Levy and Colwyn Trevarthen distinguished between the ability of each hemisphere to perform a specific task and the degree to which each hemisphere assumes control of processing and behavior.[35] They demonstrated that the hemisphere that assumed control for a task was not always the hemisphere with a greater ability for that task; they used the term *metacontrol* to refer to the neural mechanisms that determine which hemisphere will be in charge.

Joseph Hellige has argued that the concept of metacontrol is particularly important when trying to understand processing in the intact brain.[36] In many situations both hemisphere are capable of performing a task, at least to some degree, but do so in different ways. When the same information is available to both hemispheres, what determines how the information will be processed?

Hellige has approached this problem experimentally by using selected tasks that can be performed by both hemispheres but in qualitatively different ways. He and his colleagues presented stimuli in three

---

*The issue of how to compute measures of lateralization from scores on behavioral tests is important and complex. In tests where percentage correct is the dependent variable, it is possible to use difference scores (left minus right, or variations thereof) as the index of lateralization. Such scores are not independent of overall performance, however. Some investigators have claimed that a laterality measure should be independent of how well someone does; others have argued that information on overall performance may itself be related to lateralization.

different conditions: right visual field (left hemisphere) left visual field (right hemisphere) and bilateral (both visual fields simultaneously.) By comparing the performance on bilateral trials with the performances when stimuli are presented to only one hemisphere, Hellige reasoned, it is possible to determine whether the qualitative pattern of results on bilateral trials matches that of one of the other two conditions.

In several such studies, the mode of processing on bilateral trials has been identical to that observed in presentations to one hemisphere but not to the other. Moreover, the mode of processing found in bilateral trials was not always the mode used by the hemisphere with greater ability for that task, a finding reminiscent of the commissurotomy studies of Levy and Trevarthen.[37] Individual differences among subjects were also observed. In general, 75–85 percent of right-handed subjects showed the same pattern of results in any given study. The remaining 15–25 percent showed a mode of processing in bilateral trials similar to that of the other hemisphere. Whether these variations represent meaningful differences in "metacontrol" among subjects is not clear at this point.

Hellige has written, "An important challenge facing cognitive neuropsychologists is to account for the emergence of unified information processing from a brain consisting of a variety of processing subsystems. The left and right cerebral hemispheres may be characterized as two very general subsystems with different processing properties and biases. Understanding interhemispheric interaction and the conditions for metacontrol can provide important clues about the emergence of unified information processing."[38] We agree with Hellige completely.

·········

CAN ATTENTIONAL BIAS
ACCOUNT FOR ASYMMETRIES?

When we introduced tachistoscopic and dichotic-listening work, we argued that asymmetries reflected the initial lateralization of stimulus input to the hemisphere best able to deal with the material. This type of explanation has been characterized as a "wiring" account of the difference, because the asymmetries result from the wiring of the nervous system and the processing differences between the hemispheres. Information lateralized to the hemisphere not specialized for it was at a disadvantage because it had to traverse callosal pathways to get to the more appropriate hemisphere, or be processed by the less able hemisphere.

Another quite different explanation has also been offered for these results. Marcel Kinsbourne proposed that asymmetries observed in dichotic-listening and tachistoscopic studies reflect covert shifts in attention to one side of space following the activation of one hemisphere.[39] He argued that the hemisphere specialized for a particular task becomes differentially active, or "primed," when appropriate material is presented to a subject and that this priming "spills over" to the centers controlling attention to the opposite side of space.

For example, in Kinsbourne's view, the right-ear advantage in tasks with dichotically presented speech is a consequence of the activation of the left hemisphere, followed by greater attention to the contralateral, or right ear. A left-ear advantage in a dichotic music task would reflect differential right-hemisphere involvement and a concomitant shift of attention to the left side of space.

Kinsbourne's attentional model of asymmetries is similar to the wiring account in that it begins with the assumption that there are basic functional differences between the hemispheres. It differs from the wiring model in its explanation of how hemispheric differences give rise to the performance differences that are studied in behavioral tests.

Kinsbourne and his colleagues have shown that tasks not normally displaying a visual-field asymmetry can be made to show a right-side advantage if subjects are asked to rehearse subvocally a short list of words while they view the laterally presented stimuli.[40] The rehearsal is presumed to activate the left hemisphere and produce a shift in attention to the right side, a process resulting in more accurate performance in that visual field.

Similarly, the right-ear advantage in speed of responding to certain dichotically presented syllables becomes a slight left-ear advantage when the subject is required to compare a brief melody presented immediately before each syllable pair with a melody presented immediately after.[41] An attentional view would claim that the musical stimuli "primed" the right hemisphere, thereby producing a shift in attention to the left ear, which would cancel out the shift to the right ear that ordinarily occurs when speech is presented.

A number of studies have provided support for the activation-orienting hypothesis,[42] as the attentional model is also known, although few investigators believe it is a complete explanation for asymmetries observed in lateralized testing. At the same time, many researchers question the adequacy of the "wiring" account and are inclined to think that both views may play some role in the phenomena we have been considering. Both models can be combined if we assume that priming one hemisphere serves to facilitate the processing of stimuli that are presented directly to it.[43]

....

LEFT-LOOKERS AND RIGHT-LOOKERS

In the course of his practice, clinical psychologist M. E. Day noticed that patients tended consistently to look either to the left or to the right when answering questions. Day suggested that the direction of these lateral eye movements (LEMs) might be associated with certain personality characteristics.[44] Paul Bakan has extended this idea and suggested that cognitive activity occurring primarily in one hemisphere would trigger eye movements to the opposite side and, therefore, eye movements could be viewed as an index of the relative activity of the two hemispheres in an individual.[45] Bakan's hypothesis is based on the well-established fact that eye movements to one side are controlled by centers in the frontal lobe of the contralateral hemisphere.

Bakan viewed the direction of lateral eye movements as a stable characteristic of each individual, reflecting the individual's hemisphericity—the tendency to rely on the processing of one-half of the brain. Later investigations considered the role played by the type of question used to elicit eye movements.[46] Questions requiring verbal analysis, it was reasoned, will tend to activate the left hemisphere in most right-handers; questions involving an analysis of spatial relationships will activate the right hemisphere. The differential activation of the halves of the brain would then be reflected in right LEMs and left LEMs, respectively.

To engage the left hemisphere, subjects have been asked to interpret proverbs, spell words, and solve logical problems (Al is smarter than Sam, and Al is duller than Rick. Who is smarter?). Questions involving visualization (How many edges are there on a cube?) and musical skills (identifying piano melodies) have been used to activate the right hemisphere. When differences in direction are found, right LEMs predominate in response to questions in the first group, and left LEMs follow questions of the second type.[47]

Other studies have suggested that the location of the experimenter affects the outcome of LEM studies. Specifically, it has been reported that when the experimenter was facing them, subjects looked to one side only regardless of the nature of the question. When the experimenter was positioned behind the same subjects, their eye movements were linked to the type of question posed.

...

Do LEMs Really Measure Brain Activation?

What exactly is the evidence linking LEMs to hemispheric asymmetry? A recent review of the work in this area has noted that the link is an indirect and weak one, based primarily on investigators' conceptions of what constitutes a left-hemisphere or a right-hemisphere question.[48]

Especially troublesome is the fact that approximately half of the studies in this area have failed to find the predicted differences. A priori, the questions used in these studies seem just as "left hemisphere" or just as "right hemisphere" as those employed in the studies reporting success. The logical problem of establishing a relationship between eye movements and brain asymmetry becomes circular if one must define left- or right-hemisphere activity in terms of the questions that produce the expected results.

In the absence of independent verification that eye movements are related to differential hemispheric cognitive activity, it would be wise to interpret the results of LEM studies cautiously. A review for which Bakan was a coauthor claimed that converging evidence from a variety of techniques support the LEM model.[49] The evidence is weak, however, leading us to conclude that it is premature to postulate conclusions about brain asymmetries and the processing of different kinds of questions on the basis of the direction of eye movements.

....

DOING TWO THINGS AT ONCE:
Mapping functional cerebral space

We all know that certain combinations of tasks are relatively easy to do together, whereas other tasks seem to interfere with each other. For example, many people can listen to music and read simultaneously, although the same people are unable to follow a conversation as they read. Intuitively, it seems as though tasks that call on very different areas of the brain show less interference when performed together than tasks that rely on the same general areas.

Marcel Kinsbourne, using such observations, has investigated what he referred to as "functional cerebral space."[50] He proposed that the distance between brain areas controlling different movements is reflected in the extent to which there is competition or cooperation when several movements are attempted simultaneously. In one study, right-handed subjects were asked to balance a dowel rod on their index fingers in silence or while repeating short sentences. Results indicated that when the subject was speaking, the right hand could not maintain balance as well or for as long as it could when the subject was silent. This was not the case with the left hand, however, which performed equally well in both conditions.[51]

Although there are no direct connections between the speech-control center and any limb-control center, Kinsbourne assumed that the control region for speech is closer to the control center for the right arm than to the left-arm control center. Therefore, there was greater disruption when speech accompanied dowel balancing by the right hand.

A later study showed that more difficult material produced shorter right-hand balancing times than easier material; left-hand balancing times were unaffected by difficulty. Interestingly, left-handers showed disruption in the balancing times of both hands under the verbalization condition, in keeping with evidence suggesting that left-handers as a group have less clearly lateralized verbal functions.[52] Other studies using a dual-task/time-sharing approach with different tasks have provided further support.[53]

Although the dual-task interference experiments are clever and quite interesting, some important reservations remain about this approach. For example, there is no validation of functional space that is independent of the study used to demonstrate it. If two tasks interfere with each other, they are assumed to be closer in functional space than two tasks that interfere less or not at all. By itself, this type of reasoning is too circular for comfort.

In addition, there have been numerous reports of failures to replicate basic findings. The reasons some investigators have been unsuccessful are not clear, but it is obvious that the outcome of dual-task interference studies is influenced by many factors. More research is needed before the interpretation and value of this approach can be assessed.

·········

NEW DIRECTIONS

The development of increasingly sophisticated models of higher level functions in normal subjects has contributed to the increased interest in neuropsychological investigations in normals. What we have learned from clinical populations should help in the development of models of normal functioning, and neuropsychological investigations in normals allow direct tests of some of the ideas generated from clinical work.

The appeal of work with normal subjects is unmistakable. First, the limitations placed on clinical and split-brain research by the scarcity of subjects are avoided. Second, work with neurologically normal subjects offers investigators more freedom in the kinds of experiments that can be devised. Third, and perhaps most important, work with normal subjects permits the study of asymmetries in the same system one is ultimately trying to understand: the normal human brain.

Although visual-field and dichotic-listening studies have been the most widely used, other approaches are also now gaining attention. As we shall see in the next chapter, electrophysiological and brain-imaging techniques offer an opportunity to observe directly correlates of brain activity in normal subjects during an ongoing task. By observing patterns of brain activity as a function of cognitive activity, investigators using these paradigms hope to build a clearer understanding of the processes involved in higher level mental acts.

FOUR

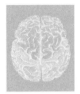

MEASURING THE BRAIN AND ITS ACTIVITY: Physiological Correlates of Asymmetry

Perhaps the most direct way to investigate differences between the hemispheres is to measure the activity of the brain itself. This strategy contrasts with the approaches considered in Chapter 3, where inferences about the brain were drawn from behavior in special testing situations. More direct measurements of brain activity bypass the need for many of the assumptions that are made in traditional behavioral studies. They also make it possible to study special groups of subjects, such as infants or animals, who might not be able to respond in the manner required by behavioral tests.

There are many different ways to measure brain anatomy and to monitor brain activity. Perhaps the most obvious is to measure the size and shape of the hemispheres. New techniques have made it possible to study anatomical asymmetries *in vivo,* that is, in living subjects.

The activity of the brain is very complex, encompassing various chemical and electrical processes along a continuum from microscopic to macroscopic function. Microscopic electrochemical communication between millions of neurons results in more global patterns of electrical activity that can be recorded from electrodes at the scalp. The "brain waves" recorded at various sites on the head and even weak magnetic fields produced by neural activity can be studied for differences within and between hemispheres.

The microscopic metabolic processes of neurons require that blood bring oxygen and glucose to brain tissue and remove waste products. Measurements of blood flow to the two sides of the brain, as well as differences in the metabolism of specific nutrients, can provide useful measures of brain activity on each side or within small regions of the brain. Recent technical developments have allowed increasingly sophisticated "imaging" of such activity and of the distribution of some of the chemicals involved in neuronal signal transmission. The rapidly growing field of "functional neuroimaging" is capturing the imagination of those who view such research as looking at the mind at work. Others feel that expectations for what can be achieved with brain imaging may be exaggerated.

In this chapter we shall first review evidence bearing on anatomical asymmetries in the brain and on electrical activity recorded from the brain. We shall then review some of the current work examining cerebral organization with imaging technology and try to present a balanced view of the potential of this exciting work that studies more directly the activity of the left brain and the right brain.

·········

ANATOMICAL ASYMMETRIES IN THE
TWO HEMISPHERES

A 1968 report by Norman Geschwind and Walter Levitsky demonstrated unequivocal anatomical asymmetries in the two hemispheres of the human brain in the regions important for speech and language.[1] Published in a journal widely read by scientists in a number of different disciplines, their paper generated a great deal of excitement among those interested in hemispheric asymmetry of function.

Geschwind and Levitsky were not the first investigators to notice such asymmetries in the brain, however. Asymmetries had been reported sporadically as far back as the second half of the nineteenth century, at which time the differences generally were considered trivial and insufficient to account for functional differences between the left brain and the right brain.

By the late 1960s, however, the time was ripe to reconsider the possibility that functional asymmetries between hemispheres might have a physical basis on a nonmicroscopic, anatomical level. Since the publication of Geschwind and Levitsky's paper, several other investigators have studied the problem, extending the search for asymmetries to neonates and nonhuman primates.

In this chapter we shall review the evidence pointing to asymmetries in the adult human brain. We shall reserve discussion of work with neonates and nonhuman primates for Chapter 9.

...

Measuring the Hemispheres

The asymmetries found by Geschwind and Levitsky were in the lengths of the temporal plane (planum temporale), the upper surface of the region of the temporal lobe behind the auditory cortex. Of the 100 brains measured at postmortem, 65 were found to have a longer temporal plane in the left hemisphere than in the right, 11 had a longer temporal plane in the right hemisphere, and the remaining 24 showed no difference. On average, the temporal plane was one-third longer on the left than on the right. Figure 4.1 shows the location of these asymmetries.

Although the size of these asymmetries is impressive, their location is more significant. The temporal plane is part of Wernicke's area, a region named after Karl Wernicke, who first noted that damage to this area frequently results in a variety of aphasic symptoms. Geschwind and Levitsky suggested that the asymmetries they observed were compatible with the functional asymmetries believed to be controlled by this region.

Several studies using various procedures to measure the temporal plane have confirmed Geschwind and Levitsky's observations.[2] Seventy percent of 337 brain specimens (including the 100 brains studied by Geschwind and Levitsky) showed asymmetry favoring the left hemisphere in length or area of the temporal plane.

Does the left get bigger or the right get smaller? In a recent reevaluation of the anatomical data used by Geschwind, neurologist Albert Galaburda and associates found an interesting relationship between the

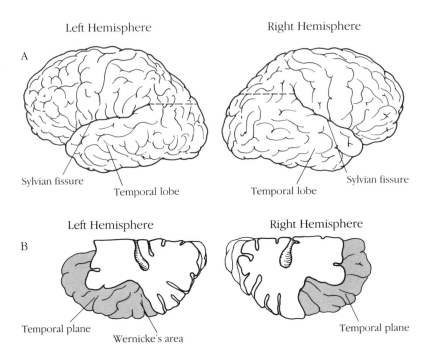

FIGURE 4.1   Anatomical asymmetries in the cortex of the human brain. A. The sylvian fissure, which defines the upper margin of the temporal lobe, rises more steeply on the right side of the brain. The dotted lines represent the plane of section for B. B. (viewed from above) The temporal plane, which forms the upper surface of the temporal lobe, is usually much larger on the left side. This region in the left hemisphere is considered part of Wernicke's area, a region involved in language. [From Geschwind, "Specializations of the Human Brain," *Scientific American, Inc.*, 1979. All rights reserved.]

degree of asymmetry and the size of each temporal plane. Geschwind previously had assumed that the asymmetry he observed was a result of greater or more rapid development of the left side. He predicted that symmetrical brains resulted from a less developed left side.

Galaburda, however, found that the left planum (temporal plane) remains roughly constant in size (corrected for variability in total brain size) but that the right planum is larger in symmetrical and smaller in asymmetrical brains.[3] Thus, symmetrical brains tend to have two large plana, whereas most asymmetrical brains have a large left and a small right planum. Galaburda speculated that whatever factors play a role in the development of these asymmetries act by controlling the extent of development of the right side in most individuals.

...

Measurements in the Living Brain

The anatomical studies considered up to this point have involved measurements taken from brains examined at postmortem. Other evidence suggests that it is also possible to find asymmetries in the living brain. Such techniques are particularly valuable because they permit investigators to correlate anatomical findings with performance measured in living subjects.

Cerebral Angiography   One technique takes advantage of the fact that the paths of the large blood vessels in the brain reflect the anatomy of the surrounding brain tissue. In particular, the middle cerebral artery courses through the language-critical region of the temporal lobe. For many years, neurologists have used a procedure known as cerebral angiography to visualize this major blood vessel to determine whether the brain regions surrounding it have been damaged. A dye injected into the internal carotid artery in the neck (the same artery used in the Wada procedure) flows into the middle cerebral artery, making the artery visible when a skull X-ray is taken. Majorie LeMay and her colleagues have evidence suggesting that left-right asymmetries consistent with those found in postmortem brain measurements may be observed with the angiographic procedure.[4]

Computerized Tomography   Another technique used to measure asymmetry in the living brain is computerized tomography (CT scanning). In a CT scan, an X-ray source is revolved in a plane around the head as detectors continuously monitor the intensity of the X-ray beam passed through to the other side. A computer stores this information and then uses it to reconstruct an image of a slice of brain. Figure 4.2 shows representative CT scans.

This technique has been used for many years now to pinpoint the locations of lesions in cases of brain damage. LeMay and her colleagues have also been active in using CT scan data to study asymmetries, with some success.[5]

Magnetic Resonance Imaging   Cerebral angiography and CT scanning techniques depend on X-ray radiation. A brain-imaging technique called magnetic resonance imaging (MRI) is capable of generating fine cross-sectional images of brain structure without using penetrating radiation. The technique uses the principle of nuclear magnetic resonance, often abbreviated NMR. In the NMR procedure, a combination

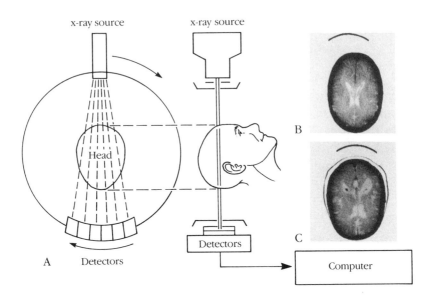

FIGURE 4.2   A. A computerized tomography (CT) scan uses an X-ray beam and an array of detectors involving around the subject's head to calculate the density of tissues in a particular slice of the brain. A computer reconstructs a two-dimensional picture of the brain in the plane swept by the X-rays. The CT pictures shown here are (B) normal, with no evidence of pathology, and (C) abnormal, with enlargement of the ventricles (fluid-filled spaces—the light central areas), especially on the right, moderate atrophy, and right frontotemporal infarct (stroke).

of radio waves and a strong magnetic field (generated by a large electromagnet) are used to detect the distribution of water molecules in living tissue (the hydrogen atoms in the water "resonate" as a result of the combined effect of the radio waves and the magnetic field). In this way, brain tissue densities can be very accurately calculated, and a fine pictorial image can be generated by computer.[6] Figure 4.3 shows an example of the resolution achieved by an MRI scan.

...

What Do Anatomical Asymmetries Tell Us?

Much of the interest in techniques that can measure asymmetries in the living brain concerns the basic problem of interpreting anatomical asymmetries. Are the asymmetries that have been identified related in a meaningful way to functional asymmetries between the hemispheres?

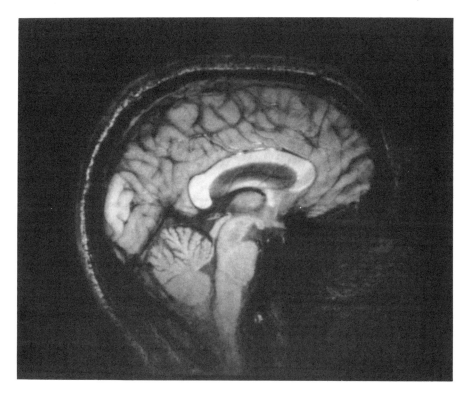

FIGURE 4.3 Nuclear magnetic resonance (NMR) scan. A computer-reconstructed image of a cross-section of a normal brain, using data derived from the NMR of hydrogen in the water molecules of a subject's head. [Courtesy of Dr. Hoby Hetherington, Center for Nuclear Imaging Research, University of Alabama at Birmingham.]

At this point, we do not know. Most of the data on anatomical asymmetries have come from postmortem measurements, where often nothing is known about the kinds of functional asymmetries that may have existed before death. In many cases, even the handedness of the individuals is not known.

Procedures that permit measurements in the living brain offer us a way to collect much crucial information. Batteries of behavioral and electrophysiological tests designed to study the distribution of functions between the hemispheres can be used along with measurements of brain asymmetry in the same individuals to see whether there is a relationship. Data indicate that, overall, left-handers show less anatomical asymmetry than right-handers.[7] It is clear, however, that investigators have only begun the process of studying how anatomical asymmetries, functional asymmetries, and cognitive abilities are related.

·········

ELECTRICAL ACTIVITY IN THE LEFT BRAIN AND THE RIGHT BRAIN

In 1929 the Austrian psychiatrist Hans Burger discovered that patterns of electrical activity could be recorded from electrodes placed at various points on the scalps. These patterns were called the electroencephalogram (EEG), literally meaning "electrical brain writing." Although the EEG is monitored from the scalp, Burger was able to demonstrate that some of the activity it records originates in the brain itself and is not simply due to scalp musculature.

Devices to record the EEG soon became commonplace in clinical settings as investigators demonstrated that brain abnormalities such as epilepsy and tumors are accompanied by distinctive patterns of electrical activity. Its potential as a research tool was also quickly recognized, and innumerable studies looking for EEG correlates of personality, intelligence, and behavior were undertaken.

···

Using the EEG to Study Asymmetry

Until the late 1960s, EEG recordings were typically made from electrodes placed at different points along the top of the head or only on one side of the head. It was assumed that activity would be identical on the two sides. A few studies did report EEG asymmetries, however, when electrodes were placed on both sides. The asymmetries seemed to be related to hand preference, but not in any simple way. David Galin and Robert Ornstein, of the Langley Porter Neuropsychiatric Institute in San Francisco, were two of the first investigators to study these asymmetries in detail and to relate them to the nature of the task performed by the subject while the EEG was being recorded.[8]

Galin and Ornstein recorded EEG activity from symmetrical positions on either side of the head while subjects performed verbal tasks, such as writing a letter, and spatial tasks, such as constructing a memorized geometrical pattern with multicolored blocks. Results were analyzed in terms of the ratio of right-hemisphere EEG power (R) to left-hemisphere EEG power (L). Electroencephalogram power is simply the amount of electrical energy being produced per unit of time. They found that the R/L power ratio in the verbal tasks was significantly greater than in the spatial tasks.

At first glance these results seem to be the precise opposite of what one would predict, because letter writing is a left-hemisphere task and should produce relatively more left-hemisphere activity than a task involving blocks. This "problem" is readily resolved, however, by considering that several different rhythms of activity have been identified as constituents of the EEG record. The first one discovered is also the most famous: the alpha rhythm. Alpha activity is a rhythmic cycling of electrical activity occurring from 8 to 12 times per second. It is the predominant activity present in the EEG when the subject is resting quietly with closed eyes. Other rhythms that are part of the EEG are also identified by Greek letters. Figure 4.4 shows EEG waveforms for five different brain states.

An analysis of Galin and Ornstein's results showed that the predominant rhythm in the EEG records was alpha. Because alpha reflects a resting brain state, less alpha activity would be expected to follow greater involvement in a particular task. Thus, the left hemisphere should show relatively less alpha when a subject is performing a language task in contrast with the amount of alpha activity present when the subject is doing a spatial task like the block-design problem. This is precisely what was found.

...

Advantages and Disadvantages of the EEG

Electroencephalographic measures of asymmetry have been popular with many investigators. Because they do not rely on an overt response from the subject, they can be used to study brain asymmetries in infants, aphasic patients, and other subjects from whom it might be difficult to obtain such responses. In addition, EEG is a continuous measure over time and can be used to study ongoing activity in the brain while the subject performs long, complex tasks.

Although the latter feature of the EEG measure is quite useful in some studies, it is difficult to see changes in the EEG that relate to the occurrence of specific stimulus events. In fact, the complex EEG waveforms do not appear to change very much during different kinds of sensory input but, instead, seem to reflect the general arousal level of the brain.

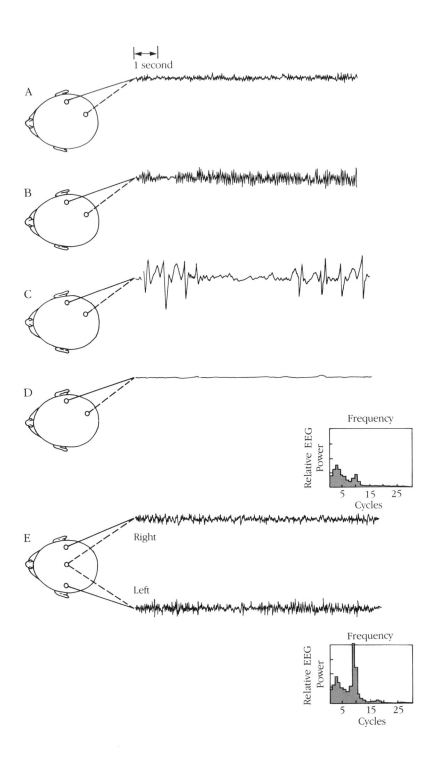

FIGURE 4.4 *(Left)* Typical electroencephalograms. The "head" to the left of each record shows the appropriate placement of the electrodes. A. At rest with eyes open. B. At rest with eyes shut. The large-magnitude waves occurring at a frequency of 8 to 12 per second are the alpha waves. C. The dramatic spiking associated with an epileptic seizure. D. "Brain death" or "cerebral death." Even though the heart may be beating, the electrically quiet record shows that the patient is clinically dead. E. Simultaneous recording of left- and right-temporal EEG activity while the subject performs a block-design task. The graph to the right of each hemisphere's record is an analysis of the relative "power" of various frequencies in the EEG waveform. Notice that the left recording contains a greater amount of alpha, evident from the 8- to 12-cycle peak in the frequency graph. During speaking and writing, more alpha is recorded on the right. The degree and direction of asymmetry varies with the task. [Part E adapted from Galin and Ornstein, "Lateral Specialization of Cognitive Mode: An EEG Study," Fig. 1, p. 417, *Psychophysiology* (1972) 9 (The Society for Psychophysiological Research, 1972) and from Doyle, Ornstein, and Galin, "Lateral Specialization of Cognitive Mode: II. EEG Frequency Analysis," Fig. 1, p. 571, *Psychophysiology* (1974) 11 (The Society for Psychophysiological Research). Reprinted with permission from the publisher.]

...

The Evoked Potential

A careful analysis of the EEG, however, reveals that specific changes do occur in response to the presentation of a stimulus such as a flash of light, but they are hidden by the overall background activity of the brain. To make visible the change in response to a specific stimulus, a computer is used to average the waveform records following repeated presentations of the same stimulus. Electrical activity that is random with respect to the stimulus presentation will be canceled out by this process, whereas electrical activity occurring in a fixed time relation to the stimulus will emerge as the potential evoked by the stimulus.

The evoked potential (EP) consists of a sequence of positive and negative changes from a baseline and typically lasts about 500 milliseconds after the stimulus ends. Each potential can be analyzed in terms of certain components or parameters, such as amplitude and latency (the amount of time from the onset of the stimulus to the onset of the activity).

The nature of the stimulus (auditory, visual, somatosensory) is one of the factors that affects the precise form of the evoked potential. In addition, the region of each hemisphere generating maximum activity differs for each type of stimulus. Figure 4.5 shows typical EPs to stimuli in different modalities. Of primary concern to us here is whether the EP

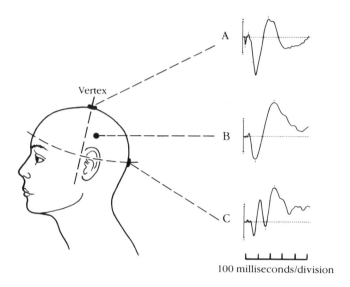

Vertex

A

B

C

100 milliseconds/division

FIGURE 4.5   Typical evoked potentials for (A) auditory, (B) somatosensory, and (C) visual stimulation. The dotted lines indicate the approximate location on the scalp from which the most pronounced peaks are recorded. [Adapted from Thompson and Patterson, eds., *Bioelectric Recording Techniques* (New York: Academic Press, Inc.)]

generated by a stimulus is the same when recordings are made from equivalent locations on the two sides of the head.

Psychologists Dennis Molfese and colleagues have collected extensive data on EPs to speech and nonspeech stimuli.[9] In one study, they found that the amplitude of part of the EP to speech stimuli was greater in the left hemisphere than in the right hemisphere. This difference was seen even when the subject merely listened to the stimuli and did not try to identify them. Nonspeech stimuli, however, produced activity of larger amplitude in the right hemisphere.

Several studies have also looked at how asymmetries are affected by the task the subject is performing while the EP is recorded. In one such study, subjects were presented with a sequence of synthetically produced spoken syllables that could differ in initial consonant ("ba" versus "da") or in pitch (high or low).[10] In one-half of the trials, subjects were instructed to listen for each occurrence of "ba," regardless of its pitch. In the other half, the subjects were instructed to listen for high-pitched syllables, independent of their names.

Evoked potentials to the high-pitched "ba" were recorded from the left and right hemispheres in each case. This procedure enabled the investigators to study the effect of two different mental activities on EP asymmetry while maintaining exactly the same stimulation conditions. Results showed a difference in the EPs produced during the naming and pitch-discrimination tasks, but only in the left hemisphere. These findings led the researchers to suggest that there are hemispheric differences in the ability to identify a syllable but no differences in the ability to determine the pitch of the syllable.

...

Probe Evoked Potentials During Mental Activity

Standard EP experiments were limited to recording responses to short, usually simple stimuli. The probe evoked potential is a more recent development that greatly expanded the applications of EP methods to studying brain-behavior relationships involving more complex mental activity. Instead of examining the response to repeated stimulation against a resting-state background, the experimenter asks the subject to perform a task, during which some irrelevant "probe" stimulus (for example, a click or a light flash) is repeatedly introduced. What is of interest is to what extent the EP, which is normally excited by the probe stimulus, is suppressed by activity or the task the subject is performing.

It is presumed that the brain can do well on only a limited number of simultaneous tasks. Thus, the more complex the background task, the greater the reduction of the brain's normal response to some intermittent probe stimulus. Probe EPs can be recorded from different regions of the brain simultaneously. The change in the probe EP amplitude is thought to be determined by how demanding the task is and by what areas are involved in the task performance.

In one study using this approach, the relative engagement of temporal and parietal regions of the left and right hemispheres was monitored during an arithmetic task and a visuospatial task by recording EPs to a probe tone presented through earphones.[11] In all conditions, the subjects viewed the same series of stimuli, consisting of fragmented segments next to a whole geometric shape, with numbers printed inside each fragment and inside the complete shape. In the visuospatial run, the subjects signaled with a finger movement if the fragments would create the intact geometrical shape presented next to them. In the arithmetic trials, the subjects signaled if the numbers inside the fragments added up to the number inside the completed shape.

The amplitude of the EPs to the tone probes varied according to which task the subjects were performing. Probe EPs were significantly reduced, compared with controls, in the left temporal area during arithmetic calculations. The visuospatial task resulted in greater probe reduction in the right parietal region.

These results confirm, of course, left-hemisphere involvement in "serial-analytic" operations, such as those involved in speech and calculation, and right-hemisphere involvement in certain visuospatial processes. In addition, this study is a good example of an experimental design in which instructions to the subject are varied in tasks involving identical stimuli and identical responses, allowing investigators to better isolate the changes in brain function that result from differences in psychological or mental function.

Similar experiments have been used to carefully investigate hemispheric involvement in recognizing emotional tone in speech.[12] Subjects listened to the same conversations under two task conditions, one in which they had to report, at the end of the presentation, how many times the syllable "na" occurred. In the other condition, they reported the emotions communicated by each speaker during the conversation. The reduction in probe EPs to a repeatedly presented click was greater in the left hemisphere during the syllable-detection condition and greater in the right during the emotional-tone judgments. Thus, the same conversation was shown to be processed to a greater extent by the left hemisphere when attention to speech sounds was required and by the right hemisphere when emotional-tone judgments were necessary. (Further discussion of the role of the right hemisphere in emotion is found in Chapter 7.)

...

How Far Can Scalp Recordings of Brain Electrical Activity Take Us?

In recent years Alan Gevins and colleagues have taken EEG and evoked-response measurement to a new level of sophistication by recording from as many as 125 scalp electrodes placed over a subject's entire head. Through complex computer analysis of the EEG changes in all electrode locations associated with various stages of repeated task conditions, Gevins has reported a number of findings regarding cerebral regions activated by different cognitive operations.[13] Most of these findings are reported in terms of the "covariance" of multiple cerebral regions with each other during stimulation, response, or decision-making. The regions that change together in an EEG are identified as part of the neural "network" involved in the task or particular task stage.

This work is controversial but has promoted several innovative concepts, including a search for correlations in cerebral activity changes as opposed to simple identification of locations of maximum activity change. We shall return to this concept when we discuss metabolic imaging studies later in this chapter.

Many electrophysiologists maintain that scalp recordings are not sufficient to isolate brain electrical activity with any precision and that different techniques are necessary to make inferences about such activity in multiple cerebral regions. The development of magnetoencephalography was spurred by such considerations.

·········

MAGNETOENCEPHALOGRAPHY

Neural activity not only generates electrical fields but also produces magnetic fields. In recent years it has become technologically possible to record and isolate the magnetic fields that accompany the electrical fields generated by neuronal activity within specific regions of the brain. Magnetic fields created by the activity of single neurons are extremely small, but under certain conditions the magnetic fields of a number of simultaneously active neurons combine to produce fields that are sufficiently strong to be measured at the surface of the head. Such a recording is called a magnetoencephalogram (MEG), the magnetic counterpart of the EEG.

Calculations based on MEG measurements permit three-dimensional localization of the cell groups generating the measured field. Thus, a major advantage of this technique over the EEG is its ability to better localize within the brain the source of the activity being recorded. Figure 4.6 illustrates the equipment.

Special superconducting coils are needed to pick up the very weak brain magnetic fields, and measurements routinely are done within elaborate magnetically shielded rooms. The heart of a MEG probe is a sensing instrument called the superconducting quantum interference device (SQUID), which is immersed in liquid helium. By either moving a single probe or using multiple probes placed in different positions, the MEG procedure creates "isocontour maps," that is, charts with concentric circles representing different intensities of the magnetic field (see Figure 4.7). From such maps, a three-dimensional location of the neurons generating the field can be calculated.

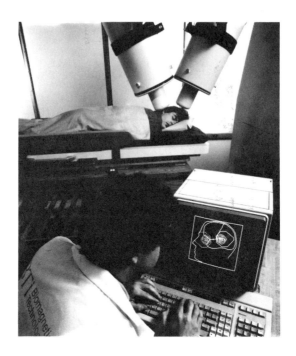

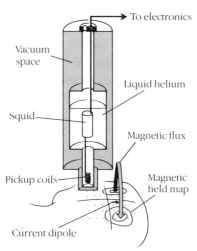

FIGURE 4.6   A. A patient undergoing a brain scan, using a 14-channel neuromagnetometer. The process tracks the electrical function of the brain by detecting magnetic fields generated by the electrical current within the brain. [Courtesy of Biomagnetic Technologies, Inc., San Diego, CA.] B. Brain magnetic fields are measured by using a superconducting amplifier (SQUID; see text) coupled to special coils. The liquid helium keeps the system at a low temperature, necessary for superconductivity. [Courtesy of Dr. Jackson Beatty, University of California, Los Angeles, CA.]

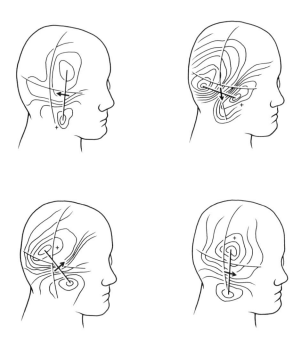

FIGURE 4.7   Examples of isocontour maps displaying the magnetic fields generated by epileptic activity in a patient's right hemisphere. Such MEG recordings allow precise localization of the sources of the seizure activity. This patient's recordings indicated multiple sources within the right temporal lobe. [From Beatty, Barth, Richer and Johnson, "Neuromagnetometry," Figs. 2-10, p. 38, in *Psychophysiology*, ed., Coles, Donchin, and Porges (New York: Guilford Press, 1986).]

Researchers initially attempted to use MEG to establish the location and depth of the electrical currents underlying discharges in epileptic tissue with greater accuracy than was possible with EEG alone. They were very successful; for example, in one patient epileptic activity was localized to an exact region 10 to 11 millimeters beneath the subject's scalp.[14]

...

Evoked Fields

Response to external stimulation can be measured with MEG by using an analogue of the EP. We have seen how a repeated auditory, somatosensory, or visual stimulus will generate a measurable response or change in averaged EEG waveforms. The same stimulus results in a characteristic waveshape in the magnetic field recorded over specific cerebral regions, the source of which is much more localizable than the source of an EP. For example, the source of magnetic-field patterns evoked by repeated clicks (evoked fields, or EFs) has been clearly localized to the auditory temporal cortex of each hemisphere.[15]

Further study determined the sources of activity within a hemisphere associated with stimulation of the ear either on the same (ipsilateral) side or on the opposite (contralateral) side of the head. The magnetic evoked fields to left-and right-ear stimulation were recorded in the right hemisphere in eight subjects, and the resulting source coordinates were projected onto the structural MRI images of each subject's head.

Not only did MEG show the activity source to fall in the vicinity of the auditory cortex in each subject, it also showed that the source was slightly different for ipsilateral and contralateral stimulation, a result indicating that adjacent but separate regions in the right auditory cortex are activated by left- versus right-ear stimulation. The investigators suggested that these results point out the potential precision and applicability of MEG in the study of human sensory motor and cognitive processes.[16]

Magnetoencephalographic research is currently being extended to study both basic physiology and more complex mental function. Because of technical complexities and costs, most MEG instrumentation has typically consisted of 7 or 14 channels contained within one or two holding assemblies, a factor limiting the regions of the brain that can be studied simultaneously. New MEG instrumentation, however, provides many more channels and even includes a version that covers the whole head with over 100 separate SQUID assemblies. These instruments will allow better studies of interhemispheric processes during complex cognitive activity, including the measurement of hemispheric asymmetries.

·········

BLOOD FLOW IN THE HEMISPHERES

The flow of blood through the tissues of the body varies with the metabolism and activity in those tissues. The blood flow, which provides necessary nutrients and removes waste products, turns out to be very sensitive and responsive to minute changes in cellular activity. In fact, changes in the activity in various regions of the brain appear to be reflected in the relative amount of blood flowing through those regions.

This discovery has made it possible to identify and study the interaction of various areas of the brain during ongoing human behavior by measuring regional changes in blood flow.

A technique for measuring regional cortical blood flow in an awake and functioning human was developed by Niels Lassen, David Ingvar, and others.[17] They injected a special radioactive isotope—xenon-133—into an artery leading to the brain and monitored the flow with a battery of detectors arranged near the surface of the head. The technique, originally used with patients requiring the test for medical reasons, has since been refined to the point where subjects can breathe a special air-xenon mixture and have their blood flow monitored by placing their heads next to a machine housing the special detectors.[*]

The results of studies measuring cerebral blood flow during different kinds of physical and mental activities have been impressive. Classic predictions about brain areas involved in psychological functions have been corroborated. The regions of each hemisphere involved in vision, for example, show increased blood flow if the subject is looking at a moving pattern. Speech stimuli increase blood flow in the auditory areas of each side.

Blood-flow investigators Lassen, Ingvar, and Skinhoj reported that they were impressed by the similarity in the blood-flow patterns in the two hemispheres, even during highly lateralized activities such as speech.[18] The most striking changes during tasks and mental activity appeared to take place along the anterior-posterior dimension of the brain, rather than left to right.

Differences between the hemispheres were nevertheless found by using techniques that permit the study of regional blood flow in the two hemispheres simultaneously. In an early study, Jarl Risberg compared the blood-flow pattern of right-handed male volunteers during two tasks, one a verbal analogies test and the other a test of perceptual "closure." In the closure task, the subjects had to view very sparsely drawn pictures and figure out what they represented.[19]

Small but highly significant hemispheric differences in blood flow of about 3 percent were found in the two conditions. As expected, the mean left-hemisphere flow was greater during the verbal analogies task, and the mean right-hemisphere flow was greater during the picture-completion task. Risberg was able to measure which regions within each hemisphere contributed the most to interhemispheric blood-flow differences. The largest differences were found in the frontal, frontotemporal, and parietal regions for the verbal tests. In the resting state,

---

* The low level of gamma radiation emitted by the isotope is not considered harmful and washes out of the bloodstream within 15 minutes.

differences between corresponding regions of the hemispheres were very small.

Another series of experiments compared several tasks thought to involve primarily right-hemisphere processing.[20] Nineteen right-handed subjects performed three tasks: judgment of line orientation, mental rotation of three-dimensional cube arrays, and a fragment-puzzle task. Examples of the visually presented stimuli are shown in Figure 4.8.

In the rotation condition, subjects judged whether projected drawings of two three-dimensional arrays of cubes were identical but only rotated in space. In the puzzle task, subjects judged whether fragmented figures could form a simultaneously presented whole figure. In line orientation, a slide showing a line pair was presented for 4 seconds, followed by presentation of a fan-shaped array of lines with arrows pointing at two. The subject had to decide whether the angle formed by

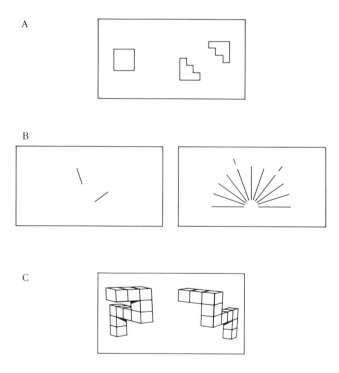

FIGURE 4.8 Examples of test material used in a cerebral blood-flow study comparing three visuospatial tasks. A. Fragment-puzzle task. (Will the fragments on the left form the figure on the right?) B. Line-orientation task. (Is the angle formed by the two lines the same as the angle formed by the lines at which the arrows point?) C. Mental-rotation task. (Mentally rotate either of the two figures to see if they are identical.) [From Deutsch, et al., 1988]

the lines at which the arrows pointed was the same as in the previously presented pair.

Asymmetries in hemispheric flow (right side greater) were observed only in the line-orientation and mental-rotation conditions. The magnitude of the asymmetry was greater in the rotation task in which blood-flow increases were especially prominent in parietal areas. On the basis of these results, the authors suggested that mental rotation uses more exclusively right-hemisphere "skills" than did the other tasks surveyed. Whether the nature of these skills is revealed more by the rotation task than by the line-orientation task, of course, is another issue. Mental rotation involves "mental manipulation" in space, a concept mentioned previously in the context of right-hemisphere superiority for certain tasks attempted with split-brain patients (see Chapter 2). In Chapter 8 we shall consider cerebral blood-flow data showing sex differences in mental rotation.

Another study examined data from 121 regional cerebral blood-flow studies conducted under a variety of conditions involving different stimuli, response modes, and task requirements.[21] These scans were compared with scans conducted while subjects were at rest, during which blood flow is very closely coupled in homologous regions of the two hemispheres. Significant hemispheric differences were found in the frontal regions when all tasks were combined. Right flow was greater than left, especially in the more demanding tasks. The study concluded that the right frontal activation observed may be due to general attentional demands and not limited to tasks usually thought to involve the right hemisphere. This finding suggests a very general role for the right hemisphere in attention or vigilance and is especially interesting in light of the clinical data on the neglect syndrome and other disorders associated with right-hemisphere lesions (see Chapter 7).

·········

IMAGING BRAIN METABOLISM:
PET and other technologies

Xenon cortical blood-flow techniques do have some limitations as measures of brain activity. The studies described above do not provide accurate information about the deepest regions of the brain. Most of the observed patterns are at cortical levels.

Newer technologies are now providing ways of "imaging" or visualizing cerebral blood flow throughout the brain, as well as monitoring other aspects of cerebral metabolism in an alive and functioning brain.

...

Emission Tomography

Emission tomography is a visualization technique that yields an image of the distribution of a radioactively labeled substance in any desired cross section of the body or head. In single photon emission tomography (SPECT), biochemicals of interest are labeled with radioactive compounds that emit gamma rays in all directions. These substances, called radiopharmaceuticals, are injected into the bloodstream of subjects. As the radiopharmaceuticals reach the brain, detectors surrounding or rotated about the head pick up these emissions, and computer programs are used to "reconstruct" what the distribution of the labeled substance must have been to generate the pattern of emissions sensed by the detectors. So far, SPECT procedures have been used to measure cerebral blood flow and blood volume in three-dimensional cross sections of the brain.

...

HMPAO SPECT Studies of Cerebral Blood Flow

Most current brain SPECT uses the radiopharmaceutical ^{99}mTc-Hexamethylpropyleneamine oxime (HMPAO) as the "tracer" that is injected intravenously and crosses into brain tissue (and gets trapped) at a rate proportional to the cerebral flow rate. Emission tomography scanning of the gamma photons emitted by the compound allows the investigator to visualize the distribution of the HMPAO tracer, which reflects cerebral blood flow at the time of injection. Because the amount and location of the tracer trapped in brain tissue is based on cerebral blood flow at the time of injection, this technique allows investigators to "lock in" the brain activity state at that time. As a result, it has been possible to capture the cerebral blood flow during an epileptic seizure by injecting HMPAO during the seizure and scanning the patient later.[22] Figure 4.9 shows that precisely localized seizure activity onset.

In a similar fashion, the effects of stimulation or mental activity can be locked in while the subject is performing a task and then scanned afterward. This property was recently used to study subjects while they

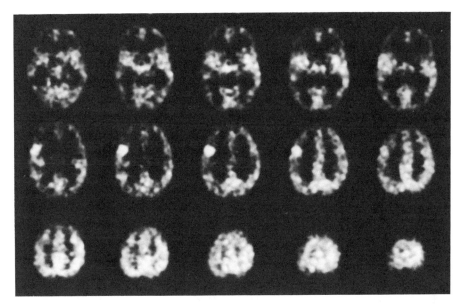

FIGURE 4.9   SPECT images of cerebral blood flow capturing a seizure onset in an epilepsy patient. Brain images are horizontal cross sections starting at a middle level of the brain (upper left hand corner) and proceeding to the top of the brain (lower right hand corner). Four cross sections in the middle row show seizure onset, indicated by high blood flow (bright spots) on the left side. This corresponds to the patient's right motor cortex, since the image orientation is as if viewed from the patient's feet. No abnormalities were evident in this region on ordinary structural scans (e.g. CT or MRI). (Courtesy of Drs. James M. Mountz and Ruben Kuzniecky of the University of Alabama at Birmingham.)

performed the mental rotation task described earlier.[23] A subject was injected while lying in a darkened room and performing the task presented on a screen. A half-hour later, the subject was scanned while relaxing and lying still. The scan showed greater activity in the right parietal region compared to a scan of the same subject injected with HMPAO during rest.

These results are similar to those shown in previous studies of cortical blood flow conducted during task performance, and they serve both to reinforce the previous findings and to validate this intriguing use of HMPAO SPECT. The lock-in-a-state property of the HMPAO SPECT technique will be quite useful for studying tasks or states (e.g., sleep) that cannot be easily done while the subject is in a scanner. It also affords a better opportunity to study patients who cannot normally be scanned without sedation, such as autistic children. Injecting HMPAO prior to sedation and scanning should allow investigators to visualize the cerebral activity as it was before sedation.

The same locked-in property of the HMPAO tracer that makes it very useful for pursuing certain questions also limits SPECT scans to the study of only one condition at a time, because it takes two days for the tracer to clear from the head. Several methods are being examined to get around this limitation of SPECT studies of cerebral blood flow. However, most current imaging studies of multiple tasks or conditions are investigated by using the much more costly positron emission tomography (PET) procedure.

...

Positron Emission Tomography

Positron emission tomography (PET) utilizes the properties of the special radiation generated by positron-emitting substances, which generate pairs of photons traveling in exactly opposite direction. The simultaneity and directionality of positron emissions allow investigators to accurately determine the location of any specially labeled substance. Positron emission tomography is the only technique developed so far that can produce regional three-dimensional quantification of glucose and oxygen metabolism in the living human brain.

Glucose metabolism is a more direct measure of the function of neural tissue than cerebral blood flow, especially in patients with cerebral injury or disease that may affect normal vascular regulatory mechanisms. Initial work with PET scanning of glucose metabolism was conducted during simple sensory stimulation. PET images clearly delineated areas in the temporal cortex associated with auditory stimulation and areas in the occipital lobe that are active during visual stimulation (Figures 4.10 and 4.11).

Investigators have started to use PET to study higher mental function. Unfortunately, the incorporation and scanning of positron emitter-labeled glucose compounds takes about 40 minutes, too long a period during which to maintain a reliable mental state or most task conditions. Newer radiopharmaceuticals, including the use of positron-labeled oxygen (^{15}O), allow the measurement of regional cerebral oxygen consumption and blood flow with PET in a matter of several minutes.

One study attempted to distinguish brain areas activated by specific language functions by repeated PET scans during a four-level progres-

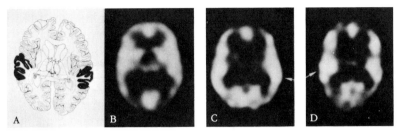

FIGURE 4.10   A. The primary auditory cortex is schematically indicated in black on the brain outline. B–D. Positron emission tomographic images of the brains of (B) an unstimulated control subject; (C) a subject listening to a factual story with the left ear; (D) a subject similarly stimulated in the right ear. Bright areas correspond to regions of higher cerebral metabolic rate for glucose. The regions of activation in C and D seemed to extend beyond the primary auditory cortex (arrows). [From Reivich and Gur, "Cerebral Metabolic Effects of Sensory Stimuli," Fig. 1, p. 332, in *Positron Emission Tomography*, ed. Reivich and Alavi (New York: Alan R. Liss, 1985).]

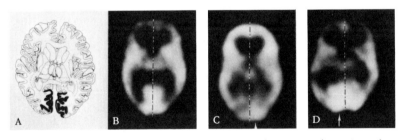

FIGURE 4.11   A. Schematic representation of a horizontal section through the brain. The striate (primary visual) cortex is indicated in black. B-D. Positron emission tomographic images of (B) unstimulated and (C, D) stimulated subjects. A dotted line defines the midline of each image. B. In a blindfolded subject, glucose metabolism in the visual cortex of the occipital pole is symmetrical. C. Left visual hemifield stimulation produces asymmetrical glucose metabolism. The right striate cortex is 25 to 30 times more active than the left. D. Right visual hemifield stimulation produces the reverse pattern. The left striate cortex has a metabolic rate 18 percent greater than a homologous area in the right hemisphere. [From Reivich and Gur, "Cerebral Metabolic Effects of Sensory Stimuli," Fig. 2, p. 332, in *Positron Emission Tomography*, ed. Reivich and Alavi (New York: Alan R. Liss, 1985).]

sion of tasks in seven normal subjects.[24] The base state was visual fixation on a symbol (+) presented on a video monitor. Observation of single nouns was the second level. Vocal repetition of cue words added motor output. In the final condition the subject had to respond to a presented object noun with a verb describing some use of the object, thus adding a semantic-processing demand to the condition.

By subtracting the blood-flow pattern measured during one level of task from that of another task level, the investigators tried to isolate some of the changes induced by relatively specific mental activity. The investigators found that vocalization produced bilateral flow increases in the sensory-motor strip and several frontal-lobe regions. The semantic task did cause an asymmetrical activation of the lower left frontal lobe compared with the control condition (vocal repetition alone). Perhaps most interesting was the fact that despite the attempt to isolate the activity due to stimulation from that of cognitive processes, the investigators still found some lateralized activity in association areas of the left hemisphere associated with "just looking" at words. The researchers suggested that the subjects were reflexively performing some linguistic analysis of the stimulus cue words even though there was no language task demand per se. The level of activity did not change in these areas of the left hemisphere during active reading/vocalization or the semantic task, a result supporting the idea that the subjects had already automatically done some form of linguistic analysis during passive presentation of the cue words.

...

PET Studies of Face Recognition

A more recent PET study used ^{15}O PET scanning of cerebral blood flow to identify the cerebral activation specific to face recognition.[25] To do so, a face-recognition condition was compared with a condition requiring the processing of another property of faces—categorizing by gender—that is not typically affected in brain-injury patients suffering from face-recognition problems, or prosopagnosia. A baseline condition involving fixating on a monitor screen, and the two conditions viewing simple patterns and viewing common objects, were also employed.

Compared with the baseline condition, cerebral blood flow changes in the simple-pattern condition were found in the primary visual cortex in the occipital lobe (striate cortex) of both hemispheres. Activation of the primary visual cortex did not change in any of the experimental task conditions.

Categorizing faces by gender resulted in activation in right-hemisphere posterior regions just outside the visual cortex. The face-identification task produced additional activation in right temporal lobe regions, the activation extending deep into the temporal lobe toward the hippocampus. Cerebral activation during an object-recognition task occurred in the left posterior temporal cortex and did not involve the right-hemisphere regions specifically activated during the face-recognition task.

This study thus provided the first evidence from normal subjects regarding the important role of central temporal regions of the right hemisphere in face recognition. Because there is conflicting data and opinion regarding the role of the left hemisphere in face recognition, the PET investigators conducted an additional study, using lateralized visual-field presentation of faces, like that used in the divided visual-field studies described in Chapter 3. They found a right-hemisphere advantage only during the first lateralized presentation of each face. Once subjects were familiarized with the faces, there was an overall left-hemisphere advantage in the task. The investigators concluded that conflicting evidence for a left-hemisphere role in face recognition is based on data gathered in artificial experimental settings involving repeated presentation and over-familiarization with testing stimuli.[26] Normal, everyday facial recognition, they contend, depends essentially on the right hemisphere, as shown in the PET results.

One of the more surprising findings of this study was the extent to which object recognition and face identification involved activity in separate cerebral regions. The organization of the cortex dissociates objects from faces, utilizing different regions—and probably strategies and physiological mechanisms—to deal with the kind of information that is gleaned by humans from these two types of visual stimuli.

...

Measuring Interregional Correlations in Activation

The studies we have been discussing are all based on analyzing increases in regional metabolism or blood flow. Although this is the most obvious way to look at changes occurring during tasks, it is not the only way—and perhaps not the best.

A recent study illustrates how hemispheric asymmetries associated with several visuospatial tasks were not evident when only examining for simple increases, but became evident when an analysis was done of the interaction of specific brain regions during task performance. Some investigators have postulated that, in addition to typically necessitating increases in activity in specific regions, proper cerebral performance depends on the interaction of specific brain regions with one another. Thus, the extent to which regions function together or change together (as opposed to what goes up most) can indicate the areas most involved in the task.

A PET study by James Haxby and associates at the National Institutes of Health used the [15]O PET technique to examine regional cerebral blood-flow changes while volunteers performed both a face-matching task and a dot-location-matching task.[27] The investigators used these conditions because both animal and clinical human neuropsychological data suggest that there are two visual systems in the brain, one dedicated to object vision and involving mostly occipital and temporal regions, and one dedicated to spatial location and including more occipitoparietal pathways.

When analysis was performed in the more traditional manner, in which a control task was simply subtracted from the more complex cognitive task condition, the investigators indeed found what they predicted: Face recognition appeared to activate the occipital and temporal region, while the location task activated the occipital and parietal areas. This activation pattern occurred in both hemispheres.

However, when a correlation analysis was conducted, examining the extent to which regions changed together during each task, another finding emerged: The posterior regions subserving face matching and dot-location matching had much stronger functional interactions in the right hemisphere than in the left. They concluded that the bilateral activation seen in the simple regional-increase analyses may in fact be due to changes that originate in the right hemisphere but, because of the corpus callosum, also activate the left hemisphere.

This conclusion suggests that perhaps many imaging studies examining task effects on brain activity miss real hemispheric asymmetries in function due to the brain's tendency to show symmetrical increases in activity even though the task is really initiated by one side much more than the other. This is a possible explanation of the surprising degree of bilateral activation seen in the xenon blood-flow studies of speech production we discussed earlier. Newer approaches, such as the analysis of covariance in activity just described, may offer ways to get around this limitation on imaging studies of hemispheric asymmetries.

...

Metabolic Imaging with Nuclear Magnetic Resonance: New Directions

The image shown in Figure 4.3 is a good example of the structural imaging capabilities of NMR. The use of NMR has more recently extended into the realm of functional imaging as well. Instead of measuring the frequencies associated with magnetically perturbed water molecules, as in structural MRI, magnetic resonance spectroscopic imaging (MRSI) "tunes to" the characteristic frequencies emitted during magnetic perturbations of other molecules found in the brain—those associated with several aspects of cerebral metabolism.

At the present time, investigators can reconstruct images of the phosphorus distribution associated with ATP energy cycles and images of aspects of glucose metabolism (glycolytic flux and lactate production).[28] MRSI is at a relatively early stage of development, and the images it produces look relatively crude compared with those obtained with structural MRI. However, the information provided is extremely valuable and is generated without the use of ionizing radiation, as in PET and SPECT. This factor opens the door to conducting multiple scans of metabolic activity under different study conditions of normal subjects, because radiation exposure is not a concern.

...

Functional MR Activation Imaging

A very recent development in functional MR imaging allows indirect but rapid visualization of cerebral activation during stimulation based on changes in the level of blood oxygenation, sometimes called BOLD (blood oxygenation-level dependent) MRI.[29] Because active areas of the brain become slightly engorged with oxygenated blood and because the magnetic properties of oxygenated blood are different from those of deoxygenated blood, special sequence MRI scans can identify cerebral regions that are activated during stimulation, motor activity, and cognitive activity. Figure 4.12 shows activation images superimposed on structural MRI of a volunteer subject performing an oppositional thumb-finger movement task with the right hand.

Still in its infancy, this technique could truly revolutionize the study of activated brain function in normal subjects, because it can provide data with a temporal resolution of several seconds, can scan activation during any task multiple times, and/or can provide almost continuous information about cerebral activity changes occurring during changing study conditions. These capabilities should allow investigators to examine factors such as habituation effects and strategy changes within individual subjects.

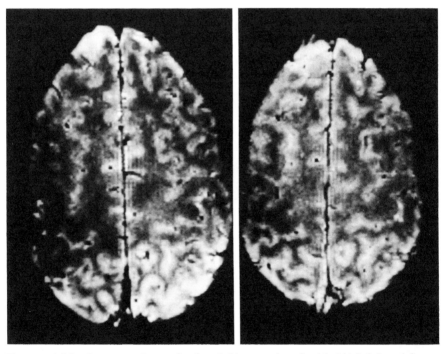

FIGURE 4.12   Increases in cerebral activity associated with (A) left hand finger movements and (B) right hand finger movements. Bright spots represent increases in blood oxygenation level as measured by functional MRI methods. These are superimposed on regular anatomical MRI images of the brain. The activated regions correspond to sensory-motor cortex in the right and left hemisphere, respectively (the image orientation is from the subject's feet, so the right hemisphere is on the left side and left hemisphere is on the right side of each brain slice). The bright area at the bottom of picture B is an artifact due to venous drainage. Courtesy of Drs. Donald Twieg and Hoby Hetherington of the University of Alabama at Birmingham Center for Nuclear Imaging Research.

·········

ISSUES RAISED BY TECHNIQUES MEASURING BRAIN ACTIVITY

Electrophysiological measures, studies of regional blood flow, and other measures of metabolic processes all offer investigators the opportunity to study relationships between brain activity and behavior. They have been of great value in validating physiologically some of the insights about brain function gleaned from psychological research with both brain-injured and normal subjects. They are also beginning to contribute new findings about cerebral organization, including hemispheric differences, not previously evident from clinical studies.

Measures of brain activity during task performance have raised some questions about the most exaggerated claims for hemispheric asymmetry. There is little evidence to support the notion that either one or the other hemisphere turns on to perform a specific task all by itself. Each of the measures we have discussed points to the involvement of many areas of the brain in even the simplest task. These findings remind us that hemispheric differences are but one of several different organizational schemes in the brain. There are asymmetries in activity between the hemispheres, to be sure, but they can be very subtle, a fact that should lead us away from thinking about hemispheric specialization in overly simple terms.

···

Limitations of Neuroimaging Research

Functional neuroimaging has become a powerful tool for the study of brain-behavior relationships. Being able to visualize activity in the living brain without interfering with it has opened the doors to studies of a multitude of questions concerning both normal and abnormal brain function. The possibilities seem enormous, apparently limited only by financial resources and by our ability to ask the right questions and make careful observations.

Some individuals, inspired by the early successes of seeing on screen the involvement of brain regions in tasks exactly as predicted by a hundred years of neuropsychological research, are quick to predict that we will soon have "maps" of how the brain generates most mental operations. Upon hearing this, one might start worrying that brain imaging may soon be able to expose one's innermost thoughts. This is, however, an unwarranted concern. As exciting as this field of research is, expectations for what can be achieved with functional neuroimaging need to be tempered by an appreciation of its limitations, both practical and conceptual. First, one must remember that most neuroimaging involves measuring the distribution of a tracer that, in turn, represents the relative level of some aspect of cerebral metabolism. The regional metabolism thus being traced is also only a reflection of the amount of activity in different cerebral regions and does not, in and of itself, represent the actual physiological mechanism behind the mental activity being studied. Nor does locating the region of greatest activity during a task or mental operation explain the brain processes behind the mental process. Neuroimaging provides, at best, a relatively crude map of where some events associated with a particular task take place.

It must also be remembered that all metabolic neuroimaging represents a cumulative or time-averaged "snapshot" of brain events taking place within the total time period it takes the imaging tracer to properly distribute and/or the scanning procedure to measure the distribution. This interval is at best approximately 1 minute for current PET scans of blood flow and is considerably longer for most other PET and SPECT procedures. Thus, activity changes occurring over shorter intervals are lost or averaged out. This time discrimination capability, or temporal resolution, of imaging procedures is improving, especially with the advent of functional MR imaging, but still remains very slow when compared with neuronal communication speeds and changes in brain electrical activity.

In addition, there are more serious conceptual problems involved in "timing" and localizing "thoughts" with functional imaging. Neuroimaging attempts to capture a mental operation in a snapshot—or, as technology progresses, in a series of snapshots. This procedure may work, in a limited fashion, for basic sensory-motor functions or even some specific task conditions. However, it will probably never be adequate to characterize the cerebral activity associated with a personal stream of thought, much less provide the brain imaging investigator with information sufficient to "read" the thought.

Researchers have to rely on averaging many repetitions of the same task or on using many subjects performing the same task to separate some aspect of cerebral activity that is common to the task from a plethora of activity associated with individual differences and much other "noise." In addition, even the simple attempts by PET researchers to isolate specific mental operations through the subtraction techniques we described earlier are fraught with many assumptions and interpretation problems.[30] Is a complex mental operation really the simple sum of simple steps that we can study in isolation? Does adding a new "stage" not affect the operations taking place in prior "stages"? Do experiences really have definable beginnings and ends? We do not really know when thoughts begin or end or whether a mental event can really be the same when repeated.

Finally, all imaging experiments aimed at establishing the brain activity underlying mental processes are naturally guided by current psychological theory and by the investigator's own view of how to partition and isolate mental operations. The actual organization of mental processes—as well as the underlying cerebral processes—is, of course, not governed by our conceptualizations of them. Even though we normally assume that poor models get thrown out or modified by the actual empirical results, in the case of psychology and neuroimaging the situation is so complex and the number of variables in images so vast, that "expected" findings can be fairly easy to tease out or "see" in the data. It is also easy to fall into the "psychologist's fallacy"—to design an experiment based on a certain view of mental function whose results will reinforce that view simply because the experimental design highly constrained the results in that direction.

These considerations are not meant to discredit functional neuroimaging research nor to imply that its potential for studying both normal and abnormal brain function is less than vast. We wish merely to acquaint the reader with some of the important constraints that make the endeavor of studying the left and the right brain with this new technology an even more challenging one.

·········

BIOCHEMISTRY OF THE HEMISPHERES

Neurons communicate through chemistry. Although electrical activity is associated with neuronal firing and interactions, the basic mechanisms generating this activity are chemical, and the mechanisms that transfer signals from one brain cell to another are also chemical. Brain cells communicate with other brain cells by using transmitter chemicals, called neurotransmitters. Many neurotransmitters have been discovered, and anatomists and chemists are busy mapping the cell groups and pathways defined by the neurons utilizing each particular transmitter chemical.

Early evidence of true neurochemical asymmetries in the human brain was gathered in 1978, when it was discovered that the neurotransmitter norepinephrine was distributed unequally in the right and left halves of the thalamus—a subcortical structure that, among other things, serves as a main relay center for sensory impulses to the cortex.[31] Higher levels of norepinephrine were found on the right side.

In 1981 a group of Italian scientists showed that there were neurochemical asymmetries at the cortical level as well. They found that an area of the left temporal lobe shows greater activity by the enzyme choline acetyltransferase (CAT) than did the corresponding area of the right hemisphere.[32] CAT is involved in chemical processes associated with acetylcholine, a major neurotransmitter defining extensive neuronal networks in the brain.

The list of neurotransmitter systems discovered in the brain continues to increase, and there is growing evidence that a number of transmitters are unequally represented in the left and right hemispheres. Dopamine, another major neurotransmitter, may also define more extensive neuronal networks in the left hemisphere.[33] There is some speculation that the extra norepinephrine-defined pathways of the right hemisphere complement the extra dopamine-defined pathways of the left in terms of the kind of attentional mechanisms they subserve, which, in turn, lead to some of the well-documented hemispheric asymmetries in function.[34]

Dopamine has been implicated in the control of fine movement, especially in the initiation of action sequences. Thus, the predominance of dopamine-defined pathways may be a basis for the specialization of the left hemisphere for complex motor operations such as speech. Conversely, norepinephrine appears to facilitate arousal to novel stimuli. Thus, the abundance of norepinephrine-defined pathways may be a basis for the specialization of the right hemisphere, for certain visuospatial-perceptual operations.[35]

Positron emission tomography, discussed earlier in this chapter, holds great promise for the study of neurotransmitter and neuroregulator levels in the living human brain. Many cerebral metabolites can be made into positron-emitting radiopharmaceuticals without altering their clinical or physiological properties. Thus, with appropriate radiolabeling, researchers are already capable of PET imaging the dopamine specific neurons and neural pathways in human subjects.[36] This type of work is only beginning and is expected to grow dramatically over the next few years. It should reveal much about the biochemistry of both the resting and the mentally active brain.

·········

PHYSIOLOGY AND PSYCHOLOGY:
Building the link

Anatomical measurements, recordings of electrical activity, blood-flow studies, and the scanning of metabolic processes offer investigators the opportunity to study relationships between mental processes, behavior, and brain activity. These techniques have at least partially validated some of the theoretical insights about brain function and hemispheric asymmetry developed in the brain-damage clinic and from psychological research with normal subjects.

Some researchers have claimed that physiological tools offer the ultimate resolution of questions that deal with relations between mind and brain; others argue against overreliance on such measures on both philosophical and practical grounds. Clearly, certain concerns must be confronted in the attempt to establish relationships between physiological processes and psychological functions. Although these concerns are important for the study of hemispheric asymmetries, their significance extends beyond any specific area of research and has applicability to the study of brain-behavior relationships in general.

One issue is the problem of selecting from among the various physiological measures available those that will prove most informative. Like all other tissues in the human body, the brain is dependent on complex metabolic processes for its functioning. A great deal of the brain's biochemistry, however, is unique and involves the communication of information between neurons. Biochemical processes operating in each cell generate electrical potentials, and biochemicals operating between cells effectively transmit electrical impulses between groups of neurons.

We do not know what aspects of this activity best reflect the functioning of the brain with which we are concerned. If, for example, we just want to know what areas of the brain are most active during particular human behaviors, we can look at cerebral blood flow, for it responds rapidly to changes in metabolic activity. Yet such measures may not be indicative of the true information-processing strategies or codes of the brain. Such codes could involve chemical pathways extending across many areas of the brain or could perhaps be reflected in patterns of electrical-wave activity. Neither would necessarily correlate with regional metabolic activity.

Even after deciding on a measure to study, we may be faced with further choices. The evoked potential, for example, may be broken down into several components and analyzed in different ways. In the absence of a comprehensive theory about the meaning of these components, investigators must decide how best to analyze their data to look for asymmetries or other effects. Anatomists, too, must decide what measurements of what regions of the brain will be most useful for the problem at hand.

Another issue involves the concept of localization of function in general. How much does attributing some psychological activity to a specific area of the brain contribute to insights about that activity? Certainly, findings on localization have been of tremendous clinical value. Furthermore, relationships between location and function may help establish the components of a complex behavior or task in terms of more basic processes. As a hypothetical example, it may be demonstrated that the memory of how to get somewhere involves linguistic processes in the left hemisphere as well as imagery processes in the right hemisphere. It is not clear, however, how far this kind of approach can take us. Ultimately, it is likely that dividing the brain in terms of "where" will not completely answer the question of "how."

Discovering brain–behavior and brain–mind relationships is not only an experimental problem and certainly not only one of localization of function. The problems are at least as much conceptual in nature: What are we trying to explain? How are we defining things? In what sense does some neurophysiological activity accompanying a mental event explain something about the event? What would constitute a satisfactory "explanation" about some mental or behavioral event?

Investigators have become more sophisticated, at least with respect to localization issues. They now talk of the "state of activity in the system," rather than "where." They realize most psychological functions should be associated with activity changes in multiple areas or defined pathways of the cerebrum. They also realize that these may be flexible and time varying, perhaps even probabilistic.[37]

More conceptual development will have to do with the nature of our questions and definitions, including a better appreciation of the levels of explanation involved. For the time being, it does seem that the interaction of psychology and physiology should be fruitful for the study of both mind and brain. Physiological injuries of the sort studied by neuropsychologists have had an impact on the way we break down mental functions. Physiological imaging of the sort described in this chapter has the potential to reorganize it further. Psychological questions are also guiding at least some investigations into anatomy and physiological processes. Although attempts at such interactions of the two disciplines often have led to premature simplistic conclusions, we are getting better.

FIVE

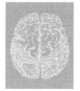

THE PUZZLE OF THE LEFT-HANDER

An overwhelming majority of human beings almost exclusively use their right hands for writing and other skilled, unimanual activities. Cross-cultural studies put the incidence of right-handedness at about 90 percent. A variety of indirect evidence suggests that this has been the case since prehistoric times.[1] Drawings of people found on cave walls and inside Egyptian tombs typically show the subjects engaged in activities involving the right hand, and an analysis of paleolithic tools and weapons suggests that they were made with, and for, the right hand.

A study of hand tracings believed to have been made by Cro-Magnon people showed over 80 percent to be of the left hand. If we assume the artists traced their own hands, these data also point to a very strong preference for the right hand in skilled activity. A study of 1,180 works of art spanning a 5,000-year period, from pre-3000 B.C. to 1950, showed that depiction of right- and left-hand use showed no significant change or trends over time, with left-hand use averaging 7 to 8 percent. Perhaps the most ingenious evidence of all for right-hand preference in early humans comes from an analysis of fossilized baboon skulls with fractures. On the basis of the locations of the fractures, the investigator concluded that the injuries were the result of blows inflicted by early humans wielding clubs with their right hands.

Why are most human beings right-handed? Conversely, why does a significant percentage of the population use the left hand, despite subtle and sometimes overt social pressure to conform to the handedness pattern characteristic of the majority?

We mentioned in earlier chapters that handedness is related in complex ways to the distribution of functions between the left brain and the right brain. Any analysis of brain asymmetry must deal with this problem if it is to be complete. What factors determine handedness? In what ways do left-handers and right-handers differ?

In this chapter, we shall consider modern theories proposed to account for variations in handedness and studies designed to examine possible differences between left-handers and right-handers. To provide a historical context for recent work, we shall briefly review some of the older ideas about handedness.

....

HISTORICAL NOTIONS OF LEFT-HANDEDNESS

...

Is There Anything Sinister About Being Left-Handed?

Webster's Third International Dictionary lists several definitions of the adjective *left-handed,* including the following:

> **a:** marked by clumsiness or ineptitude: awkward; **b:** exhibiting deviousness or indirection: oblique, unintended; **c:** obs.: given to malevolent scheming or contriving: sinister, underhand.

Left-handers are frequently referred to as "sinistrals," and *Roget's Thesaurus* lists left-handed as a synonym for unskillfulness. In other languages as well, the terms for left or left-handed have almost always contained at least one derogatory meaning, ranging from "clumsy" or "awkward" to "evil." The French word for left, *gauche,* also means "clumsy"; *mancino* is Italian for left as well as for deceitful. The Spanish idiom *no ser zurdo* means "to be very clever." Its literal translation is "not to be left-handed." Other examples abound.

Anthropologists have provided us with a number of examples of how symbolic associations with left and right are part of different cultures.[2] For example, the involuntary twitching of an eyelid is thought to be significant by the native people of Morocco. For them, twitching of the right eyelid signifies the return of a family member or other good news, whereas twitching of the left eyelid is a warning of an impending death in the family. In another part of the world, the Maoris of New Zealand at one time believed that a tremor during sleep meant that a spirit had seized the body. A right-side tremor meant good fortune, whereas a left-side tremor meant ill fortune and possibly death.

The Bible, too, reflects a bias against the left hand or side. One example from the New Testament that is especially striking is the Vision of Judgment in Matthew 5:25:

> And he shall set the sheep on his right hand, but the goats on the left.
> Then shall the King say unto them on his right hand, Come, ye blessed of my Father, inherit the kingdom prepared for you from the foundation of the world. . .
>
> Then shall he say also unto them on the left hand, Depart from me, ye cursed, into everlasting fire, prepared for the devil and his angels: . . .
>
> And these shall go away into everlasting punishment: but the righteous into life eternal.

Michael Barsley, author of *Left Handed People,* has argued that the Vision of Judgment has been responsible for "fixing the prejudice against left handers [more] than any other pronouncement, and that this prejudice has come down through the ages, adopted by inquisitors, judges, soldiers, artists, teachers, nurses, and parents as the supreme example of the association of sinistral people with wickedness and the Devil."[3] Whether or not Barsley is correct, it is clear that the association of left with bad is of very long standing.

What is the origin of this bias? At this point we can only speculate. Carl Sagan, of Cornell University, has suggested one possibility in *The Dragons of Eden,* his book on the evolution of intelligence.[4] Sagan notes that in preindustrial societies, both now and in the past, the hand has been used for personal hygiene after defecation. This use of a hand is both unaesthetic and potentially harmful because it can spread disease, but these drawbacks can be reduced somewhat by using only the other hand to eat and to greet others. Right-handed individuals would perform activities like eating and throwing weapons with the right hand, leaving toilet hygiene to the left. Sagan suggests that the left hand became associated with excretory activities, which have a long history of negative associations in human cultures. Thus, the chain linking left with bad was forged.

This explanation assumes that human beings begin with a preference to use the right hand for activities requiring fine control. We must still explain the basis for that preference. Speculation abounds on this issue, but, thanks to the tools of modern science, we now stand a good chance of resolving the question in a satisfactory way.

...

Nineteenth-Century Theories of Handedness

Let us first consider some of the ideas proposed in the nineteenth century to account for handedness. One popular theory was known as "visceral distribution." Proponents argued that the asymmetrical placement of visceral organs, such as the liver, puts the center of gravity of the human body slightly to the right of the midline, and, as a consequence, human beings are better able to balance on the left foot. This stance leaves the right hand free, so over time the muscles on the right side became better developed. This notion, however, does not explain why some people are left-handed, unless we assume a reversal in the orientation of their viscera.

Social-evolution explanations of handedness were also popular in the nineteenth century. There are several variations on this general theme, the most common being the sword-and-shield theory.[5] According to this theory, attributed to English essayist and historian Thomas Carlyle and others, most soldiers hold their shields with their left hands to protect their hearts when they are engaged in battle and use their right hands to hold their weapons. As a consequence, during eons of armed conflict, the right hand gained in manipulative ability and came to be used for other unimanual activities as well. Again, there is no attempt to explain left-handedness or the apparently high incidence of right-handedness in humans before the invention of the shield.

The idea of cerebral dominance emerged in the last quarter of the nineteenth century, and with it came yet another theory of handedness. D. J. Cunningham, a Scottish anatomist, summarized this view in 1902 in a Huxley Memorial Lecture: "Right handedness is due to a transmitted functional preeminence of the left brain. Left braineдness is not the result but, through evolution, it has become the cause of right handedness."[6] As it is stated, this view would not easily account for left-handers with left-hemisphere speech, who comprise about 70 percent of all left-handers. In addition, it fails to explain the reasons for the transmitted functional preeminence of the left brain.

....

THE DIFFICULTY OF DETERMINING HANDEDNESS

Before we consider more modern theories of handedness, it is important to consider how handedness is actually assessed. We might assume that the best way to find out whether a given individual is a left- or a right-hander is simply to ask. Unfortunately, this direct approach does not always work. Few people use one hand exclusively for all unimanual activities, and simple self-classification does not indicate how someone weighed various activities when making the determination. Another approach is to ask people which hand they use for specific activities. The researcher can then compute a handedness preference based on the same weighting scheme for everyone.

A widely used questionnaire to measure hand preference was developed at the University of Edinburgh. Subjects are asked to indicate their preferred hand, if any, and strength of the preference for writing, drawing, throwing, cutting with scissors, brushing teeth, cutting with a knife without a fork, using a spoon, holding a broom (upper hand), holding a match while striking, and holding a lid while removing it from a box. The questionnaire yields a laterality quotient that ranges from –100 for extreme left-handedness, through 0 for equal use of the two hands, to +100 for extreme right-handedness.

In a study of over 1,000 undergraduates at the University of Edinburgh, most showed a consistent preference for one hand; few showed no preference.[7] Those showing right preference, however, tended to show their preferences more strongly than those showing left preference. That is, the distribution of positive and negative scores was different. The positive scores were clustered toward the high end of the range, whereas the negative scores were more evenly distributed over the range of values. Findings like these have led some investigators to speak of right-handers and non-right-handers, rather than right-handers and left-handers.

The way in which subjects are classified into different handedness groups is critical for the outcome of research investigating handedness as a variable. Most studies using questionnaires attempt to classify subjects in terms of handedness based on their scores. Problems arise, however, because handedness is not a simple all-or-none dimension—a decision, most likely arbitrary, must be made about the placement of the boundaries between handedness group categories.

In an attempt to avoid this problem, other studies do not form groups based on test scores but use the actual scores in the handedness measure. For either of these approaches, however, different types of questionnaires may yield different classifications for a group of subjects. In light of this, it should not be surprising that experiments investigating the effects of handedness sometimes yield conflicting results. Differences in the way subjects are classified may account for much of the conflict.

....

EYES, EARS, AND FEET

Handedness is clearly the most obvious human asymmetry. Most people, however, also have a preferred, or dominant, eye, ear, and foot. What is the nature of these preferences, and what, if any, relationship exists between them and brain asymmetry? In this section, we shall briefly review some of the evidence bearing on these questions.

...

Eye Preference

Preference for one eye over the other can be measured in different ways. When acuity dominance is being measured, the dominant eye is the one that shows relatively better performance on standard tests of visual acuity (for example, the eye that can read letters further down on the Snellen eye chart). Sighting dominance can be easily measured by determining the eye used to sight down a telescope or along a pistol.

What relationship exists between eye preference and hemispheric asymmetry? Experimental evidence shows little relationship, a finding which, on further analysis, should not be surprising.[8] As shown in Chapters 2 and 3, the visual system is organized in such a way that each eye sends information to both hemispheres, from different halves of the retina. Because of these neuroanatomical arrangements, sighting preference for the left or right eye is not simply a reflection of preferential use of one hemisphere.

...

Ear Preference

Ear preference can be measured in tasks that do not permit the subject to use the two ears simultaneously—pressing an ear against a watch to hear its ticking, for example. Sensitivity of the two ears relative to each other can also be assessed. Within the normal range of hearing thresholds, there is no relationship between auditory sensitivity and ear preference in tasks requiring a choice between ears. In addition, there is little evidence for a relationship between handedness and ear preference, and only a very weak relationship between ear preference and ear asymmetry measured in dichotic listening.[9]

...

Footedness

Footedness refers to the preferred foot for such tasks as kicking a ball, grasping a small object with the toes, or stomping on a small object. Relatively few studies have looked at footedness, but those that have suggest that different measures of foot preference are highly correlated with each other. In a large-scale study of hand, foot, eye, and ear preferences[10] correlations among the four kinds of preference were all positive and statistically significant, a result showing that the various preferences were related. The largest correlation was between hand preference and foot preference, although none of the relationships was exceptionally strong.

Thus, we have seen that human beings show lateral preferences in more ways than just hand usage. In the remainder of this chapter, however, we shall be directing our attention to handedness because it appears to be the lateral preference most closely linked with asymmetries in the hemispheres of the brain.

....

IS HANDEDNESS HEREDITARY?

Is handedness, like eye color, blood type, and general body build, genetically determined? The probability of two right-handed parents having a left-handed child is 0.02. It rises to 0.17 if one parent is left-handed and to 0.46 if both are left-handed.[11] These figures are consistent with the hypothesis that genes play a role in determining handedness. The problem with interpreting the data, however, is that environmental factors can account for these differences as well.

Two left-handed parents could provide a child with different experiences relevant to the determination of handedness, just as they might provide specific genes. Nature (genes) and nurture (experience) are confounded in these figures, making it impossible to sort out the contribution of each.

...

The Environmental View

Robert Collins has taken an extreme environmental position, arguing that handedness is transmitted from one generation to the next through cultural and environmental biases. Collins based his conclusions in large part on his work with paw preference in mice. This work (discussed at greater length in Chapter 9) showed that individual mice demonstrate consistent paw preferences in reaching for food in a glass tube. These preferences are not subject to genetic selection: It is not possible to breed right-pawed mice over several generations by mating mice that show a right-paw preference. The offspring of such animals will show the same paw-preference distribution found among mice in general: 50 percent left preference and 50 percent right preference.[12] Collins also showed that young mice that have not yet shown a preference for either paw become predominantly right-pawed if they are presented with the glass tube placed toward the right side of the case, thereby making it easier to reach with the right paw than with the left paw.[13]

Collins's emphasis on the role of cultural and environmental biases in the determination of handedness is consistent with views expressed by another investigator who, after reviewing the evidence that existed up to 1946, concluded: "Preferred laterality is not an inherited trait. There is absolutely no evidence to support the contention that dominance, either in handedness or any other form, is a congenital, predetermined human capacity."[14]

The author argued that right-handedness is a learned response to a right-handed world and that left-handedness occurs when this response is not learned as a result of a physical defect, faulty education, emotional problems, or the like. An environmental model of handedness determination must account, however, for the fact that right-hand preference has been found across all cultures studied and over all time periods for which evidence is available. It remains to be explained why environments biased in favor of the left hand do not occur.

...

Genetic Models

Evidence for a genetic model of handedness, in contrast with environmental models, may be evaluated by formulating specific models of how handedness might be transmitted from generation to generation through the action of genes. Different models make different predictions of the actual figures. A good fit between the predictions of a specific model and actual data would suggest that genetic factors can account for most of the variations in handedness found among people.

One of the first genetic models of handedness proposed that handedness is a consequence of the action of a single gene that has two different forms, or alleles.[15] One allele, R, was dominant and coded for right-handedness. A second, l, was recessive and coded for left-handedness. An individual inheriting the R allele from each parent would be right-handed, as would someone with an Rl genotype (R from one parent, l from the other). Left-handers would be those individuals who inherited the l allele from each parent.

This model, however, cannot account for the fact that 54 percent of the offspring of two left-handed parents are right-handed. The model predicts that all offspring of such parents should be left-handed, because the l allele is the only one that left-handed parents can transmit to their offspring. There have been attempts to rescue this model by introducing the concept of variable penetrance, which proposes that all individuals with the same genotype do not express that genotype the same way. In this case, some individuals with the Rl genotype will be left-handed. These left-handers could transmit an R allele to their offspring, accounting for the nonzero incidence of right-handedness among the children of two left-handed parents. Even with variable penetrance built into the model, however, the model's "goodness of fit" to actual data is less than satisfactory.

Marion Annett, of the University of Hull in England, has proposed a different kind of genetic model of handedness.[16] She hypothesized that there is no gene for left- or right-handedness as such, but that there is a dominant gene (RS+) responsible for the development of speech in the left hemisphere, which, in turn, increases the chances of greater skill in the right hand. Annett refers to her theory as the "right shift" theory. She proposed a recessive form of the gene (RS−) that results in the absence of systematic bias to one side, for either speech or handedness. Chance factors would then operate independently on the direction of lateralization for speech and handedness.

If both alleles occur equally often in the population and if mating is random with respect to this gene, then 50 percent of the population will be RS+RS−, 25 percent RS+RS+, and 25 percent RS−RS−. Persons in the first two groups (RS+RS− and RS+RS+) would show a right shift (left-hemisphere language and right-handed). The RS−RS− group, however, would lack any right shift, and in Annett's view environmental effects would determine their hand preference. In the absence of any strong environmental bias, one would expect about half of this 25 percent to be left-handed and half right-handed. The value of 12.5 percent left-handed persons predicted by Annett's model is quite close to the number of left-handers actually found in the general population. The same reasoning can also readily account for the fact that about 50 percent of the offspring of left-handed parents are left-handed and for the finding that left-handers show a very mixed pattern of asymmetry on other measures such as speech lateralization and eye dominance.

Although we shall have more to say about the relationship between handedness and cognitive abilities later, we should mention here that Annett specifically proposed such a relationship. She suggested that the RS+RS+ genotype (double dose of right shift) may lead to poor performance with the left hand and to spatial deficits, whereas the RS−RS− person may be susceptible to reading disabilities. The RS+RS− genotype would be optimal, according to Annett, and would favor the continued presence of both RS+ and RS− in the population.

·········

PATHOLOGICAL LEFT-HANDEDNESS

The incidence of left-handedness in twins is about 20 percent, approximately twice that found in the singleton population. Twins also show a disproportionately high incidence of neurological and other disorders, which is believed to be a consequence of damage resulting from intrauterine crowding during fetal development.[17] It is a logical next step to suggest that the elevated incidence of left-handedness in twins is due, at least in part, to these factors.

The idea that minor brain damage may underlie much of the left-handedness in twins was first proposed in 1920.[18] Several pieces of evidence support that suggestion. First, the incidence of left-handedness is very high in populations that may have suffered minor brain injury before or during birth. In the mentally retarded, for example, the incidence is 20 percent. Left-handedness is also very common in children with learning disabilities and in epileptics. Perhaps the minor brain damage that is the cause of the problem in many of these cases is also responsible for the shift in hand preference in individuals who otherwise would have been right-handed.

Second, clinical data from sodium amobarbital work suggest a relationship between handedness and early brain damage. In one study, the majority of left-handed patients with evidence of early damage to the left brain showed evidence of language in the right hemisphere, whereas left-handers without signs of early damage had left-hemisphere language.[19] This finding suggests that damage to the left hemisphere early in life may result in a shift in the language hemisphere and in hand preference.

Paul Bakan and associates asserted that all left-handedness is essentially pathological in origin and that trauma occurring at birth, or birth stress, can account for most of it.[20] They suggested that left-handedness is the result of left-hemisphere motor dysfunction following perinatal hypoxia, or reduced oxygen supply at birth. According to Bakan, sinistrality runs in families because of an inherited tendency for difficult births or abnormal pregnancies and not because handedness per se is genetically determined.

The data relevant to Bakan's hypothesis are mixed.[21] Some studies have shown a relationship between birth complications and handedness, whereas others have failed to reveal such a relationship. However, all have been based on retrospective data, that is, information about the presence or absence of birth stress obtained from subjective reports of mothers or subjects many years after the fact. To reduce the errors inherent in retrospective reporting, Murray Schwartz undertook a longitudinal, prospective study that begins tracking children at age two and includes hospital records as well as maternal reports in assessing birth stress.[22]

The Apgar rating is a simple neonatal rating system in which low scores may reflect hypoxia and possible neurological abnormality. Of all the stress/risk factors and complications examined by Schwartz, only one—the Apgar rating measured at one minute after birth—showed a relationship to subsequent sinistrality, with a greater incidence of sinistrality associated with lower Apgar scores.

Thus, the evidence relating birth stress to sinistrality remains mixed. In any event the data fall far short of supporting Bakan's original hypothesis—that all left-handedness is the result of birth stress. Less extreme views of the role of pathology have been taken by others. Paul Satz, for example, suggested that pathological factors can account for a good deal of the elevated incidence of left-handedness among certain clinical populations, as well as some of the left-handedness in the population at large.[23] The remaining left-handers are, in his view, "natural" left-handers, whose left-handedness is genetic in origin.

Satz and his colleagues became interested in other changes that may occur in individuals who are left-handed because of early brain injury. They viewed a shift in handedness as one of several alternatives in lateral development that form what they called the syndromes of pathological left handedness (PLH).[24] We have already mentioned one of these changes—a shift in hemispheric specialization for speech. Left-handers with a history of early brain damage are three times more likely to have speech controlled by the right hemisphere than are left-handers without early brain damage.

Another component of PLH, according to Satz, is impaired visuospatial ability. He and his colleagues cited the earlier work of Herbert Lansdell with a group of left-brain-injured epileptics, work suggesting a link between early left-sided brain injury and impaired visuospatial ability.[25] Lansdell examined the association between the age at which neurological symptoms first appeared and the difference between verbal and nonverbal factors in the Wechsler-Bellevue intelligence scale. He noted that the verbal factors were affected less with early lesions, whereas the nonverbal factors suffered less with later lesions (five years). Lansdell speculated that early injury to the left hemisphere may shift language functions to the right hemisphere, thereby disrupting and displacing the visuospatial functions that otherwise would develop there. Later injury would not produce this shifting but would result in impaired left-hemisphere function and intact right-hemisphere visuospatial ability.

A third component of the PLH syndrome is failure of the right side of the body to develop fully. Satz and colleagues cited studies in the 1930s and 1940s showing that decrease in the growth of all or part of half of the body can follow from early injury to the hemisphere on the opposite side. Their own research measuring foot size has shown that epileptic patients whose seizures began before age two had a shorter right foot if the lesion was located in the left hemisphere, whereas patients with early right-sided lesions had a shorter left foot.

Much more work needs to be done before the existence of the PLH syndrome is established with certainty. Individuals with the syndrome would be relatively rare, and studies to test the hypothesis adequately would need to look for all the components at one time, not just one or two in isolation. Existing evidence, however, appears sufficient to support the more basic position that some left-handedness is pathological in origin, although few researchers would take the extreme view that all left-handedness can be explained in this way.

The popularity of the pathological model of left-handedness has led investigators to compare the cognitive abilities of left- and right-handers. The rationale for such studies is simple. If left-handedness is a consequence of brain damage, however mild, then such damage might be reflected in lowered ability in various higher mental functions. We shall review studies exploring this possibility in a later section.

....

HANDEDNESS AND FUNCTIONAL ASYMMETRY

In what ways does the brain organization of left-handers differ from that of right-handers? Both clinical and behavioral studies have helped answer this question. In Chapter 1, we noted that sodium amobarbital testing has shown that over 95 percent of right-handers have speech localized to the left hemisphere, with 70 percent of left-handers showing the same pattern.[26] Of the remaining 30 percent, most show evidence of bilateral speech representation.[27] From these figures, one might conclude that the majority of left-handers are just like right-handers.

Other clinical data, however, suggest that the picture is more complex. Several studies have reported that the prognosis for recovery from aphasia following stroke is much better in left-handers than in right-handers.[28] Many investigators believe that recovery from massive damage to the speech hemisphere is a function of the extent to which the remaining, undamaged hemisphere can take over. If this is so, it suggests that language functions may be bilaterally represented in more than just those left-handers identified by the sodium amobarbital data. Left-handers with speech controlled predominantly by one hemisphere may have the other hemisphere available "in reserve" to a much greater extent than right-handers.

Behavioral studies with normal subjects generally confirm this picture of complexity. Dichotic-listening and lateralized tachistoscopic studies that compare the performance of left- and right-handers show less evidence of asymmetry in left-handers.[29] As a general rule, any asymmetry found in right-handers will be smaller and perhaps in the opposite direction when studied in left-handers.

By themselves, however, these summary statements do not allow us to differentiate between a situation where left-handers truly show no asymmetry in these tasks and a situation where approximately equal numbers show a right or left advantage. When data from individual subjects are examined, we find that left-handed subjects show smaller asymmetries than right-handed subjects, although there are some left-handers with strong left or strong right superiorities. These findings mesh nicely with the clinical evidence pointing to greater bilaterality in left-handers.

...

The Role of Familial Sinistrality

The brain organization of left-handers appears to be more complex than the sodium amobarbital data would lead one to expect. Other clinical work has suggested that some of the variability between left-handers may be accounted for by determining whether a given left-hander has first-degree relatives (parents, siblings, or children) who are themselves left-handed.[30]

Left-handers with histories of familial sinistrality (left-handers in the immediate family) showed similar frequencies of language disturbances occurring after damage to either the left or the right side of the brain. In nonfamilial left-handers, language disturbances were almost nonexistent after right-hemisphere lesions. This difference suggests that there are at least two kinds of left-handers and that the patterns of brain organization in the two groups are different.

Studies with normal subjects have looked at the effect of familial sinistrality on performance in lateralized tests. A number of studies support the idea that left-handers with left-handed relatives differ from those without. Unfortunately, studies are not consistent in their findings about the nature of that difference.[31]

The evidence pointing to differences in brain organization between persons with and without family histories of left-handedness has been taken by some to be a sign of a genetic component to handedness. The same relationship, however, may also be viewed as support for an environmental determinant of handedness.

...

Inverted and Noninverted Writing Postures

Jerre Levy and MaryLou Reid identified another variable—hand posture—which they believed might help sort left-handers into different groups on the basis of brain organization.[32] Some left-handers write in an inverted or hooked position, holding the pen or pencil above the line of writing. Other left-handers, as well as almost all right-handers, hold their writing instruments below the line of writing.

Levy and Reid argued that the inverted hand posture means that the speech hemisphere is ipsilateral to the preferred hand. Thus, the speech of a left-handed inverter would be controlled by the left hemisphere. The speech of a right-handed inverter (these individuals are rare) would be controlled by the right hemisphere. The speech of noninverted writers would be controlled by the hemisphere opposite the preferred hand. Their view conflicts with conventional wisdom, which suggests that hand posture is due only to training.

The basis for Levy and Reid's conclusions is data from two tachisto-scopic tests involving lateralized presentation of stimuli, one requiring the identification of three-letter syllables and the other the recall of the position of a dot appearing randomly in 1 of 20 possible locations. Right-handers showed a right-visual-field superiority for syllables and a left-visual-field superiority for the spatial task. Left-handers who write with the noninverted posture showed the reverse. In contrast, left-handers with an inverted posture performed like the right-handers with a noninverted posture. The one right-hander who wrote with an inverted posture generated data comparable with those of left-handers writing in a noninverted fashion.

A number of investigators have attempted to extend these findings to other tasks and measures of hemispheric asymmetry, with generally poor results; a limited number of studies have reported supportive data, however.[33] The clinical data, unfortunately, present the same mixed picture. One set of investigators has stated that "the presence or absence of aphasia with a right or left hemiparesis has been appropriate as would have been predicted by hand posture utilized during writing."[34] These clinical data, however, have not been published. Other investigators have failed to find evidence for such a relationship in patients undergoing sodium amobarbital testing.[35]

At this point, there are too many inconsistencies in the data to conclude that hand posture is a useful predictor of brain asymmetry.

·······

HANDEDNESS AND HIGHER MENTAL FUNCTIONS

Do left-handers differ from right-handers in ways other than brain organization? The search for the relationship between handedness and brain asymmetry has led many investigators to consider the consequences of this relationship for other functions. Recall, for example, the pathological model of left-handedness. According to this view, some left-handers have suffered from very early, minimal brain damage that results in a shift from what would have been a right-hand preference to a preference for the left hand. The pathological model leads readily to the prediction that minimal brain damage will result in lowered ability on various tests of higher mental functions.

...

Evaluating the Case for Deficits in Left-Handers

Studies that compare the performances of left-handers and right-handers on tests of higher mental functions have yielded little in the way of data to support predictions of inferior performances by left-handers. One review of the literature cited 14 studies examining reading ability. Only one of them found a difference between left-handers and right-handers, and it reported that left-handers were superior.[36] Using measures of academic achievement, one study found no difference between groups, whereas another study reported that left-handers did more poorly on a college entrance exam. Three studies reported that left-handers did more poorly in perceptual tasks, although the sole study to be replicated failed to show a difference in subsequent work.

Despite a relatively meager collection of empirical evidence documenting performance differences between left-handers and right-handers, the association of left-handedness with deficit persists. This belief is most likely a result of the high incidence of left-handedness among the mentally retarded and reading disabled. This association suggests that some of the left-handedness in these groups selected for deficits is pathological in origin. The same damage that produces the impairment also might be responsible for the shift to left-hand usage. It does not follow, however, that a similar relationship holds for unselected groups of subjects obtained outside of the clinical setting.

The pathological model of left-handedness, then, has been responsible for much of the interest in the relationship between handedness and cognitive ability. Another theoretical approach to this question has been taken by Levy.[37] She noted that many left-handers show evidence of some language ability in the right hemisphere in addition to language ability in the left hemisphere. What, she asked, are the consequences of this for the visuospatial functions typically controlled by the right hemisphere in the right-hander?

She proposed that language and visuospatial functions compete for available neural tissue within a hemisphere and that language functions predominate at the expense of the others, "crowding-out" visuospatial centers. Thus, she predicted that left-handers should do more poorly than right-handers on visuospatial tasks but perform similarly on verbal tasks.

To test her hypothesis, she recruited 10 left-handed and 15 right-handed California Institute of Technology graduate students and administered the Wechsler Adult Intelligence Scale (WAIS) to them. The WAIS can be broken down into two parts, a verbal component and a performance component. The verbal subtests include general information, vocabulary, and similarities (simple abstraction). The performance subtests include block design (Koh's blocks), object assembly (puzzle assembly), and picture completion (noticing anomalies in drawings).*

Levy found that scores on the verbal component were the same for left-handers and right-handers. Left-handers scored significantly lower than right-handers on the performance score, however. Thus, Levy's prediction of a deficit in visuospatial tasks was borne out.

It is important to remember, however, that this "deficit" is only relative. Levy's subjects, both left-handers and right-handers, showed markedly superior scores on both parts of the WAIS compared with the overall population. The performance scores of the left-handers, however, were lower than their verbal scores, whereas there was no difference between the scores of the two tests for the right-handers.

Levy's work has generated considerable interest and several attempts at replication, with mixed results.[38]

...

Leonardo da Vinci Was a Lefty

Some investigators have suggested that the more bilateral distribution of language function that appears to characterize left-handers may result in superior abilities. The argument has been made that creativity might be enhanced in individuals whose brains permit a greater interplay between verbal and nonverbal abilities by virtue of their being housed within the same hemisphere. Occasional studies have reported superior performance by the left-hander, but these studies do not paint

---

* The verbal subtests seem most sensitive to damage to the left hemisphere, probably because they are so language dependent. The performance subtests are known to be quite sensitive to damage to either hemisphere, especially in the parietal region. In addition, the performance tests seem to be more sensitive than the verbal tests to brain damage in general, especially diffuse damage. They are the first to show decline with increasing age and are the tests most affected by brain trauma and diffuse pathological processes.

a picture any clearer than do those pointing to deficits in left-handers. Proponents, however, are eager to mention that Leonardo da Vinci, Benjamin Franklin, and Michelangelo were all left-handed.

It is interesting to note that the incidence of left-handedness is considerably higher among artists than among the general population. For example, in one study comparing college undergraduates with less than two years of art training with students enrolled in an art-degree program, 20 percent of the artists were left-handed, compared with 7 percent of the nonartists. Mixed-handedness occurred in 27 percent of the artists and in only 15 percent of the nonartists.[39]

The meaning of these findings is uncertain. They clearly pose problems for Levy's cognitive deficit model of left-handedness, unless one argues that the deficit in visuospatial ability occurs in only a subset of left-handers. Another interpretation is that interest in and experience with art leads to greater utilization of the left hand, instead of the brain organization of left-handers directly predisposing them to greater artistic ability.

Despite the suggestion of deficits in left-handers and the amply justified reprisals mentioned, it is evident that any differences in the cognitive abilities of left- and right-handers in general are very small and of little practical importance. Individual variation within a group is much greater than the statistical difference between groups. However, the issue of statistical differences in cognitive functioning and handedness will continue to be pursued because of its significance to theories of brain variability and organization.

....

NEW IDEAS ABOUT HANDEDNESS

This chapter has dealt with basic issues related to hand preference—their origins, their implications for human abilities, and their relation to hemispheric asymmetry of function. In this section, we discuss two relatively new and very speculative ideas about handedness.

...

Left-Handedness and the Immune System

The possible relationship between handedness and the body's immune system has been the subject of a great deal of interest and controversy since it was first proposed in the early 1980s. The idea emerged at a meeting in Boston in 1980, when Norman Geschwind commented that those interested in studying the genetics of dyslexia should not limit themselves to examining the frequency of dyslexia among the relatives of dyslexics—they should look for the presence of other conditions in these families as well.* In addition to psychologists and neurologists, the audience at Geschwind's talk was composed of large numbers of parents of dyslexic children, who told Geschwind afterward about their family histories of immune disorders and migraine. These observations led Geschwind to a series of studies with Peter Behan, studies that demonstrated an unexpected link between left-handedness and such disorders.

In the first two studies, a total of 500 strongly left-handed and 900 strongly right-handed subjects were compared.[40] The strong sinistrals had a rate of immune disorders 2.5 times greater than that of right-handers and a rate of learning disorders 10 times greater. In the second study, 652 strongly right-handed and 440 strongly left-handed control subjects were studied along with 304 patients with proven autoimmune diseases.[41] Among the control subjects, the incidence of migraine, allergies, dyslexia, stuttering, skeletal malformations, and thyroid disorders was significantly higher in the left-handed group. Among the patients with proven autoimmune diseases, the rate of left-handedness was significantly higher than in the general population in five of the eight different autoimmune disorders included in this group.

These observations led Geschwind and neurologist Albert Galaburda to develop a far-reaching theory of lateralization that would account for these findings as well as many others.[42] They proposed that a common factor may be responsible for both left-handedness and susceptibility to immune disorders. Such a factor most likely would be male related, they reasoned, because the incidence of left-handedness and of developmental disorders of language and cognition is higher in males. Because similar effects, although less marked, occur in females, the factor must also have the potential for affecting females. The male sex hormone testosterone met these criteria. Fetuses of both sexes are exposed to testosterone, although females are exposed to lower quantities.

Geschwind and Galaburda proposed that testosterone slows the growth of parts of the left hemisphere during fetal life, so that corresponding regions on the right develop relatively more rapidly. As a consequence, they argue, males will show a greater degree of shift to

---

* Dyslexia is the term applied to cases of reading disability unaccompanied by other problems such as sensory impairment. Dyslexia is discussed in greater detail in Chapter 10.

right-hemisphere participation in handedness and language and will more likely have augmented right-hemisphere skills. The delay in left-hemisphere development, in some cases, may result in a permanent developmental learning disorder, the incidence of which is higher in males.

At the same time testosterone is affecting the development of the left hemisphere, Geschwind and Galaburda believed that it may also affect the development of the immune system, thereby increasing susceptibility to subsequent immune disorders. Hence, testosterone could be responsible for both the apparent association between the incidence of left-handedness and the incidence of immune disorders.

Geschwind and Galaburda's ideas are intriguing and suggest a host of interesting possibilities. For example, they note that in some cases, the more rapid development of the right hemisphere mediated by testosterone may lead to special skills. Autistic individuals, for example, occasionally show very superior artistic ability (see Chapter 10 for further discussion). The effects of testosterone on the left hemisphere would account for the disabilities the person showed, while the accompanying enhanced development of the right hemisphere would account for the "island" of superior performance.

Such a mechanism could even account for certain types of superior performance in persons not showing cognitive deficits. In a study of a large, male-predominant group of mathematically gifted children, the subjects had five times the rate of allergies and twice the rate of left-handedness as a less gifted group.[43] Could the testosterone hypothesis account for this as well? Geschwind and Galaburda tentatively suggested that it could—depending on the precise timing and levels of testosterone present in utero, the deleterious consequences of a slowing of left-hemisphere development might be avoided, while the advantages of right-hemisphere enhancement might be realized.

It is clear that much work remains to be done to verify or falsify (and, indeed, even clarify) the predictions of the Geschwind and Galaburda theory of cerebral lateralization. A large number of studies have already been undertaken, some of which confirm and some of which disconfirm, aspects of the theory.[44] The effort will no doubt continue for a long time, given the complexity and far reaching nature of the model.[45]

···

Left-Handedness and Mortality

Another controversial set of findings comes from the work of Stanley Coren at the University of British Columbia. Coren was intrigued by his own data showing that the proportion of left handers diminished from 13 percent in 20-year-olds to less than 1 percent in 80-year-olds. Were these differences in the incidence of left-handedness real, and if so, what did they mean? Coren and his colleague Diane Halpern began by analyzing data on handedness and age at death for 2,272 baseball players listed in the *Baseball Encyclopedia*.[46] They chose these data to analyze because handedness is an important part of a baseball player's profile and would be prominently mentioned in the description of a deceased player.

Not counting any difference in the risk of dying of less than 0.5 percent, the study found no difference between left- and right-handers up to age 33. From that age on, the percentage of right handers who survive averaged about 2 percent higher than the percentage of left-handers. At the far end of the age range, differences between left-handers and right-handers become most marked. The oldest surviving left-hander was 91 years of age; the oldest surviving right-hander was 109. More than 2.5 percent of right-handers lived to be 90, whereas less than 0.5 percent of the left-handers reached that age.

Coren subsequently conducted another study with a broader sample of subjects and a different approach.[47] Information about handedness of recently deceased people was obtained from next of kin who did not know the purpose of the study. Results showed an overall advantage for being female (mean age of death for females, 77.55; mean age of death for males, 71.61). A much larger difference, however, was found as a function of handedness. The mean age of death for right-handers was 75.34 years; for left-handers, it was 66.20 years.

These findings are consistent with those obtained in the baseball study. How can they be accounted for? Earlier in this chapter we reviewed evidence that some left-handedness is pathological in origin. Perhaps the pathological factors producing left-handedness produce other conditions that affect mortality as well. We have also just considered data from the work of Geschwind and his colleagues showing an association between left-handedness and immune disorders; that link could also affect mortality.

While acknowledging the role of these factors, Coren proposed yet another possible explanation—a higher rate of accidents among left-handers. In the next-of-kin study, Halpern and Coren asked for information about the cause of death and whether accident-related injuries were involved.[48] They found that left-handers were six times more likely to die from accident-related injuries than right-handers. Separating out vehicular accidents from others, they found left-handers were about four times more likely to die in accidents while driving. Coren's analysis led him to conclude that much of the mortality difference between left-handers and right-handers can be accounted for by accidents that decrease the survival of left-handers related to that of right-handers.

Coren and Halpern's work relating left-handedness and mortality is highly controversial. The controversy lies not so much in the data themselves, although some have argued that response biases may have affected the outcome of the next-of-kin questionnaire study,[49] but in their interpretation. While Coren and Halpern concluded that left-handers are eliminated from the population through early mortality, others see differences in the mean age at death of left-handers and right-handers as an artifact of the relationship between age and the incidence of left-handedness found in the population as a result of cultural pressure.[50]

Kenneth Hugdahl and his colleagues have referred to the latter interpretation as the modification hypothesis[51] as opposed to the elimination hypothesis proposed by Coren and Halpern. According to the modification hypothesis, the differences in the incidence of left-handedness between younger and older persons are due to changing social norms—older persons were more likely to have been exposed to stronger pressure to shift from left-hand to right-hand use, resulting in a lower incidence of left-handedness in the older population. Thus there are fewer left-handers, proportionately, among older persons not because of early death, but because older persons were more likely to have had right-hand use imposed upon them in childhood.

Hugdahl and his associates have attempted to directly test the modification hypothesis by simultaneously collecting data on current hand use and hand switching in childhood in the same subjects. Working with data from almost 3000 subjects, the investigators report that the decline in left-handedness in old age was counteracted by a similar increase in subjects who had switched from using the left hand for writing to using the right hand.

Hand switching does not appear to completely account for the distribution of handedness across the age span, however, and issues of handedness and its implications for mortality continue to be of great interest. As more investigators approach the problem with increasing sophistication, we can expect to obtain better answers.

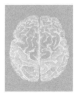

FURTHER EVIDENCE FROM THE CLINIC: Aphasia, Apraxia, Agnosia

·········

CONTEMPORARY NEUROPSYCHOLOGY

In Chapter 1 we reviewed from a historical perspective how the concept of brain asymmetries developed from data on brain-injured patients. In this chapter, we shall continue our review of the insights into brain function gleaned from studies of the effects of various injuries to the cerebral hemispheres. This pursuit is the realm of clinical, experimental, and cognitive neuropsychology. Before the days of CT scans and other brain-imaging methods, neuropsychologists emphasized the use of their clinical skills to predict the location of damage in patients showing various functional or behavioral disturbances. Modern neuropsychology still does this to an extent, when neurological and physiological techniques show questionable findings; but the emphasis is on comprehensive assessment of any mental and behavioral dysfunction accompanying evidence of brain damage, usually for clinical purposes but often also for theoretical insight.

Modern neuropsychology attempts to extend our understanding of psychological processes by examining the ways in which they break down. Sometimes a behavior thought to be a unitary mental process turns out to be a complex interaction; at other times, investigators discover that what were thought to be separate mental activities actually arise from the same brain mechanisms. Memory, language, and emotion are among the psychological processes that have been studied.

Information obtained from the brain-damage clinic must be interpreted very carefully. Neuropsychologists studying brain-behavior relationships must rely on lesions occurring naturally or on lesions created by surgeons for medical reasons. These are usually less than ideal for answering specific questions an investigator might wish to ask. Natural lesions, such as those caused by stroke, do not respect anatomical boundaries. A lesion may destroy an area of the brain involved in some psychological process, it may disconnect areas contributing to this process, or it may do both.

There are other confounding problems as well. In Chapter 1 we mentioned the brain's tendency to adjust its operations as best it can in the presence of damage. As neurologist John Hughlings Jackson pointed out a century ago, the abnormal behavior observed after a brain lesion reflects the functioning of the remaining brain tissue. This remaining tissue may compensate for the damage and thus minimize the deficit. However, it may also react adversely and operate more poorly, thus adding to the deficit—a concept called diaschisis.

...

Cognitive Neuropsychology

The advent of cognitive neuropsychology, introduced in Chapter 1, has not changed the importance of the problems discussed above, but it has more explicitly connected them to the assumptions underlying the cognitive neuropsychological approach. In Chapter 1 we briefly described an assumption of cognitive neuropsychology, namely, that of the "modularity" of mental processes, which holds that mental activity is the result of the coordinated activity of many different "modules," each of which engages its own form of processing independently of the activity in others.

Several other assumptions are also implicit in the approach taken by cognitive neuropsychologists.[1] These include the following ideas:

Neurological specificity or isomorphism: The assumption that there is a correspondence between the organization of the mind and the organization of the brain;

Transparency: The assumption that impaired performance following brain injury will provide us with a basis for determining which mode of the system is disrupted;

Subtractivity: The assumption that the performance following brain injury reflects the previous intact cognitive apparatus minus those systems that have been impaired and that the mature brain does not produce new modules.

The first two assumptions are, for the most part, implicit in all neuropsychological research, both past and present, that seeks to establish brain-behavior relationships from the effects of brain damage. With regard to the third assumption, cognitive neuropsychology is somewhat more explicit in regard to how brain injury affects the hypothesized modular organization of the brain. A very literal (or strong) form of the subtractivity assumption implies that brain injury does not affect the normal function of modules not directly damaged by the injury; therefore, performance following brain injury reflects the normal operation of all undamaged modules.

This last statement is almost certainly an oversimplification, because at least some undamaged brain is likely to adjust some aspect of its normal operation. Most cognitive neuropsychologists agree with this conclusion; however, they insist that what matters is not that old modules can be put to new use but that new modules should not come into existence following brain injury.[2] They believe that if the brain can truly reorganize its structure and generate new modules following injury, then it is not possible to learn much about normal brain function from clinical disorders. However, all indications are that most neural destruction, once it occurs, is permanent and that compensation and recovery must depend on changes in spared brain. It is relatively safe, therefore, to assume that an injured brain functions only with spared preexisting modules, although these may modify their operations as recovery progresses and new strategies are developed over time.

Despite practical and conceptual difficulties, neuropsychology has generated a substantial framework of data and theories that categorize and attempt to explain most brain-behavior dysfunctions. A discussion of neuropsychological disorders involves many concepts and definitions that have been developed over the years by notable investigators.[3] We shall not attempt to trace this development but shall present certain concepts as established and shall cite newer studies bearing on hemispheric asymmetries. The interested reader is referred to some of the excellent texts that review clinical neuropsychology in general.[4] We shall briefly discuss some of the more general concepts of brain structure-function relationships gleaned from the study of brain injury but shall concentrate on how newer data has furthered our understanding of functions within each cerebral hemisphere.

·········

DISORDERS OF SPEECH AND LANGUAGE

Language is a complex, multifaceted skill that encompasses the formation of sounds, the development of sophisticated rule systems, and the existence of a vast quantity of meaning and significance information. Linguistics, the formal study of language, has developed many concepts that deal with the structure of a language and apply to all languages.

Linguists have defined four major components of language: phonology (dealing with producing and processing speech sounds); syntax (involving the rules of word order and form, or grammar); semantics (the processing of meaning); and pragmatics (involving intonation in speech, practical significance, and context).

The term *aphasia* has become the general heading for a broad class of speech and language dysfunctions caused by neurological damage. We review here the major categories of aphasia with respect to how they arise from damage to different areas of the brain and the extent to which they shed light on the organization of linguistic processes. The study of the aphasias also provides classic examples of the theoretical controversies that can arise when psychological theories are formulated from clinical data.

...

The Aphasias

The two major categories of aphasia are expressive (motor) aphasia and receptive (sensory) aphasia. Not all investigators, however, adhere to this distinction.

Expressive (or Broca's) aphasia is a deficit involving primarily the patient's own speech; the patient's comprehension of the speech of others remains relatively intact. This type of aphasia is associated with damage to the frontal regions of the left hemisphere controlling speech output, particularly the region called Broca's area. Broca's area, shown in Figure 6.1, is located just in front of the primary motor zone for speech musculature (lips, tongue, jaw, and so on). These speech motor areas, however, are spared in cases of classic Broca's aphasia; that is, there is no paralysis of the speech apparatus.*

A patient with Broca's aphasia speaks very little. When speech is attempted, it is halting—the patient has difficulty getting the words out. There is an absence of small grammatical parts of speech and proper inflection. Such speech is often called telegraphic or agrammatic speech. For example, in response to a picture showing a woman washing dishes, an overflowing sink, and some children tipping a stool as they attempt to get a cookie jar, a Broca's aphasia patient might say, "Sink . . . water . . . b . . . boy . . . boy fall . . . step . . . ." In severe cases the patient will often be able to vocalize only one or two words over and over again in any attempt to speak or describe something.

When a patient does say a word, it is usually pronounced reasonably well. The ability to name objects is poor, but prompting helps significantly. These facts help justify the view that the deficit is not simply at the level of articulation. Most Broca's aphasics seem to understand spoken or written language, so the problem is considered to be at the motor output stage of language rather than in comprehension. Patients also seem to be aware of most of their errors. Some investigators have argued, however, that the comprehension of Broca's aphasics is not as intact as many have believed. Edgar Zurif claimed that many such patients understand a sentence only by inferring what makes sense from a sampling of its major nouns and verbs.[5] When the syntactic structure of a sentence is more complex, comprehension seriously falls off.

---

* Impairment of speech (such as slurring) due to partial paralysis of the speech musculature is called dysarthria.

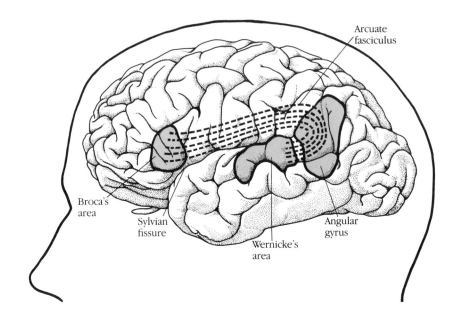

FIGURE 6.1   The areas of the left hemisphere in humans associated with speech and language. The arcuate fasciculus is a nerve-fiber bundle beneath the cortex, connecting Broca's and Wernicke's areas. [Adapted from Geschwind, "Language and the Brain," *Scientific American, Inc.,* 1972. All rights reserved.]

Patients seem unable to properly utilize the information conveyed by complex grammatical structure.

Receptive (or Wernicke's) aphasia is a disturbance in which the patient has great difficulty comprehending speech. It is associated with damage to the posterior region of the first temporal gyrus, or Wernicke's area (see Figure 6.1). The speech of a patient with receptive aphasia is much more fluent than that of an expressive aphasic, but, depending on the extent of damage, it may vary from being slightly odd to completely meaningless. Patients often use inappropriate words (paraphasias) or nonexistent words (neologisms). In some cases, the patient's output sounds like complete jargon or "word salad," although the rhythm and flow of speech seem to be preserved. One patient, when asked how he was, responded, "I felt worse because I can no longer keep in mind from the mind of the minds to keep me from mind and up to the ear which can be to find among ourselves."[6] In severe cases, it may consist mostly of meaningless utterances yet sound fluent, as in the following exchange [examiner's interjections in brackets]:

Examiner: How did you get sick?

Patient: Eeh, oh malaty? Eeeh, favility? Abelabla tay kare. Abelabl tay to po stay here. [stay here?] Aberdar yeste day. [yesterday?] and then abedeyes dee, aaah, yes dee, ye ship, yeste dey es dalababela. Abla desee, abla detoasy, abla ley e porephee, tee arabek. Abla get sik? [get sick?][7]

Such patients often seem unaware that their speech is defective or meaningless and continue to talk as if nothing is wrong.

Reading and writing are comparably impaired. There are aphasic patients who will go through the motions of reading a book out loud but produce only gibberish. Some investigators believe that Wernicke's aphasia results from damage to verbal or semantic memory stores,[8] as distinct from a defect in syntactic and articulatory mechanisms involved in Broca's aphasia.

...

Beyond the Expressive-Receptive Distinction

Although relatively pure forms of expressive and receptive aphasia do occur, the division of aphasia into these two categories implies a more clear-cut distinction than is generally the case. Patients often show symptoms attributed to both types of aphasia, and some investigators feel the distinction is too artificial—not truly representing how language is organized in the brain. We shall review some of these criticisms later but must first consider several other categories of aphasia. Beyond the expressive-receptive distinction, investigators have labeled other forms of aphasia, according to both patterns of brain damage and patterns of language deficits. Some of these categorizations are controversial, yet many neuropsychologists and speech pathologists argue that they truly represent distinct, recurring clinical syndromes.

Besides the receptive aphasia named after him, Wernicke predicted another type of aphasia that he claimed would arise from a lesion interrupting the neural pathways connecting the centers for speech production (Broca's area) and speech comprehension (Wernicke's area). This aphasia, now labeled conduction aphasia, is characterized by a patient's inability to repeat aloud what is heard. In addition, spontaneous speech may be meaningless, fluent jargon (as in Wernicke's aphasia), but unlike comprehension in Wernicke's aphasia, comprehension of spoken and written material remains largely intact.

These symptoms can be explained as arising from a disconnection of the receptive and expressive language centers of the brain. In fact, damage to the neural tract called the arcuate fasciculus, connecting Broca's and Wernicke's areas (see Figure 6.1), has been implicated in such cases.[9] Stuart Dimond has claimed that the arcuate fasciculus, along with some subcortical structures (the thalamic region), is involved in integrating the input and output aspects of speech.[10] He also suggested that these neural tracts and associated structures form a storehouse of linguistic information and may act as language generators.

The anatomical model for conduction aphasia was elaborated further by Norman Geschwind to explain several other combinations of symptoms observed in aphasic patients.[11] The transcortical aphasias involve lesions that spare the speech areas and their main interconnecting pathways but, in a variety of ways, isolate these areas from the rest of the brain. Depending on whether brain damage isolates Wernicke's area (transcortical sensory aphasia), Broca's area (transcortical motor aphasia), or both (transcortical mixed aphasia), there are various degrees of comprehension and spontaneous speech problems. Such patients, however, are able to repeat quite well what is said to them. Transcortical aphasics, in extreme cases, may echo everything they hear, a condition known as echolalia. This sparing of repetition ability is what distinguishes transcortical aphasia from Broca's, Wernicke's, or conduction aphasia, where repetition is disturbed. Several additional aphasia types should also be mentioned.

Word deafness results from a lesion disconnecting Wernicke's area from auditory inputs. Comprehension is impaired for spoken language only; the ability to hear sounds in general is not affected. Comprehension of writing is normal, as is verbal and written expression, although the patient's speech may eventually also suffer because the patient lacks adequate feedback from his own speech.

Anomic aphasia involves difficulty in naming objects. Although this condition is present in most aphasics, a "purer" or isolated form results from damage limited to the cortical area at the junction of the temporal, parietal, and occipital lobes—the area called the angular gyrus (see Figure 6.1). A purely anomic patient will have normal comprehension and be able to speak almost normally in spontaneous casual conversation. When confronted with objects, however, or when trying to think of a word or a name, the patient will falter badly. It has been suggested that this impairment is a result of disruption of associations involving different sensory modalities (and, hence, different regions of the brain) that are part of the naming act.

Global aphasia refers to severe impairment of all language-related functions. Comprehension as well as production of speech are defective or absent in global aphasia. Communication may be attempted with a symbol system—for example, by learning to use plastic objects to stand for words—but even this approach is difficult and sometimes unsuccessful. Global aphasia results from widespread damage to the left hemisphere involving most of the areas thought to play a role in language.

...

Theoretical Issues Arising from Aphasia Classification

The view that there are discrete cerebral centers performing specific aspects of language processing has been called the localizationist-connectionist view.* It has served to categorize the variety of language disorders seen in clinical settings and, to an extent, to predict the kind of disorder one might expect to see after specific types of brain damage. Evaluating a patient's language disorder can also do the reverse, that is, predict where the damage might be.

The localizationist approach has been criticized, however, by investigators who claim it is overly simplistic in its "flow diagram" view of the brain and the organization of language. Such criticisms can be traced back to the nineteenth-century holistic view of brain function, when neurologists such as Jackson argued that all aphasia is associated with defective comprehension, that is, that sensory aphasia underlies all others. Some present-day investigators have contended that the localizationist view places too much emphasis on independent components or depots interconnected by neural wiring.[12]

Cognitive neuropsychologists have not faulted the idea of independent components itself; rather, they have placed an emphasis on the need to reorganize our conceptions of what the components or "modules" really are.[13] Most neuropsychologists have agreed, however, that the actual situation is more dynamic than the traditional connec-

---

* *This view is sometimes called localizationist-associationist, in the sense that most modern concepts that attribute functions to specific areas of the brain also place importance on the interactions between these areas in any complex mental activity.*

tionist view, involving simultaneous interactions of many areas for any language function. The evidence mentioned for comprehension deficits in Broca's aphasia supports such a viewpoint.

Neurologist Jason Brown proposed an alternative to the standard cortical localizationist view.[14] Synthesizing the work of several earlier theorists, he described the organization of the brain in terms of evolutionary layers modified by maturational growth.[15] Broca's and Wernicke's areas are only the last stage "tips," not only in terms of the brain's evolution, but also in terms of brain function and language formation. Speech and language emerge at these cortical areas simultaneously from more primitive linguistic stages operating below. Thus, cortical lesions do not so much disconnect the cortical flow of information necessary for language as force the language system to operate at a more primitive, incomplete level.

Some support for such a hierarchical view of language organization comes from evidence that certain subcortical structures, particularly the thalamus, play an important role in language.

...

Subcortical Aphasia: The Role of the Thalamus

Lesions to brain structures deep within the brain, especially the thalamus, can result in language disturbances. The thalamus, as shown in Figure A.1 in the Appendix, is also divided into right and left halves. Damage to the left thalamus has been reported to affect verbal fluency, creating word-finding hesitation as well as perseveration (repeating the same sound or word several times).[16] As mentioned in the discussion of conduction aphasia, it has been suggested that the thalamus is an integrating center between frontal and posterior cortical language areas.

Neurosurgeon George Ojemann reported on the effects of electrical stimulation of the thalamus, using a procedure similar to the cortical stimulation tests described in Chapter 1. Left thalamic stimulation typically led to speech arrest or to problems with object naming coupled with perseveration of the initial syllable of the word a patient was attempting to say. Ojemann also reported that there was a general slowing, slurring, and distortion of speech. He suggested that the thalamus has two general functions in speech: (1) to serve as an alerting mechanism to direct attention to verbal information in the environment as well as to retrieve verbal information properly from verbal memory;

(2) to control, at least in part, some of the physical substrates of speech, such as respiration and the speech musculature.[17]

...

Left Hemispherectomy

Hemispherectomy, or removal of one-half of the brain, is a rare operation and, despite the name, usually involves removing only the cortex of the hemisphere. It is sometimes performed in infants suffering from serious cerebral birth defects. Because of their age, such children often recover and develop remarkably well after the operation. We shall discuss childhood hemispherectomy in Chapter 9.

Hemispherectomy is performed very rarely in adults, usually for removal of malignant tumors. The operation is almost never performed on the dominant hemisphere, because of the very severe consequences. Nevertheless, left hemispherectomies offer investigators the opportunity to examine the functions of the right hemisphere in isolation. Neuropsychologist Aaron Smith and others have extensively studied such patients.[18] Several patients made significant recoveries, although they initially showed markedly impaired language function. They were eventually able to produce short, relatively grammatically correct sentences. Most left-hemispherectomy patients show a surprising amount of verbal comprehension, although their voluntary speech, reading, and writing abilities remain severely impaired.

An important case for our understanding of how the two hemispheres may interact when one is damaged was described by Smith in 1969, when a patient underwent surgery to remove most of a damaged right hemisphere.[19] The patient's language improved after the surgery! This outcome suggests that the damaged right hemisphere hindered the potential of the left hemisphere. It is very probable that normal communication between the hemispheres involves a substantial number of inhibitory signals, an exchange that serves to coordinate function and prevent unnecessary duplication or competition. When one hemisphere is damaged, its inhibitory effects on the other may become pathological or, at least, inappropriate for recovery of function. The extent to which this is true makes interpretation of the effects of focal brain damage that much more difficult. It is also possible that understanding pathological inhibition eventually may allow surgeons to develop a rationale for when to remove damaged brain tissue for therapeutic reasons.

...

Reading and Writing

Disorders of reading and writing accompany some types of aphasia, especially aphasias resulting from posterior lesions. We mentioned, for example, how some Wernicke's asphasics go through the motions of reading aloud but produce only jargon. Reading and writing, however, can be selectively impaired; that is, a reading deficit or a writing deficit can be the primary problem after certain brain injuries even though speech production and comprehension remain relatively intact.*

Most reading and writing disorders involve either direct damage to the left angular gyrus or damage to adjacent regions. As mentioned in the discussion of anomic aphasia, the angular gyrus is located at the junction of the parietal, temporal, and occipital lobes and is thought to integrate the sensory, auditory, and visual information processed by these regions, respectively. This central position adjoining the major sensory and language-comprehension systems of the brain seems to make the left angular gyrus fundamentally important to reading and writing.

Investigators have subdivided disorders of reading and writing into two main categories: alexia with agraphia (inability to read and write) and alexia without agraphia (inability to read, but with writing spared). Alexia with agraphia almost always involves damage to the angular gyrus. In addition to deficits in reading and writing, it is often accompanied by some aphasic deficits, such as difficulties in word finding and naming. Alexia without agraphia is a rather astonishing condition to observe, for patients with this disorder can write a sentence properly, either spontaneously or from dictation, but when this writing is shown to the patients, they cannot read it.

Alexia without agraphia has been explained as a "disconnection" between certain visual processing areas of the brain and the angular gyrus. It seems to arise when lesions damage the left occipital lobe and a part of the neural tracts forming the corpus callosum. The lesion to the corpus callosum disconnects the intact right occipital lobe from the left angular gyrus, leaving little, if any, visual information flow to the language processing areas.[20] Thus, these patients cannot read, although they can still see. Writing is preserved because the angular gyrus is intact and because writing can proceed with only minimal visual feedback.

Our discussion of reading and writing disorders here concerns only those acquired following injury, after a person has developed the skills. Some developmental disorders in children will be discussed in Chapter 10.

A more controversial form of alexia, labeled deep dyslexia, has been described and is believed to demonstrate some right-hemisphere reading skills.[21] (The nature of right hemisphere language skills will be discussed in the next section.) When asked, for example, to read aloud the printed word *table,* some alexic patients with left-hemisphere damage will respond with "chair." This type of error is called paralexic and involves a wrong response that is nevertheless meaningfully relative to the target word. It has been proposed that brain lesions have entirely inactivated the normal reading mechanisms of the left hemisphere in such patients. The right hemisphere, having some semantic (meaning) skills, understands the word and communicates some meaning information to the left hemisphere. The left hemisphere then forms the pronunciation of a word with a related meaning, because it does not "know" exactly what word the right hemisphere saw. The semantic information conveyed by the right hemisphere is not enough to distinguish among synonyms or closely related words, and thus the paralexic errors are made by the speaking left hemisphere.

As part of the evidence that supports this theory, patients who make paralexic responses in attempting to read do so to concrete words such as object nouns, whereas they show little or no response to abstract words. As we shall see, there is evidence that right-hemisphere comprehension abilities are limited to words that describe objects.

·········

THE ROLE OF THE RIGHT HEMISPHERE IN LANGUAGE

Semantic processing, the comprehension of word meanings, is severely disrupted in patients with damage to posterior regions of the left hemisphere, like that found in Wernicke's aphasia. No similar disruption can be demonstrated with right-hemisphere lesions. However, as mentioned in our discussion of split-brain patients in Chapter 2, investigators have demonstrated that the right hemisphere can show comprehension of certain words, especially object nouns. Some research with normal subjects suggests that the extent to which a word's meaning is understood by the right hemisphere depends on how concrete (as opposed to abstract) it is.[22] Thus, correct comprehension of words such as *justice,* *harmony,* and *hate* seems to depend more exclusively on left-hemisphere processing than does comprehension of words such as *table, car,* and *hospital,* which the right hemisphere can also understand.

The right hemisphere's ability to understand certain words, however, probably does not contribute much to our speech and language skills, because the left can do the same and more. But does the right hemisphere make any unique contributions to our language communication skills? The answer, based on observing many patients and several studies with normal subjects, appears to be yes.

...

Intonation

Communicating through speech and language involves many subtle nuances that are not an obvious part of the structure and content of sentences. Intonation patterns and emotional tone play an obvious, important role.

Many left-hemisphere-damaged aphasic patients can discriminate the purpose of an utterance. Broca's aphasics, despite their problems with verbal output, attempt to use the correct pattern to produce a statement (as opposed to a question).[23] Patients with right-hemisphere damage, however, often speak with a flattened intonation; they also have difficulty judging the emotional tone of the speech produced by others.[24] Right-hemisphere-damaged patients have been known to add parenthetical phrases to their speech to emphasize their feelings—for example, "I am angry (and mean it)."[25] This behavior occurs after the patients realize that their speech is not sufficiently forceful or emotional to evoke the desired response.

Neurologist Elliot Ross has developed a model of how lesions of different areas of the right hemisphere result in the disruption of the rhythmic and intonational aspects of language ("prosody") in a manner analogous to the way in which left-hemisphere lesions disrupt the syntactic and semantic aspects of language. Thus, Ross claimed that there is a "conduction aprosodia" and a "transcortical sensory aprosodia" and so on.[26] This model, although supported in part by the general evidence for a right-hemisphere role in intonation, remains controversial in terms of its finer distinctions.

...

Melodic Intonation Therapy

The preservation of intonation and singing that often occurs in aphasic patients (see Chapter 1) has been exploited in therapy designed to teach such patients phrases through song. The program, called melodic intonation therapy, has been successful with certain patients who have reasonably good comprehension but poor speech production, such as Broca's aphasics. Word sequences are first incorporated in a song, and the melody is deemphasized gradually until the patient can speak the phrase without singing. It is presumed that the intact right hemisphere learns the phrases this way and, as a result, develops more language production skills that compensate, to a degree, for the left-hemisphere deficit. The program's developers claimed that some aphasic patients, after not having had any meaningful speech for over a year following a stroke, are able to carry on short, meaningful conversations after a month or two of therapy.[27]

···

Metaphor and Humor

There are several other language-related skills in which the right hemisphere appears to be involved. These skills are demonstrated by deficits found in right-hemisphere-injured patients, but not in aphasic (left-hemisphere-injured) patients, and seem to involve more conceptual aspects of language communication. For example, right-hemisphere-injured patients tend to be overly literal in their interpretation of words, stories, and cartoons. Given a choice, they often pick literal interpretations of metaphorical statements ("sour grapes") and popular sayings ("A penny saved is a penny earned.").[28] They also very frequently pick totally inappropriate endings to cartoon strips, as if the humor is in a surprise ending.[29]

We see again that the right hemisphere contributes in important ways to language communication. In addition to possessing some comprehension abilities, as discussed earlier, it truly complements left-hemisphere speech and language processing through more subtle, but definitely important, communication skills. Emotional intonation, aspects of metaphor, and some qualities of humor seem to depend on right-hemisphere abilities. The extent to which the right hemisphere enriches other language skills remains to be determined.

···

The Right Hemisphere in Recovery from Aphasia

Partial or complete recovery from initially severe deficits after stroke or head injury is not uncommon. Reports generally show that most improvement occurs during the first 6 to 12 months, depending on a number of factors such as age, cause, and severity of the original symptoms. The fact that recovery does take place raises a number of issues concerning the mechanisms responsible for it and the plasticity of the central nervous system.

One of the hypotheses offered to explain the recovery of language after left-hemisphere damage is that structures of the intact right hemisphere become more involved in language processing. Wernicke was probably the first to propose this idea, which has continued to be entertained by investigators to this day. The hypothesis is supported by several lines of evidence. In the late 1800s it was observed that recovered aphasics who had sustained left-hemisphere injuries relapsed after new lesions developed in the right hemisphere.[30]

Much more recently, Marcel Kinsbourne studied the effect of intracarotid injection of barbiturates (the Wada procedure) in three patients recovering from aphasia due to left-hemisphere lesions.[31] He found that, although injection into the left carotid artery did not worsen speech, right carotid injection resulted in arrest of speech in two of the three patients.

Other evidence for right-hemisphere involvement in recovery of language, although indirect, comes from the study of left hemidecortication or hemispherectomy in infants and very young children who develop apparently normal language (see discussion in Chapter 9), as well as from case studies such as that of a 54-year-old patient who recovered from global aphasia although he had sustained total destruction of the temporal-parietal regions of the left hemisphere.[32]

Several recent studies have examined such recovery by using more direct physiological measures of brain activity. One probe evoked potential study showed greater than normal participation of the right hemisphere during a language task[33] in patients who had recovered from aphasia.

Some cerebral blood-flow data also supports increased participation of the right hemisphere in recovery from aphasia.[34]

Another possible mechanism for recovery of function has to do with the resolution of "diaschisis." We briefly mentioned diaschisis earlier in discussing how brain tissue that is not directly affected by an injury or stroke may nevertheless react adversely and operate more poorly. It is thought that this occurs because the injury interrupts neural pathways and information that normally stimulates the area involved. Functional neuroimaging scans have recently shown this to indeed be the case in cerebral regions outside the lesion in some stroke patients: Some areas of the brain outside of the stroke are less than normally active despite an adequate blood supply. Thus, diaschisis immediately poststroke may account for some of the patient's deficits and, as the area recovers, may also account for the recovery of those deficits.[35]

The "resolution of diaschisis model" and the "unaffected hemisphere taking on new functions model" are competing but not necessarily mutually exclusive explanations of recovery. Both probably occur in many cases.

....
DISORDERS OF PURPOSEFUL MOVEMENT

Our daily activities involve many movements that have become almost automatic. We perform many complicated acts without having to think about how to do them, from picking up a pen, to drinking from a cup, to putting on perfume. Patterns of complex learned movements are organized in terms of both position and timing and follow intricate sequences established through experience. Apraxia is the inability to perform certain learned or purposeful movements despite the absence of paralysis or sensory loss. This breakdown in movement can occur in a number of ways.

Kinetic (or motor) apraxia is most frequently associated with lesions of the premotor area of the frontal lobe on the side opposite the affected side of the body. This form of apraxia affects the finer movements of one upper extremity, such as properly holding a pen or placing a letter in an envelope. Reaching out and properly grasping an object consists of a largely unconscious series of movements that depend on a built-up memory of acts similarly performed. Kinetic apraxia may be regarded as a breakdown in the program or "memory" of the motor sequences necessary to perform some basic act.

Ideomotor apraxia is usually due to damage in the parietal lobe of the left (dominant) hemisphere, but it seems to have bilateral effects behaviorally. Patients are unable to perform many complex acts on command, although they may perform them spontaneously in appropriate situations. The difficulty is especially noticeable when patients are asked to use pantomime, for example, when asked to "Pretend you are brushing your teeth." or when asked "How do you strike a match?" or "How do you wave goodbye?" Patients seem to know what they have been told to do but are unable to do it. Given the actual objects and appropriate context, patients will usually perform much better. The main disturbance seems to be in voluntary recall of some action, not in its actual execution. Therefore, it seems that the motor memory of the action is not disturbed, as it is in kinetic (motor) apraxia. Ideomotor apraxia is considered to be a result of the interruption of pathways between the center for verbal formulation of a motor act and the motor areas of the frontal lobe necessary for its execution.

Ideational apraxia involves an inability to formulate an appropriate sequence of acts or to use objects properly. Patients seem to know how to perform isolated movements, such as striking a match, but will do them inappropriately. For instance, given a candle and a book of matches, they may strike the candle against the matchbook cover. Sometimes complex sequences are done out of order: Patients may start the hand motions involved in writing before picking up a pen.

The patients' appreciation of what they are doing often seems to be defective, so it has been suggested that such apraxia is a form of agnosia, a deficit in knowing or perceiving the object properly. The assigned locus of damage in such disorders is controversial. A classic view was that ideational apraxia arose from lesions in the parietal lobe of the left (dominant) hemisphere or in the corpus callosum. It is most frequently found, however, in cases of diffuse bilateral damage, such as that following disruption of the oxygen supply to the brain (anoxia).

Constructional apraxia involves a loss in the ability to reproduce or construct figures by drawing or assembling. There seems to be a loss of visual guidance or an impairment in visualizing a manipulative output, although basic visual and motor functions appear to be intact. It is seen in certain cases of damage to the occipital and parietal cortex, and perhaps to pathways between them.

Although the incidence of deficits called constructional apraxia by various investigators seems to be the same for either left- or right-hemisphere lesions, later reviews show that there are characteristic differences in the quality of performance on constructional tasks between left- and right-hemisphere-injured patients.[36] For example, when the left hemisphere is damaged, patients draw pictures that preserve the overall configuration of objects but tend to lose detail; this result supports the view of the right hemisphere as better at perceiving overall spatial relationships. When the right hemisphere is damaged, patients draw pictures that include much detail but lack an overall coherence. Proportion and spatial relationships are often quite poor.

...

The Role of the Hemispheres in Apraxic Disorders

As noted above, ideomotor apraxia and, possibly, ideational apraxia much more often involve lesions of the left hemisphere than of the right. The anatomical model for ideomotor apraxia explains it as a disconnection between posterior brain areas for verbal formulation of an act and those areas of the frontal lobes that generate the motor output.

There is some question as to the extent of verbal involvement in apraxic disorders in general, in the sense that "internalized speech" may mediate many kinds of movement. There is a high incidence of apraxia in aphasic patients, but the fact that the two disorders can occur relatively independently suggests that apraxic disturbances involve motor memories that in some case can be separated from the speech system. It is intriguing to speculate, nevertheless, that there is a similarity in the mechanisms required to produce speech and those required to produce fine motor movements of the limbs. We shall return to this topic and its relationship to handedness in Chapter 12.

Constructional apraxia, as we have seen, appears to be not one but many different disorders involving either or both hemispheres. Neuropsychologist Arthur Benton has provided some perspective on constructional apraxia in the context of distinguishing among various kinds of visual deficits.[37] He separated visuoconstructive, visuoperceptive, and visuospatial deficits and argued that the right hemisphere is most involved in the latter two disorders. For visuoconstructive tasks—those involving block designs and construction and figure drawing—both hemispheres are usually involved, although in different ways, as demonstrated in our brief discussion of constructional apraxia. For visuoperceptive tasks—those involving separating a figure from a complex ground, recognizing deformed objects, discriminating between faces—the right hemisphere plays a greater role than the left. Finally, for visuospatial tasks—those involving judgments of depth, line orientation, and matching simple patterns—the right hemisphere plays an almost exclusive role.

·········

PERCEPTUAL DISORDERS

Our interaction with the external world depends on intact sensory and perceptual processes in the two hemispheres. We are all aware that damage to the peripheral organs of our senses, such as our eyes or ears, effectively destroys the use of a sensory modality. In a similar fashion, damage to areas of the brain receiving neural information directly from a sensory organ leads to blindness, deafness, and so on. However, there are many other more subtle injuries to our perceptual systems, injuries that result in symptoms such as not understanding what one is seeing. We shall review how some of these disorders have been categorized and what has been learned from them about the workings of the left brain and the right brain.

...

Agnosia

Agnosia is usually defined as failure of recognition that is due neither to impairment of the sensory input nor to a naming disorder of the kind seen in aphasia.* For example, agnosic patients would not be able to tell what they are looking at, although one could demonstrate that the patient could see the object and have no trouble naming it if they held it. Definitions of agnosia suffer from an inability to carefully specify the difference between sensory loss and "higher level" loss of recognition, because in fact there is no clear-cut dividing line. For the most part, the distinction is based on some of the practical differences observed in patients with various kinds of perceptual problems. Various agnosias have been classified according to the sensory modality that is affected and the type of objects or sounds that cannot be recognized.

Visual object agnosia, as mentioned, is a failure to recognize objects for reasons that cannot be attributed to a defect of visual acuity or to intellectual or language impairment. Not all clinicians insist that good visual acuity has to be demonstrated, as is the case in the "purer" forms of visual agnosia. Certain cases of mixed sensory and perceptual loss have also been called agnosia. The decision as to whether a visual deficit is purely a sensory or a higher level perceptual problem is often very difficult to make. Most cases fall somewhere in between. Most severe agnosias for objects occur after bilateral damage to parietal-occipital regions of the brain or after damage involving these areas in the left, dominant hemisphere coupled with damage to interhemispheric pathways. The latter situation is thought to mimic bilateral damage by disconnecting any remaining intact visual processing areas from the language centers of the left hemisphere. A patient with visual agnosia may still be able to recognize objects tactually, although extensive parietal damage often leads to problems in both modalities.

A distinction has often been made between "associative" object agnosia and "apperceptive" object agnosia. In associative agnosia a patient demonstrates form (or shape) and detail perception as evidenced by the ability to copy a drawing, for example, but this patient is still unable to recognize or identify objects. In apperceptive agnosia the

---

* *The patient's failure technically should also not be due to a general intellectual impairment, such as that seen in dementia.*

patient is not only unable to recognize objects but also demonstrates problems in form perception and copying. So defined, apperceptive agnosia appears as a more basic deficit in perception, perhaps of vision, than associative agnosia, which appears as a deficit in a later stage in object recognition.

Auditory agnosia is a condition in which patients with unimpaired hearing fail to recognize or distinguish what they hear. These sounds may include musical tones or familiar noises, such as a telephone ring or running water. They may also be limited to speech sounds, but such an auditory agnosia—known as word deafness—is usually considered to be a type of aphasia, as noted earlier in this chapter. Auditory agnosia is associated with damage to regions of the temporal lobe in the left, dominant hemisphere, although these disturbances are more severe when the injury is bilateral.

Astereognosis is a breakdown in tactile form perception (stereognosis). The patient cannot recognize familiar objects through touch or palpation, even though sensation in the hands appears to be normal. This condition usually results from damage to regions in the parietal lobe adjacent to the somatosensory projection areas (see Figure A.3 in the Appendix). It is thought that such damage interferes with tactile-kinesthetic memories that have been acquired and stored over the years and built up into perceptions of form, size, and texture. Evidence from clinical studies suggests that the right hemisphere plays a particularly important role in tactile form perception. Several studies have reported astereognostic conditions in patients with right posterior lesions.[38]

...

The Right and Left Hemispheres in Perception

Of the agnosias just discussed, only astereognosis results from right-hemisphere lesions alone. Our discussion of visual object agnosia did not implicate the right hemisphere in this disorder but, instead, pointed to damage to the left or to both hemispheres. This association may be surprising to the reader, considering the general visuospatial nature attributed to the right hemisphere. In fact, one should not assume that the term *visuospatial* refers to vision or visual perception. Both hemispheres are completely equipped to deal with most types of visual information. Although admittedly vague, the term *visuospatial* implies more complex operations on visual stimuli, such as those presented in Figure 1.4 in Chapter 1, or tasks involving judgments of spatial relationships.

Further evidence from the clinic, as well as from functional neuroimaging studies, does suggest several interesting differences in hemispheric contributions to perception. Some of this evidence comes from the study of patients with a selective agnosia for faces.

Prosopagnosia   We can recognize a familiar face almost instantly, despite the infinite number of expressions and orientations it can have, and we can distinguish it from hundreds of similar faces in a crowd. Patients with prosopagnosia, however, will not be able to recognize a previously known face and, in some cases, have difficulty recognizing their own face in a mirror. The patients have no trouble, however, recognizing that the face is in fact a face. Originally thought to be a right-hemisphere deficit, prosopagnosic symptoms were later described as involving lesions to both hemispheres.

Arthur Benton shed some light on the controversy by distinguishing between two forms of failure to recognize faces.[39] One is agnosia for familiar faces, or true prosopagnosia, and the other is a defect in discriminating between unfamiliar faces or in learning new faces. Benton claimed that true prosopagnosia is largely due to right-hemisphere deficits but also involves the left hemisphere. The parietal-occipital regions of both hemispheres must sustain damage for the deficit to clearly manifest itself. Defective discrimination of new (unfamiliar) faces, however, a much more common disorder, can result from just posterior right-hemisphere damage.

These findings naturally raise the question of whether there are specialized mechanisms for facial discrimination and what their relationship to other right-hemisphere abilities might be. It is frequently speculated that facial recognition is accomplished so quickly because it involves some global or holistic analysis as opposed to feature-by-feature processing. This is, of course, what many have speculated is the difference in the processing strategies of the two hemispheres.

In Chapter 4, we described a PET brain-imaging study that reported an almost exclusive right-hemisphere role in a face-recognition task. Justine Sergent, the primary investigator in that study, also reported that divided-visual-field studies showed a right-hemisphere advantage for face processing only the first time the faces were presented—afterward they showed a left-hemisphere advantage.[40] These data are clearly consistent with Benton's suggestion that hemispheric differences in face processing are based on the familiar versus unfamiliar distinction.

The same PET study also found that visual object categorization appeared to almost exclusively require increases in left-hemisphere activity. These findings are consistent with clinical neuropsychological data that associates visual object agnosia mostly with left-hemisphere lesions. So, should the roles of the left and the right hemispheres in visual perception be characterized in terms of object recognition and analysis of new faces, respectively? Other evidence indicates this to be too simple a view as well as one that does not identify more general principles in hemispheric specialization that are really behind these differences.

New Views of Visual Agnosia   A recent examination of several prosopagnosic patients, none of whom had damage in the posterior left hemisphere, showed that they were all defective at recognizing objects seen from an unusual perspective—identifying a bucket or a hat viewed from the top, for example—whereas they recognized the same objects perfectly well when viewed from more typical perspectives.[41] This finding suggested that the contribution of the right hemisphere to object recognition becomes much more crucial when perceptual operations involving corrections, transformations, or rotation of the stimulus have to be performed.

Some related observations are found in the descriptions of visual agnosia categories by neuropsychologist Elkonon Goldberg.[42] Goldberg identified apperceptive agnosia as a loss in the ability to recognize an object as the same object when it is viewed under different conditions.[*] The patient does not necessarily have a problem in identifying what an object is (for example, "It is a hat.") but will not be able to identify it as "the same hat" if the object is viewed from another orientation or perspective.

In contrast, the skill impaired in typical left hemisphere damage-induced visual agnosia is recognizing the object as a member of a generic category. Goldberg suggested that, because face recognition is clearly a matter of specific physical identification (that is, to identify the specific John Smith as opposed to Bob Taylor), it is therefore more dependent on right-hemisphere function.[43]

We shall return in Chapter 12 to some of these distinctions, and how they may reflect even more general differences in hemispheric function, when we consider several theoretical models of cerebral lateralization.

...

A Cognitive Neuropsychological Perspective

Some cognitive neuropsychologists view distinctions, such as that between apperceptive agnosia and other agnosias, as only a starting point.

---

[*] *Apperceptive agnosia, as we stated earlier, has also been used to describe disruption of an early, more sensory stage in object recognition, occurring before meaning and understanding are achieved.*

They believe that a richer type of theory is necessary to account for some of the issues raised by modern studies of agnosia. They have pointed out, for example, additional ways in which failures in object recognition could occur. One patient may be unable to perceive the shapes of objects properly. Another patient may perceive shapes without a problem but fails to form an integrated representation that combines specific and global features of the object. Yet another patient may recognize and even mime the use of seen objects but be unable to verbally identify them. Thus, complex abilities such as object recognition are organized as a number of separable functional components or modules, any one of which may be impaired selectively.[44]

Cognitive neuropsychologists have constructed a model of object recognition that accounts for some of the deficits we discussed in agnosic patients in a somewhat different way. Visual recognition of objects is thought to proceed through a sequence of three types of representation: (1) an initial representation or "primal sketch" in which brightness changes and the two-dimensional geometry of the object is generated; (2) a "viewer-centered representation" in which the spatial locations of the object's surfaces, as visible from the viewer's position, is internally generated (this representation lacks generality because it describes the object only from the observer's viewpoint—sometimes called a "2½-dimensional" sketch; (3) an "object-centered representation," or truly three-dimensional representation is generated.[45]

Object recognition is effected by comparing viewer-centered and object-centered representations to stored structural descriptions of known objects. The object's semantic representation, or "meaning," is accessed when the visual representation of a seen object corresponds to a description of an object in the stored structural descriptions of known objects.

Thus, cases of agnosia in which the patient has a severe impairment of form perception and inability to copy seen objects would involve impairment of the ability to construct the viewer-centered representations. Patients who have problems identifying unusual views of objects would have impaired object-centered representations. Impairment of object-centered representation formation would, however, not interfere with the ability to recognize objects from a more standard or prototypical view because the separate viewer-centered representation module would be intact.[46]

The latter case, that of impaired object-centered representation, essentially describes the situation Goldberg discussed as apperceptive agnosia and which he linked to right-hemisphere damage. The former case, that of impaired viewer-centered representation, is a more severe situation in which the patient's visual processes appear to be disturbed at an earlier and more elementary stage. It is the situation more traditionally described as apperceptive agnosia—and one that is not specifically associated with damage to any one hemisphere.

It is interesting to note how, despite some differences in approach and even definitions, a good deal of modern research is neuropsychology is yielding similar distinctions about how cerebral processes are organized. As work progresses, including that based on a more modular view of brain organization, we expect to see new distinctions, some reorganization of questions, and hopefully new and accurate findings about the cerebral processes involved in perception.

Because there is a very close relationship between the cerebral systems used in perception and those involved in memory storage, we shall return to the topic of perception when we discuss amnesia and human memory in the next chapter.

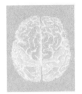

FURTHER INSIGHTS FROM THE CLINIC:
Neglect, Amnesia, Music, and Emotion

....

THE NEGLECT SYNDROME

A patient in a rehabilitation hospital wakes up in the morning and proceeds to shave his face. When he puts the shaver down to go eat breakfast, one notices that he shaved only the right side. While eating breakfast, the patient starts to look feverishly for his coffee cup until someone points out that it is just slightly to the left of his dish. At lunch or dinner, he may leave the food on the left half of his plate untouched while asking for more, only to be reminded that there is still food on the plate. If asked to draw a clock, the patient will draw a circle correctly but then crowd all the numbers into the right half. If asked to draw a person, he will draw only the right side of the body, leaving out the left arm and leg. If questioned about the drawings, the patient states that they look all right to him.

This phenomenon, known as neglect or hemispatial inattention, is observed in stroke or accident victims who have fairly extensive damage to the posterior (parietal or occipitoparietal) regions of the right hemisphere.[1] It sometimes occurs after similar damage to the left hemisphere, but much less frequently and in milder form. The impression one gets in observing such patients is that they behave as if the whole left side of space, and sometimes even the left side of their own body, does not exist. Figure 7.1 shows drawings made by a patient with neglect.

Several questions have long been asked about the syndrome. Why is there such blatant inattention to one-half of space? To what extent is it related to damage in the visual system? Why are patients with damage to the right hemisphere much more likely to show long-lasting neglect symptoms than patients with equivalent damage to the left hemisphere? The answers are still not clear, but the phenomenon of neglect provides some valuable clues about the working relationship between the left brain and the right brain.

Although they may be initially unaware of it, many neglect patients are actually blind in their left visual fields. Because information from the left half of visual space is initially processed in the visual area of the right hemisphere, damage there can produce a hemianopic (literally, "half-blind") observer who cannot see any object to the left of the point of fixation. This half-blindness, however, does not solely explain the inattention of neglect patients.

Many examples can be found of patients who are blind to half of the visual field but do not show neglect of that side of space. Patients in whom damage is restricted to the optic-nerve pathways or to the primary visual areas of either hemisphere typically compensate for their half-field blindness through eye and head movements. Patients with damage to the left hemisphere who are blind in the right visual field rarely display the kind of persistent functional neglect of one-half of space shown by right-hemisphere-injured patients.

Moreover, some neglect patients are not hemianopic at all. In testing situations, they can accurately report simple visual stimuli flashed alone in the left visual field. However, when stimuli are presented simultaneously in both visual fields, experimentally or in everyday situations, they will report only the items in the right half of visual space. Input

Model   Patient's Copy

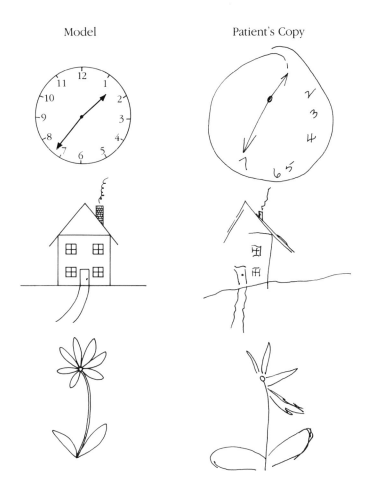

FIGURE 7.1   Drawings by a neglect patient.

from the right field reaching the undamaged left hemisphere appears to interfere with the brain's ability to process input from the left field coming into the damaged right hemisphere. The left half of the stimulus is "extinguished" by the right, but the patients see the left half of the pattern clearly if it is presented alone.

The extinction effects seen in these patients may explain at least part of the neglect patient's inattention to the left half of the world. Events in the right visual field may continuously extinguish information in the affected left field and consequently lead to orientation only to the right.

What happens to extinguished left-field information? Is it truly lost? Or is it present in the nervous system but unavailable to conscious experience? Several lines of research have addressed this question. Some investigators have found that, under certain circumstances, the patients are able to report what appeared in the left field even when there was simultaneous stimulation in the right. If forced to guess from among several choices, they perform much better than chance, although they may never acknowledge having actually seen the pattern in the left visual field.[2]

In a somewhat different line of research, patients who normally extinguished the left-field stimulus when two discrete patterns were presented did not do so when a single large pattern crossing the midline between the left and right fields was used, even though relying only on the information in the right half of the drawing would not have provided them with enough information to recognize it.[3]

Information in the left field is apparently not processed to the same extent as that in the right but is nevertheless available at some preconscious level. Some have speculated that neglect is basically the result of limited visual capacity (due to right-hemisphere damage) coupled with a left-hemisphere tendency to rationalize what it sees. There is some parallel to this in work with split-brain patients, where it has been shown that the left hemisphere often "completes" partially drawn figures when reporting what it saw in a tachistoscopic presentation or even confabulates incorrect verbal responses based on that part of the visual information available to it.[4]

Other explanations have been proposed for the asymmetrical nature of the neglect syndrome. One possibility is that mechanisms controlling selective attention or even arousal are lateralized to the right hemisphere. Another possibility is that the right hemisphere is more spatially adept in general and thus, in its absence, the left does a poor job of comprehending space.

Attentional theories of neglect postulate an asymmetry in the extent to which each hemisphere controls orientation to stimuli in extrapersonal space, that is, to events occurring outside the body. Marcel Kinsbourne proposed that each hemisphere has a directional field of attention into contralateral space that can also inhibit the other hemisphere. The directional tendencies of each hemisphere thus oppose each other but are not equal in strength, the left hemisphere having the stronger directionality (into right space).[5] As evidence, Kinsbourne found that newborns tend to turn to the right, adults tend to veer to the right, and normal subjects prefer pictures with the informational content on the right. Severe neglect of events on the left occurs after right-brain damage because the normal directionality advantage of the left hemisphere into right visual space becomes even more exaggerated.

Kenneth Heilman has proposed a different attentional explanation. He suggested that the right hemisphere is dominant for attention and arousal.[6] The left directs attention contralaterally, but the right is able to direct attention to both contralateral and ipsilateral space. Evidence for this model consisted of an impressive assortment of findings from the EEG literature, blood-flow studies, and other physiological experiments showing activation of the right parietal region during task conditions involving orienting or attending to events in both the left and the right sides of space. Left hemispatial neglect occurs, according to this view, because right parietal damage leaves only the attentional mechanisms of the left hemisphere intact, and these only direct attention to the right side of space.

Using tests of visual scanning and tactile exploration, Sandra Weintraub and Marcel Mesulam found that many right-hemisphereinjured patients not only show neglect of the left side of space but also have significant neglect of events in the right—they miss considerably more items on the side ipsilateral to the lesion than do left-hemisphere-damaged patients. Weintraub and Mesulam believed these data provided pivotal support for the model that the right hemisphere is involved in the distribution of attention within both sides of space.[7]

Our discussion of hemianopia and extinction emphasized the sensory and perceptual components of neglect. The other studies and models just reviewed emphasize the role of attention and of explora-tory factors, such as those measured by visual-scanning and manualexploration tests. Some investigators have expressed the opinion that thinking about neglect in perceptual and even attentional terms does not capture all its manifestations nor perhaps the real basis of the problem.[8] An anecdote about a neglect patient serves to illustrate this point.

An Italian neglect patient was asked to imagine entering a well-known plaza in Milan, called the Piazza del Duomo, from the north end and to describe what he saw. The patient had been very familiar with the plaza before his stroke. He proceeded to describe all the buildings to the west—that is, to the right—of where he would have entered, but he failed to mention any of the buildings to the east. He was then asked to imagine entering the plaza from the south and to describe what he saw. The patient proceeded to describe all the buildings in the eastern half of the plaza.[9]

This story suggests that neglect can be independent of real sensory events, because it even affects the recall of images from memory. Can neglect be an attentional disorder or a disorder in higher perceptual processes? There is no final answer yet, but additional insights may be forthcoming from new investigations into memory and its relationship to perception, a topic we shall discuss in the next section.

·········

AMNESIA AND LOCALIZATION OF MEMORY

Concepts of localization in the brain have long included the idea that specific storage sites exist for human memories. The search for the engram, the storage unit of memory, has continued for decades. Karl Lashley, following extensive experiments with rats whose brains were lesioned in a systematic fashion with respect to location and size, concluded that memory was critically affected by the amount of cortex removed (principle of mass action) but not by the area removed; that is, all areas of the cortex were equally important for memory (principle of equipotentiality).[10] Lashley was unable to reduce significantly a rat's performance on a learned task following removal of small areas of brain tissue from any of a great many regions of the brain. However, in destroying a rather large portion anywhere in the brain, he significantly affected the rat's memory of what it had learned.

Human clinical data over the years have provided evidence that aspects of what we loosely term memory are organized in both diffuse and focal ways in the brain. Electrical stimulation studies by Wilder Penfield and his associates, some of which are described in Chapter 1, were used to support the concept of the localization of long-term memories.[11] Interesting responses were obtained from stimulation of points in the temporal lobes, including the hippocampus and the amygdala (see Figure 7.2), structures deep within the temporal lobes. Patients at times reported experiencing vivid visual or auditory memories, as though they were being lived over again. However, excision of the whole area did not seem to erase any memories. This and other evidence has led to the view that most memory impairment after brain damage to a particular region is not so much a removal of localizable engrams as an interference with mechanisms involved in forming or retrieving memories.

Most neurological disorders affecting higher mental function have some impact on memory. Diffuse neurological damage, such as that often observed in accidental head injury, typically results in prominent memory disorders. Memory loss in these and many other kinds of patients involves amnesia for events prior to the accident (retrograde amnesia) and loss of new learning capacity (anterograde amnesia). Retrograde amnesia usually diminishes in an orderly fashion, with oldest memories coming back first. Both types of memory loss typically diminish simultaneously during recovery. Ultimately, it is only the recall of certain events after the accident that may seem to be lost.

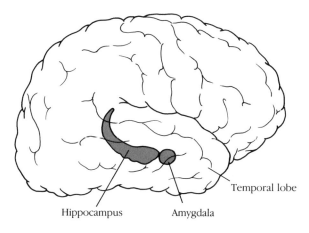

FIGURE 7.2   Areas of the human brain involved in memory disorders. Certain memory processes appear to be associated with structures on the inner surface of the temporal lobes, such as the hippocampus and amygdala. Unilateral lesions of these structures have been reported to impair memory selectively, depending on which hemisphere is involved. Bilateral lesions have been known to cause severe memory disorders.

Alzheimer's dementia is a disease that most frequently affects the elderly. There is diffuse degeneration of cerebral tissue and an accentuation of the degeneration in the posterior temporal lobes, which result in a very prominent memory disorder.[12] Although the "senile" symptoms of this disease involve most intellectual functions, deficits in orientation and memory are the most obvious impairments. Dementia patients usually retain older memories—that is, memories of people and events they encountered earlier in their lives—until the later stages of their disease.

...

Isolated Memory Disorders

In addition to the memory loss that can frequently occur in neurological disorders affecting other functions, striking disorders of memory can occur in isolation, that is, out of proportion to any other deficit of higher function. Such isolated disorders are associated with damage to relatively specific areas of the brain, notably the temporal lobes, the hippocampus, and several other structures deeper within the brain (see Figure 7.2). Patients with some damage to these structures can appear normal under casual observation and may have normal intellectual capacity. Their defect is primarily in acquiring and retaining new memories. Many remember their past histories and earlier events to various degrees.

Most amnesic syndromes do not convincingly show a true obliteration of long-term memories. When older memories are affected, there is evidence that the defect is in accessing the memories, for most do, indeed, "come back" when patients recover. Prompting or cuing an amnesic patient can also bring back many memories.

...

Partitioning Memory

Different physiological processes are thought to underlie two basic forms of memory representations, short-term memory and long-term memory. Material in short-term memory can be retained only for a brief period of time and can contain a very limited amount of information.[13] Remembering a telephone number for a few seconds is an example. One is always very conscious of information in short-term memory. Material in long-term memory, in contrast, is stored over a long duration and can represent very large amounts of information. We are normally not aware or actively conscious of this information unless it has been activated and probably reintroduced into short-term memory.

The concept of "working memory" was proposed to describe what must take place during most mental tasks. Mental arithmetic, reading, problem-solving, and reasoning in general, all require not only some form of temporary storage but also an interplay between information that is stored temporarily and a larger body of stored knowledge.[14] Thus, working memory corresponds to the activated information in long-term memory, the information in short-term memory, and the decision process that manages which information is activated.[15] The decision-making system that selectively activates information in long-term memory and "swaps" information in and out of short-term memory as needed to perform a task is believed to involve the frontal lobes.

The pattern of impairments and sparings of memory observed in brain-damaged patients has led investigators to "divide up" memory processes in a number of additional ways. These include episodic versus semantic, explicit versus implicit, conscious versus unconscious, and declarative versus nondeclarative.

These distinctions do not necessarily conflict with one another, but each does stress somewhat different aspects of memory. Most were devised to account for certain dissociations in what was typically affected (first item in each pair) versus what was spared (second item in each pair) in most amnesic patients. Much of neuropsychological memory research has been concerned with confirming or disproving such distinctions.

Episodic Versus Semantic Memory; Cortical Versus Hippocampal Lesions   Many memory researchers have agreed to recognize two types of long-term memory: episodic and semantic. Episodic memory records information about specific events within the context of other events in a person's lifetime—for example, having the memory of learning to play soccer when in first grade. Semantic memory concerns our permanent knowledge of the world; that is, it primarily concerns facts, concepts, rules, and meanings.* It contains the information necessary for perceptual recognition and complex motor skills, including speech (for all of us) and playing the piano or typing (for some of us).

The cerebral cortex is thought to subserve much of semantic memory. The loss of meaning information in certain aphasias and the loss of object recognition in certain agnosias can be viewed as loss of semantic memories resulting from damage to the language regions and the perceptual regions of the brain, respectively. Thus, the memory loss associated with damage to cortical regions can be relatively specific, as in Wernicke's aphasia, where left temporal-lobe damage appears to interfere with language knowledge.

In contrast with the role of the cortex in semantic memory, the hippocampus (and associated structures) is thought to be primarily involved in episodic memory, because bilateral hippocampal lesions that occur in conjunction with deep damage to the middle of the temporal lobes produce a severe loss for new episodic information.[16] Patients with such damage quickly forget events in their daily lives: where they are, what they had for lunch, where they put their checkbooks, or if, in fact, they wrote a check. Their verbal skills, however, may remain intact, and they are able to have normal conversations, at least about events that occurred before their injuries. When damage is restricted to the hippocampus, patients can learn to perform new tasks, such as playing a new card game. They will be able to use their knowledge of the rules and play correctly when tested at a later time, without remembering how or when they learned the game.

---

* In this context, the term semantic has a broader definition than it has in linguistics, where it refers to word meanings. Semantic memory refers to a more general kind of knowledge encompassing perceptual codes, motor skills, and other "how" and "what" information.

Explicit Versus Implicit Memory   Most direct or "explicit" testing of memory in amnesic patients reveals profound deficits in the conscious recollection of events, faces, new facts, and so on. However, careful testing of a patient's performance generally reveals that previously presented information does in fact have some permanent, although unconscious, impact on the patient.

"Implicit" tests of memory make no reference to the past but do evaluate whether there is any evidence for memory for an item or any training by inferring it from performance. For example, after not being able to remember any words presented in a prior testing trial, a patient may be asked to come up with endings to word stems, for example, to complete "sho____". Amnesic patients will often use an ending that creates a word related to one of the words they were exposed to (but could not "remember") in the prior memory test. They may say "shower", for example, because they have just previously been exposed to the word "bath," instead of coming up with many other equally probable endings.

This effect is called semantic priming, because the meanings or categories of previously presented information influences or "primes" choices made on subsequent tests. Other types of priming effects are also commonly tested, including a simple form of priming in which the primers are the actual words that may later be useful for completing word stems—for example, presenting "shower" before a task involving completion of "sho____".

Implicit forms of memory are also revealed by an amnesic patient's ability to perform a skilled task or play a game learned in a prior testing session, despite the fact that the patient may not recollect that the session ever took place, as we described above.

Other neuropsychological disorders, such as neglect and aphasia, have also come under scrutiny in terms of the explicit-implicit testing distinction. Because the explicit-implicit distinction appears to yield similar results across multiple disorders, it is now thought to hint at a general organizing principle of the brain. Many researchers feel that explicit and implicit testing basically reveal conscious and unconscious cerebral processes, respectively.

Conscious Versus Unconscious Memory; Modular Versus Central Processes   In almost all cases, amnesia is now described as an impairment only of conscious recollection of recently acquired information, not as a global failure to retain it.[17] The level of brain function that is damaged in these patients can best be revealed by carefully analyzing these disorders in terms of interruptions of unconscious versus conscious stages of the task performance.

Neuropsychologist Morris Moscovitch has elaborated a theory of memory that encompasses the conscious-unconscious distinction. Moscovitch distinguished "modular" and "central" processes in the brain. Modular processes apply to more automatic and often elementary stages of cerebral operations. The actual processes involved may be quite complicated but are "shallow" in the sense that they are stages that occur automatically without conscious effort or modification. Modules operate strictly within one domain (e.g., visual input), deal with a limited type of information, and have an output not amenable to conscious manipulation.[18]

In the case of memory, multiple modules are thought to represent the input stages of different sensory modalities. These input modules are modified by stimulation: specific aspects of events create "records" in the input modules via modification of neural circuitry in response to stimulation. The hippocampus, damage to which, as we have said, plays a major role in producing amnesic disorders, is also considered to be modular in organization and operation. The hippocampal retrieval process is automatic and results in the often-described experience of a memory automatically "popping" into one's mind once some cue is provided. We do not have conscious access or awareness of most of the process leading to this. (The fact that no conscious strategies or modifications are involved is one reason Moscovitch considered the hippocampal system modular, with "shallow" output.)

Most tasks, however, including any real recollection of past events, do involve conscious strategies and assessments of which we are often aware. These are thought to involve the "central systems" of the brain, most notably the frontal lobes. Moscovitch contended that patients with frontal-lobe lesions provide a dramatic demonstration of how memory might operate if it relied only on the "shallow" output of the hippocampal system. Such patients appear to confabulate extensively because the stories they generate have no temporal order or spatial context. The stories are not pure fabrication,[19] however, but appear to be because they are often completely out of context, in terms of both when and where events took place and are mixed up in terms of the order of events.

Many other investigators agree that the frontal lobes play a crucial role in guiding conscious memory-retrieval operations. We mentioned earlier, for example, that the frontal lobes are thought to control what information in long-term memory was brought into short-term memory to form working memory.[20] Whether the frontal-lobe functions in memory represent modular processes or not is partly a question of definition that should be resolved as cognitive neuropsychologists refine their approach and conceptualizations based on the basis of new experimental findings.

...
Hemispheric Differences in Memory

Differences have been reported for many years in the kinds of memories lost after production of either left or right temporal lobe lesions. The most striking asymmetries related to memory function were observed in cases involving surgical removal of one temporal lobe. These unilateral temporal lobectomies were performed to remove tissue responsible for epileptic seizures or tumors. Left, or dominant, temporal lobectomy led to difficulty in the learning and retention of verbal material. This deficit was always· evident, whether the material was presented visually or through auditory means, and occurred when memory was tested either by straight recall or by recognition procedures.[21]

Right temporal lobectomy led to difficulties with nonverbal material, whether visually or auditorily presented.[22] ("Nonverbal material" involves stimuli that are difficult to name or encode verbally, such as abstract patterns.) In addition, Brenda Milner showed that patients with right temporal lobe removals have difficulty with maze learning, whether by visual or proprioceptive (exploratory touching) means.[23]

Thus, memory deficits resulting from lateralized lesions, such as unilateral temporal lobe removals, seem to involve loss in specific semantic memory skills. They are often coupled with some impairment of the contextual (episodic) information involving the hippocampus, however, because this structure deep in the temporal lobe may also be damaged.

Analysis of split-brain patients has supported the evidence from lesion studies of some differences in the memory processes of the two hemispheres. As mentioned in Chapter 2, cutting the corpus callosum alone seems to have negligible effects on a patient's memory when tested in a conventional manner. However, when the hemispheres are tested separately, there is a clear difference in the kinds of information each can learn and remember.[24] With lateralized testing procedures, it is primarily language information that is retained best by the left hemisphere and primarily visuospatial information that is retained by the right hemisphere. Cerebral blood-flow studies have also shown greater right temporal lobe activation during recognition tasks involving visuospatial information.[25] These differences, of course, are expected on the basis of other data we discussed in previous chapters concerning what types of information each hemisphere is best equipped to deal with.

Other studies undertaken from a cognitive neuropsychological perspective have also shown asymmetries in how memory is affected by hemispheric lesions. For example, short-term phonological memory storage appears to be selectively impaired by damage to the lower ("inferior") region of the posterior left parietal lobe.[26] Short-term visuospatial memory has been shown to be selectively impaired by lesions of specific areas in the posterior right hemisphere.[27] Additional data bearing on a recent model of memory function is presented in the next section.

...

Neuroimaging Studies of Declarative Versus Nondeclarative Memory

The earlier listing of attempts at partitioning memory included the declarative-nondeclarative distinction. This classification scheme is an effort at modifying the older episodic-semantic dichotomy, which did not always appear to account for all the ways in which memory broke down. Declarative memories are memories of specific facts and events and are, in effect, explicit memories. Declarative memory thus encompasses all episodic memory but also includes some semantic knowledge in the sense of memory for faces, words, objects, and so on. Nondeclarative memory underlies stimulus-response habits (conditioning) and various motor and cognitive skills that have essentially become automatic. It is, in effect, implicit memory and is revealed by implicit testing procedures such as those examining the indirect effects of testing sessions on subsequent sessions. Unconscious motor skills and priming effects are examples.

Neuropsychologist Larry Squire and colleagues, who have promoted the declarative-nondeclarative distinction, recently conducted PET scan studies of normal subjects at several stages of memory testing. According to Squire, the results of these studies, combined with findings from related electrophysiological studies, indicate that declarative and nondeclarative memories are associated with neuronal activity in different brain locations and in different hemispheres.

The PET study provided direct evidence for the importance of the right posterior cortex, just outside the primary visual (or striate) cortex, in word priming. Priming was measured by having subjects rate words in terms of likes and dislikes, followed by the presentation of a word stem completion task in which the stems could be completed by using words from the previous task.[28] The cerebral blood flow in a region of right extrastriate cortex during word stem completion with prior priming was significantly lower than that during a control condition in which subjects without prior priming also completed word stems.

One explanation for the reduced activity during priming is that, for a time after a perceptual stimulus has been presented, less neural activity is required to process the same stimulus. Squire proposed a physiological or neural role for the key psychological feature of priming—that less information is needed to perceive and identify a stimulus the second time it is presented.[29]

The investigators also measured explicit memory by using word stems as cues to recall previously presented words. They found activation of the right hippocampal regions during this recollection task. In addition, the overall increase in cerebral blood flow was significantly greater during the cued recall condition than during priming.

Recent electrophysiological studies of event-related potential (ERPs) in normal subjects also point to different brain systems for declarative and nondeclarative memory.[30] Event-related potentials related to declarative memory (word recall or recognition) had a different amplitude, latency, and scalp distribution than do ERPs related to word stem completion priming or perceptual identification priming. In one study the ERP associated with recollection was largest at a latency of 500–800 milliseconds, whereas the ERP associated with priming was largest at a latency of 400–500 milliseconds. The ERP related to recollection was greater at left anterior electrode placements, whereas the ERP related to priming was greater at posterior electrode placements.

Taken together, the PET and ERP experiments provided evidence for a role of the posterior right hemisphere in memory priming conditions. The recollection condition, however, resulted in two different findings: a right-hemisphere locus of activation in the PET study and a left hemisphere locus in the electrophysiological study. Both studies, however, found that the recollection condition resulted in activity distinctly different from the priming experiment.

Squire maintained that these studies strongly support the idea of multiple forms of memory and the position that declarative and nondeclarative memory are indeed associated with distinct and separate neural processes. Priming effects, he believed, can be supported by right posterior cortex functions that operate prior to the analysis of meaning. Later stage memory processes involve the hippocampus and more widespread cortical areas and result in truly conscious recollection—the item is remembered declaratively, that is, in relation to the item's meaning and in relation to the context in which the item was presented.[31] These studies await replication and further clarification of the findings, but it is intriguing to see evidence that stages in memory formation may break down along hemispheric lines.

...

Memory and Perception, the New Synthesis

The discovery in the 1960s by physiologists David Hubel and Thornton Wiesel that many neurons in the visual cortex respond only to extremely selective aspects of visual stimuli, such as a specific line orientation, and that there is a hierarchical organization of these neurons leading to ever increasing specificity of response, has led to a relatively one-directional information processing view of perception and even brain function in general. In this view, "early" or "low level" sensory neurons pick out relevant details from a myriad of real world data and send summaries up to "high level" neurons. The information gets refined and integrated as it proceeds up this chain of hierarchical processing. The final product, which is stored in memory, consists, in some way, of the "distilled yet complete essence of an experience," something like a finished movie.[32]

This view, although perhaps accurate in its account of the earliest phase of the analysis of sensory data, suffers from several problems. One is that it seems to assign the art of "perceiving" to something like a little person (or "homunculus") looking at the finished movie. Another is that, if each experience is individually coded in totality and separately stored, then our mental library would have to be impossibly vast.

There is an alternative view: Instead of storing every possible image at high brain centers, the brain attempts to reconstruct them by reactivating sensory fragments in different patterns. Current perspectives emphasize the close relationship between the locus of storage and the locus of the processing systems that are engaged during the perception, processing, and analysis of the material being learned.[33] The contributions to memory of a given brain structure are usually closely related to its nonmnemonic functions.[34] For example, lesions of the lower posterior temporal cortex, an area important for visual discrimination, impair visual recognition and associative memory.[35] Lesions of the superior temporal cortex, an area important for auditory discrimination, impair auditory recognition memory.[36]

Several PET studies have attempted to image the extent to which sensory cortex is activated during imagining and recall and have indeed reported significant increases in activity in brain regions considered to be devoted entirely to sensory processes.[37] Subjects were asked to imagine or visualize events, with eyes closed. Cerebral blood flow increases were observed not only in higher level association areas of the brain but in primary sensory cortex (see Appendix for a further explanation of these regions). These data support the view that recollection of events involves some cerebral activity in the regions utilized in the original sensory analysis and perception of the event.

...

Perceptual Convergence Zones and Memory

Neurologist Antonio Damasio has expanded on the above idea by suggesting the existence of a specific type of hierarchical cortical organization that could be efficiently utilized in reconstructing memories. He proposed the term *convergence zones* for regions that combine the constellation of details needed to distinguish one object from another as opposed to storing memories of individual objects. In the case of prosopagnosia, Damasio suggested that patients have lost convergence zones for any unique visual image (of a face, and in many cases, of specific car types). The lower zones that link the smaller number of features one needs to tell that a face is a face remain unchanged. Higher zones that link diverse features such as gait, voice, face, and name are also intact. What is damaged are intermediate zones that distinguish one face (or car) from another.[38]

Based on his brain-lesion data from many patients, Damasio proposed that similar hierarchies of convergence zones cover the cerebral cortex—convergence zones for generic knowledge feeding into zones for more specific knowledge. Convergence zones store only information that links knowledge fragments, not the fragments themselves. The fragments—for example, the color of the eye or the shape of the nostril—remain scattered in the separate sensory cortices. To recall an image, convergence zones must reactivate the various fragments. Damasio noted that this idea reconciles the fluidity of mental images with the limited storage capacity of the brain.[39]

The technology to help address such issues has only recently come into place. Our concepts of memory are still somewhat vague and ill-defined: A useful understanding of the brain processes behind memory functions requires, at the least, additional conceptual clarification of the many psychological functions we refer to loosely as memory. Neuroscientists believe that such clarification will come from further analysis of memory disorders.

·········
MUSIC AND THE HEMISPHERES

In Chapter 1 we presented some evidence for the role of the right hemisphere in music. Patients who had suffered left-hemisphere strokes that affected their speech were often unaffected in their ability to sing. Conversely, right-hemisphere strokes often resulted in the loss of musical abilities while leaving speech unimpaired.

Early research was consistent with the idea that most aspects of musical perception are right-hemisphere functions. Pre- and postoperative testing of musical skills was performed on patients undergoing excision of either the left or the right temporal lobe to remove epileptic tissue.[40] It was found that removal of the right hemisphere significantly increased errors on tests of melodic pattern, loudness, sound duration, and timbre. Left-hemisphere removal did not result in a change in performance. The ability to sing was also investigated in patients undergoing temporary anesthetization of the right hemisphere with the Wada procedure. Singing was grossly disturbed, and, although rhythmic elements were preserved, melody was reduced to a monotone.[41]

Evidence from other clinical cases, however, has suggested that the right-hemisphere predominance in music is not always complete. Additional studies using sodium amobarbital have revealed a more complex picture: as expected, interference with singing followed right-side injection; however, interference, although less severe, also followed left-side injection.[42] A review of the literature on musical perception following brain damage by Robert Zatorre showed that deficits in the processing of patterns of pitches and in the processing of timbre differences accompany right-side damage most consistently.[43] Left-side damage, regardless of whether or not there is aphasic impairment, causes problems with the naming or identification of familiar tunes.

Musicians who have sustained left-hemisphere stroke have shown documented impairment of at least some of their skills. Composer Maurice Ravel (1875-1937) suffered a stroke (presumed to be in the left hemisphere) and developed a Wernicke's type of aphasia while at the peak of his career. Many of Ravel's musical skills remained intact; he could recognize melodies, pick up the smallest mistakes in performed music, and judge how well a piano was tuned. In contrast to these preserved skills, however, Ravel experienced a substantial loss in ability to identify (label) notes and recognize written music. He also could not play the piano or write music, even by dictation.[44]

Although one could argue that most of Ravel's musical deficits seem related to his language disorder (as in his loss of writing and dictating skills) and to some motor output problems (as in his inability to play the piano), research with normal subjects points to left-hemisphere involvement in certain aspects of musical processing. In a dichotic-listening study looking at the detection of pitch and rhythm changes, the right ear proved more accurate in detecting changes in rhythm as well as in pitch in five-note sequences.[45]

Other investigators have reported findings suggesting that laterality differences in music perception are a function of training.[46] In a memory recognition task, nonmusicians showed a left-ear advantage, whereas listeners with musical training showed a right-ear superiority. The investigators suggest that naive listeners focus on overall melodic contour, whereas experienced listeners perceive a melody as an articulated set of component elements. These results are controversial, however, because of conflicting findings in subsequent work.[47]

Overall, however, the data on music and the hemispheres suggests that, just as all of the components of language do not appear to be equally lateralized to the left hemisphere, all aspects of musical skill do not reside exclusively in the right hemisphere. Those aspects of musical processing that require judgments about duration, temporal order, sequencing, and rhythm differentially involve the left hemisphere, whereas the right hemisphere is differentially involved when judgments about tonal memory, timbre, melody recognition, and intensity are required.

...

Modules in Musicians:
Evidence from PET Studies of Cerebral Blood Flow

Justine Sergent of the Montreal Neurological Institute recently conducted an ambitious PET imaging study of cerebral blood flow in ten classically trained musicians.[48] The main experimental condition consisted of the presentation on a TV monitor of a little-known score, which each subject played on a keyboard with the right hand while listening to their own performance. In addition, PET scans were conducted during six other "control" conditions that included simple visual fixation of the lighted TV monitor, listening to musical scales, playing scales on the keyboard with the right hand, making simple manual responses to a dot presented on the screen, reading a musical score presented, and listening to its performance.

The scans of all subjects in each of the testing conditions were averaged and then compared as pairs of conditions (task minus control) to isolate the component operations of the successively more complex tasks. Each of the three components of the main experimental task (playing, listening, and reading) engaged specific cortical areas. Activation related to listening to musical scales was detected in the auditory cortex of both hemispheres (as expected from auditory stimuli) and in the superior temporal region of the left hemisphere, regardless of whether the scales were played by or to the subject. Listening to a musical piece activated the same areas but also engaged the right superior temporal region, a result showing bilateral temporal lobe activity not evident in simple scale listening.

Just reading a musical score activated visual cortex in both occipital lobes (as expected of visual stimuli) but did not engage additional areas normally activated by visual processing of words. Instead, an area at the junction of the left occipital and parietal lobes involved in spatial processing was activated. Sergent suggested that, in contrast to word reading, the relevant information in musical notation is derived through analysis of the spatial location of notes on the staff (which is directly related to pitch intervals).

When both reading and listening to a score are done conjointly, areas are activated in the lower parietal lobe of both hemispheres that are not engaged when either condition is done separately. Sergent suggested that these areas perform a mapping between musical notation and its corresponding sounds or melodies. Similar visual-to-sound mapping functions are performed by the parietal lobes in the case of word reading, not in the identical region but in adjacent areas.[*] Thus, "the mapping of printed musical notation and its auditory representation takes place in areas distinct from, yet adjacent to, the structures underlying the mapping of visual and auditory representations of words."[49]

Finally, two additional regions were activated when the main experimental task was performed. One involved the superior parietal lobe in both hemispheres. This activity was thought to represent transformations from the musical notation to the visually guided finger positioning involved in executing the musical piece. The other area of activation involved the region in the left frontal lobe immediately above Broca's area. Because Broca's area plays a critical role in organizing the motor sequencing underlying speech production, Sergent suggested that a similar role is played by the adjacent area during keyboard performance. This study indicated that reading music and performing it results in activation of cortical areas distinct from but adjacent to those underlying similar verbal operations. Sergent felt that this result explains why some musicians suffering from left-hemisphere injury and aphasia also

---

[*] *As based on the damage observed in cases of alexia without agraphia, which we discussed in Chapter 6.*

have their musical skills impaired. Sergent also suggested that these findings are consistent both with a modular view of cerebral organization, emphasizing the unique competencies of specific cerebral regions, and with a distributed view, made necessary by the multiple processes involved in musical performance and most other forms of human expression.

....

EMOTION

Emotion involves many kinds of human mental states, reactions, and attitudes, some related in terms of the brain mechanisms involved, others not. Emotional information is reflected in our facial expressions and in other less noticeable physiological signs. Emotional information may be conveyed directly in speech, or it may be superimposed in the tone by which other information is conveyed in speech. As in other studies of brain-behavior relationships, the answers to where and how emotional processes take place in the brain depend, to a great extent, on what aspects of emotional behavior one is investigating.

...

Models of Emotion

Three significant models have been proposed to explain the basis for emotional feelings.

Visceral Feedback   The visceral feedback or James-Lange theory proposes that emotion-provoking stimuli induce bodily or "visceral" changes and that the experience of these changes as they occur is essentially the emotion.[50] For example, the "sick feeling in the gut" associated with anguish and certain upsetting situations or the "adrenaline rush" sensations in the upper torso associated with danger or fright are considered to represent visceral changes that we read as emotional states.

Although this theory has been around for 100 years and has been ridiculed or dismissed by many psychologists, some modern research does demonstrate that different bodily reactions can be associated with different emotions[51] and that certain drugs that only affect the body (and do not cross into the brain) may reduce anxiety and fear in humans and animals.[52] Furthermore, there is some evidence that patients with very high spinal cord lesions, disconnecting their viscera from their brain, report experiencing fewer emotional states than patients with lower spinal cord damage.[53]

The visceral feedback or "somatic" theory may not be a comprehensive model of emotion but it does identify an important, often overlooked, aspect of emotional experience.

Cognitive Arousal   The cognitive arousal or Maranon-Schacter theory proposes that a cognitive state must interact with arousal to produce emotion.[54] Psychologist Stanley Schacter claimed to disprove the James-Lange visceral feedback theory by showing that drug-induced physiological arousal did not produce an emotional state in and of itself. In Schacter's experiment, subjects attributed different emotions to the same arousal state (induced by an adrenaline injection), depending on differences in their mental state at the time, which was manipulated by variations in the way the investigators prepared each subject for the experiment.[55]

This highly cited study has recently been criticized for the broad generalizations made on the basis of very limited methodology, including the use of only one drug.[56] Nevertheless, some neuropsychologists believe that the cognitive arousal theory is consistent with clinically observed effects on emotion of left- and right-hemisphere damage.

Central Theories   Central theories of emotion hold that feelings or subjective emotions depend entirely on activity in the central nervous system, that is, on brain activity alone and not on physiological changes in the body. Cannon proposed in 1927 that the thalamus, a deep brain structure, was the critical structure.[57] He felt that signals emanating from the thalamus not only were important for the expression of emotion but also, upon reaching the cortex, were responsible for subjective emotional experience. Since Cannon's time, other brain "centrist" theories of emotion have moved the major organ of emotion to the hypothalamus,[58] another deep brain structure, and then to a larger circuit also involving the hypothalamus, hippocampus, and cortex.[59]

It is highly likely that a comprehensive model of emotion or emotional experience will have to include a role for central brain structures and an assessment of the extent to which our emotional experience depends on our body state. Clearly, the visceral reaction emphasized by the James-Lange theory is determined by the brain also, but this seems to occur in an automatic, almost instantaneous manner. Thus, both the cognitive appraisal and visceral changes associated with an emotion-provoking situation are controlled by the brain. The questions are,

What comes first, the visceral changes or cognitive appraisal? and What is the relative importance of each? Another question is, Are specific regions of the brain responsible for emotion-related changes, whether visceral or cognitive? Most research on hemispheric asymmetries related to emotion has stressed the latter question and has simply looked for any differences accompanying left- versus right-hemisphere damage or evidence for asymmetries in emotional expression and perception in normal volunteers.

...

Emotional Responses to Hemispheric Injuries

A number of investigations have focused on the emotional behavior of patients with unilateral brain lesions. Left-hemisphere-injured patients have been reported to display feelings of despair, hopelessness, or anger (often referred to as a catastrophic-dysphoric reaction), whereas right-hemisphere damage produces what is known as an indifference-euphoric reaction, in which minimization of symptoms, emotional placidity, and elation are common. A frequently cited study, for example, compared the frequencies of the catastrophic and indifference reactions in 150 patients with unilateral brain lesions. Of the patients with left-hemisphere lesions, 62 percent showed a catastrophic reaction, whereas that response was observed in only 10 percent of right-lesion patients. The incidence of indifference reactions, however, was 38 percent among those with right lesions and only 11 percent among those with left lesions.[60]

Extreme emotional reactions have also been reported after unilateral injection of sodium amobarbital into the carotid artery (the Wada test). Several investigators have observed dysphoric reactions, frequently accompanied by crying, after left-side injections.[61] Indifference-euphoric reactions were found in significantly fewer patients. One researcher described the catastrophic reaction in the following way: "the patient especially when spoken to despairs and expresses a sense of guilt, of nothingness, of indignity and worries about his own future or that of his relatives."[62] After right-side injection, however, indifference-euphoric reactions were more common than dysphoric reactions, with patients sometimes breaking out into peals of laughter as the effects of the sodium amobarbital wore off. The same investigator describes the indifference reaction that occurs as "a complete opposite emotional reaction, a euphoric reaction that in some cases may reach the intensity of a maniacal reaction. The patient appears without apprehension, smiles and laughs and both with mimicry and words expresses considerable liveliness and sense of well being."[63]

Although not all investigators have reported results that are this consistent,[64] the findings we have just reviewed strongly suggest that the two sides of the brain differ in the emotional states they subserve. However, there are two problems with this interpretation. First, the reported emotional changes accompanying insults to either half of the brain might not result from disruption of brain mechanisms underlying emotion but, instead, might be a consequence of the patient's reaction to the deficits resulting from the brain insult. Thus, the catastrophic reaction following left-hemisphere injury or inactivation can be viewed as a reaction to the inability to speak and not as representing the lateralization of emotion per se. Although an analogous explanation to account for a euphoric reaction after right-hemisphere injury is not as intuitively obvious, it is possible, nevertheless, that both the dysphoric and euphoric reactions are secondary manifestations of other deficits and not the direct result of alterations to the lateralized mechanisms subserving emotion.

The second problem deals with the relationship of the two sides of the brain to the emotional states under discussion. For example, damage to one side of the brain might produce emotional reactions through its effects on the same hemisphere, or it might exert its influence on the side contralateral to the damage, perhaps through the destruction of regions that normally inhibit certain activities of the other hemisphere. To understand the nature of hemispheric asymmetry for emotion, it is important to determine which of these two actually occurs.

Psychologist Harold Sackheim and his colleagues looked at cases of pathological laughing and crying in which patients show spontaneous uncontrollable displays of emotion that are uncorrelated with objective events.[65] Their review showed that patients with pathological laughing were three times more likely to have right-side lesions than to have left-side damage, whereas pathological crying was more than twice as frequent in patients with left-side damage. Sackheim argued that pathological laughing and crying often precede the appearance of other deficits and are often the first signs of a lesion. Therefore, they concluded, these data support the hypothesis that the two sides of the brain do differ in subserving positive and negative emotional states.

Sackheim then looked at cases of uncontrollable emotional outbursts of laughing and crying that sometimes accompany epileptic seizures. Of the 91 patients showing outbursts of laughing, a left-side focus was twice as likely as a right-side focus. Many fewer cases of crying were found. In the six cases of crying that were reported, however, a different pattern was observed. Four patients were judged to have a right-side focus, with one left-side, and one indeterminate.

In brain-lesion cases, pathological laughing was strongly associated with predominantly right-side lesions. In the case of epilepsy-induced uncontrollable laughing, however, the epileptic focus was more often left-side than right-side. Similarly, results were reversed in the few cases of pathological crying and epilepsy-induced crying that were studied.

Although the results may appear to conflict, they are actually quite consistent. Seizures are associated with hyperexcitability in the regions included within the focus, whereas lesions involve destruction of tissue. These data suggest that uncontrollable outbursts of laughter may result from excitation within the left half of the brain (as occurs in epilepsy) or disinhibition of the left side resulting from damage to the right (as occurs in the case of brain injury). The conclusions regarding uncontrollable crying are more tentative because of the small number of cases. However, the data that exist are consistent with the idea that uncontrollable crying results from excitation within the right half of the brain, or disinhibition of the right hemisphere following left-hemisphere injury.

The notion of disinhibition, as used here, implies that ordinarily the two halves of the brain exert inhibitory effects on each other in the area of emotional expression, thereby resulting in a normal balance that is free of uncontrollable outbursts of any kind. In the event of damage to one side, however, this mutual inhibition is disrupted and the damaged side no longer exerts the same degree of inhibition on its partner; hence, the other hemisphere is disinhibited.

The model of hemispheric control of emotional experience that emerges from this review, thus, is one in which the left side of the brain typically subserves positive emotions, whereas the right side typically subserves negative emotions. The model is a useful working hypothesis that helps explain a good deal of the data just reviewed, although it is far from being complete and universally accepted.

...

The Perception of Emotion

Clinical Data   As mentioned in the discussion of language disorders, clinical evidence has suggested a role for the right hemisphere in the processing of emotional information. Kenneth Heilman and his colleagues, for example, reported that patients with damage in the right hemisphere have greater difficulty picking up on the emotional messages conveyed by speech intonations than do patients with damage in the left hemisphere.[66]

Patients sat in front of pictures of four faces—one happy, one sad, one angry, and one indifferent—and listened to sentences read in different tones of voice. The sentences were neutral; emotional information was conveyed only by the way in which the examiner read the sentences. The patients' task was to point to the face that best illustrated the emotional tone that the examiner was expressing on each trial. Aphasic patients, even one global aphasic, did quite well—often flawlessly—on the task. In contrast, patients with right-hemisphere lesions had great difficulty.

Another study was designed to address the question of whether this failure on the part of right-hemisphere patients was due to an inability to identify emotional expression—that is, a perceptual loss—or to a loss in the concepts of what different emotions mean—that is, a cognitive loss. The investigators required patients with right-hemisphere lesions to discriminate between pairs of sentences that had the same words but were spoken with either the same or different intonations. The patients did not have to identify the emotion but merely had to tell whether the sentences sounded the same or different.

The right-hemisphere patients, like those in the Heilman study, performed more poorly on this task than did aphasic controls. But when right-hemisphere patients were tested on whether they could identify the emotion conveyed by the contents of a story, they performed as well as controls. These results have been interpreted as showing that right-hemisphere patients have not lost the concept or comprehension of different emotions but do exhibit difficulty with standard perceptual cues to emotion.[67]

More recent studies have generally (but not unanimously) continued to support the idea that right-hemisphere damage interferes with the perception of emotion more than does left-hemisphere damage. One study found that right-brain-damage patients were significantly more impaired on discrimination and identification tasks involving emotional words than on parallel tasks involving nonemotional words.[68] Left-hemisphere-injured patients and normal controls did not show the same dissociation. However, another recent study, examining comprehension of emotional tone (or prosody) in various speech stimuli, reported equivalent deficits in left-and right-hemisphere-damaged patients.[69]

Joan Borod, in her review of recent emotion research, suggested that many apparent discrepancies in the literature can be resolved by more closely examining what "processing mode" (expression or perception), what "communication channel" (facial, prosodic or lexical), and what "emotional valence" (positive or negative) is being studied.[70] She asserts that, overall, research findings indicate that the right hemisphere is dominant for emotional perception of facial or lexical (i.e., emotional vocabulary) information, independent of whether positive or negative emotions are involved. The situation with studies examining emotional expression is more complex, with positive or negative aspects of the emotion, as well as whether it is facial communication or not, often playing an important role. In general, she felt that the concept of right-brain dominance for both positive and negative emotional expression is supported by studies of the production of appropriate intonation in speech (prosody). Conclusions about the site of control of emotional facial expressions, however, depends more on whether one is examining positive or negative emotions, as we shall see below.

Behavioral Tests in Normal Subjects   Studies with normal subjects also support a major role for the right hemisphere in the perception of emotion. In a study looking at possible asymmetries in the expression of emotion, full-face photographs and their mirror reversals were split down the mid-line.[71] Composites were put together from two left sides or two right sides. Subjects were asked to rate the intensities of emotional expression evident in a series of such pictures depicting different emotions. Figure 7.3 shows one such face and the composites formed from it.

Left-side composites were judged to express emotion more intensely than right-side composites. The researchers noted the preponderance of contralateral projections controlling facial muscles and argued that these results point to greater involvement by the right hemisphere in the production of emotional expression. A number of subsequent investigations have produced similar results.

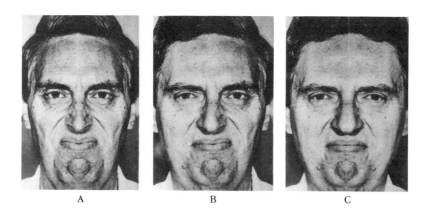

A   B   C

FIGURE 7.3   Comparison of the intensity of emotional expression in composite faces. A. Left-side composite. B. Original face. C. Right-side composite. [From Sackheim, "Emotions Are Expressed More Intensely on the Left Side of the Face," Fig. 1, p. 434, *Science* (1978) 202. American Association for The Advancement of Science.]

Findings are conflicting, however, when the expressions are divided into positive and negative categories. Some investigators have reported differences in the pattern of asymmetry for positive and negative expressions. Joan Borod and her colleagues, for example, found that negative expressions were consistently and significantly expressed on the left side, whereas positive expressions were not systematically lateralized.[72] Other studies, however, have shown left-side effects for both positive and negative stimuli under certain conditions.[73] Still others reported different facial asymmetries in response to positive and negative emotional arousal: positive stimuli resulted in more obvious changes on the right side of the face, whereas negative stimuli resulted in stronger left-sided facial expressions.[74]

Other tests of neurologically normal subjects have shown a pattern of results in which it is the right hemisphere alone that appears to be specifically involved in the recognition of emotional states, while the left hemisphere plays no special role. In a dichotic listening study using nonverbal human sounds, such as laughing and coughing, a small left-ear advantage was found. And a study asking subjects to identify both the emotional intonation and the verbal content of dichotically presented sentences found a slight left-ear advantage in identifying the emotional tone of the sentences.[75] A study using visual stimuli presented to the left and right visual fields also showed evidence of differential hemispheric involvement. The stimuli were five cartoon characters, each with five emotional expressions—extremely positive, mildly positive, neutral, mildly negative, and extremely negative—presented briefly one at a time in the left or the right visual field. The subjects' task was to judge whether the emotional expression was the same as that of a second cartoon presented in the center of the visual field. Results showed a left-visual-field superiority, consistent with right-hemisphere superiority for the task.[76]

...

Concluding Comments:
Is the Right Hemisphere Dominant in Emotion?

Overall there appears to be a good case for believing that the right hemisphere is more involved in both the processing of emotional information and in the production of emotional expressions than is the left. One can only speculate as to why this would be the case. Joan Borod suggested that "emotional processing involves strategies and functions for which the right hemisphere is superior: strategies termed nonverbal, synthetic, integrative, holistic, and Gestalt, and functions such as pattern perception, visuospatial organization, and visual imaging."[77] Howard Gardner suggested that the right hemisphere's critical role in emotional processing is a spatial one, that is, it has a sensitivity to relationships among emotions that determines which behavior is appropriate for a particular situation.[78]

Kenneth Heilman has suggested that the right hemisphere is more "in touch" with the subcortical systems that are important for arousal and intention.[79] The high incidence of hemispatial neglect arising from right-hemisphere lesions, discussed earlier in this chapter, lends some support to this view. Other supporting evidence comes from reports of an association between right-hemisphere pathology and abnormal heart rate response and skin conductance changes, both autonomic nervous system components.[80]

Heilman suggested that the cognitive arousal theory (which he terms the self-attribution model of emotion) appears to be consistent with the finding that patients with right-hemisphere lesions tend to have flattened affects and patients with left-hemisphere disease tend to be depressed and have catastrophic reaction.[81] Because right-hemisphere-damaged patients have difficulty comprehending the intonation of speech and recognizing emotion in facial expressions, these deficits could interfere with developing an appropriate cognitive state to interpret or interact with any physiological arousal occurring in the patient himself. The situation would be further exacerbated by indications that arousal itself is reduced after right-hemisphere damage.[82]

Conversely, patients with left-hemisphere damage should have no trouble interpreting intonation or facial expressions nor in properly interpreting their own physiological states. In addition, they should have increased arousal as a result of the release of right hemisphere arousal mechanisms from left-hemisphere control and thus be susceptible to catastrophic reaction.

As interesting as these speculations are, it is important to keep in mind that the laterality of emotion is far from determined-the data reviewed earlier pointing to a specialized role for the left hemisphere in the expression of positive emotions is just one case in point. To speak of the right hemisphere as the one specialized for emotion clearly oversimplifies what we know about hemispheric asymmetry as well as what we call emotion. Adding even more to this picture of complexity are the data reviewed in Chapter 10, dealing with a possible role of hemispheric differences in psychopathology. We look to future research (and perhaps some reconceptualization of what is being studied) to provide clues about how it all fits together.

EIGHT

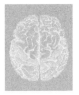

SEX AND ASYMMETRY

Consider the following simple experiment. In one condition, subjects are asked to mentally run through the alphabet and count the number of letters, including the letter *e*, that when pronounced contain the sound "ee." In a second condition, subjects are asked to count the number of letters that contain curves when they are printed as capitals. In both conditions, the subjects must perform the task "in their heads." Writing or speaking out loud is not permitted. Participants are told to do each count as quickly as possible because the results are scored for speed as well as for accuracy.

Which task is harder, counting sounds or counting curves? The outcome of this study depends on whether male or female subjects are being tested. Males are more accurate and slightly faster in the shape task; females do better in the sound task.[1]

This study is one of many pointing to sex differences in certain human abilities—in this case, verbal and spatial skills.[2] Considerable evidence suggests that females, on average, are superior to males in a wide range of skills that require the use of language, such as verbal fluency, speed of articulation, and grammar. Women also tend to be faster than men at tasks involving perceptual speed (the ability to rapidly identify matching items), manual precision, and arithmetic calculation. Males, on the other hand, perform better on average in tasks that are spatial in nature, including maze performance, picture assembly, block design, mental rotation, and mechanical skills. In addition, males do better than women in mathematical reasoning and in finding their way through a route. They are also more accurate in guiding or intercepting projectiles. Figure 8.1 shows some of these differences.

It is intriguing to note that the types of abilities that differ by sex appear to be roughly the same ones that differentiate the hemispheres in terms of function. Are sex differences in cognitive abilities related in some way to sex differences in the organization of the brain? Are there differences between men and women in hemispheric asymmetry? In this chapter we shall review the fascinating and frequently conflicting evidence bearing on sex differences in brain organization and how they might be related to cognition.

·········

BRAIN DAMAGE, ACTIVITY, AND ANATOMY:
Evidence for sex differences

If the hemispheres of the brain are organized differently in men and women, one would expect to find some evidence of those differences reflected in the effects of brain injury. Herbert Lansdell, working at the National Institutes of Health, was among the first investigators to note that the consequences of damage to one-half of the brain appeared to differ for males and females.[3] Lansdell was interested in studying the effects of the removal of part of the temporal lobe on one side of the head in patients operated on to alleviate epileptic seizures. A wealth of earlier research had led him to predict greater deficits in visuospatial

FIGURE 8.1 (*Right*)   Verbal and spatial tasks for which there are sex differences in performance. [From Kimura, "Sex Differences in the Brain," *Scientific American, Inc.*, 1992. All rights reserved.]

Problem-Solving Tasks Favoring Women

Women tend to perform better than men on tests of perceptual speed, in which subjects must rapidly identify matching items—for example, pairing the house on the far left with its twin:

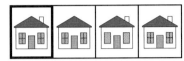

In addition, women remember whether an object, or a series of objects, has been displaced:

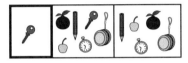

On some tests of ideational fluency, for example, those in which subjects must list objects that are the same color, and on tests of verbal fluency, in which participants must list words that begin with the same letter, women also outperform men:

L _ _ _	Limp, Livery, Love, Laser, Liquid, Low, Like, Lag, Live Lug, Light, Lift, Liver, Lime, Leg, Load, Lap, Lucid ...

Women do better on precision manual tasks—that is, those involving fine-motor coordination—such as placing the pegs in holes on a board:

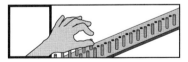

And women do better than men on mathematical calculation tests:

77	$14 \times 3 - 17 + 52$
43	$2(15 + 3) + 12 - \dfrac{15}{3}$

Problem-Solving Tasks Favoring Men

Men tend to perform better than women on certain spatial tasks. They do well on tests that involve mentally rotating an object or manipulating it in some fashion, such as imagining turning this three-dimensional object

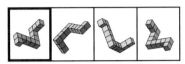

or determining where the holes punched in a folded piece of paper will fall when the paper is unfolded:

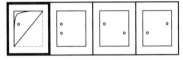

Men also are more accurate than women in target-directed motor skills, such as guiding or intercepting projectiles:

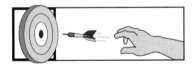

They do better on disembedding tests, in which they have to find a simple shape, such as the one on the left, once it is hidden within a more complex figure:

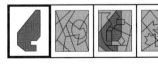

And men tend to do better than women on tests of mathematical reasoning:

1,100	If only 60 percent of seedlings will survive, how many must be planted to obtain 660 trees?

tasks after operation on the right hemisphere and greater deficits in verbal tasks following left-hemisphere surgery. His predictions were borne out, but only for male patients. These unexpected findings led Lansdell to speculate that some physiological mechanisms underlying visuo-spatial and verbal abilities might overlap in the female but be located in opposite hemispheres in the male brain.

Later work has pointed to the same conclusions. For example, psychologist Jeannette McGlone reported data from 85 right-handed adults with damage to the left or the right side of the brain.[4] Most had suffered a stroke, although some were tumor cases. Each patient was given a battery of psychological tests, including the Wechsler Adult Intelligence Scale (WAIS) and an aphasia test, to determine whether the pattern of verbal and nonverbal deficits that emerged was a function of both sex and side of damage.

The results for language impairments were striking. Aphasia after damage to the left hemisphere occurred in males three times more frequently than in females. Even when patients showing signs of aphasia were excluded from the analysis, deficits in higher verbal tasks in the remaining patients continued to be more common and more severe in males.

In contrast, performance on the nonverbal subtests of the WAIS did not show any significant differences due to sex or side of damage. When performance on the nonverbal tests was compared with performance on the verbal tests, however, differences by sex and side of lesion again appeared. The relevant measure is the difference between the score on the nonverbal IQ items and the verbal IQ score. For men, left-hemisphere damage impaired verbal IQ more than nonverbal IQ, and right-hemisphere damage lowered nonverbal performance relative to verbal. Women showed no effect of side of lesion. Their verbal and nonverbal IQ scores were not significantly different for damage to the left or the right side. These data also support Lansdell's speculation that both language and spatial abilities are more bilaterally controlled in females than in males.

...

Have Sex Differences Always Been Present?

How can these findings be reconciled with almost 100 years of clinical investigations of hemispheric asymmetry that did not report sex differences? One explanation is that many of the older studies included patient populations that were predominantly male. Patients in veterans administration hospitals have been extensively studied, and they are almost exclusively male. Patients suffering from war-related brain damage have also been the object of much research; they too are overwhelmingly male. Populations having surgery on the temporal lobe are biased as well. Most surgery of this type is done to alleviate epilepsy, a disease that is much more common among males.

Another important factor in explaining the failure of early work to notice sex differences is simply that no one looked for them. There is tremendous variation from patient to patient (even within one sex) in the effects of unilateral brain damage. Damage to the left hemisphere of some right-handed people can produce a massive disruption of language skills, whereas comparable damage in other individuals has a minimal effect. This variability in the effects of brain damage within groups of males and females makes it difficult to find differences between males and females unless the investigator is working with a large subject population and is specifically looking for differences.

With these ideas in mind, James Inglis and J. S. Lawson have performed an interesting reanalysis of a number of older studies that investigated the effects of unilateral brain damage on verbal and spatial abilities without looking for sex differences.[5] Inglis and Lawson predicted that those studies reporting significant verbal and spatial deficits in groups with left- and right-brain damage, respectively, would be found to contain many more male than female patients. Those studies that failed to find this pattern of deficits would be expected to contain more female patients, they argued, because reduced laterality effects in women would mask the stronger effects found in men. The reanalysis strongly supported these hypotheses and has provided additional evidence for the importance of sex differences in the study of brain injury and brain lateralization.

···

Differences in Brain Anatomy

In Chapter 4 some of the evidence pointing to anatomical differences between the hemispheres was reviewed. Mounting interest in sex differences in lateralization has encouraged investigators to see whether sex is a factor in these asymmetries, and findings have begun to appear suggesting that it is.

Although data on sex have not been reported in some studies, one large investigation obtained gender information for most of the brains that were examined postmortem.[6] Results were reported as ratios of the length of the right temporal plane to the length of the left temporal plane for each brain. Overall, this ratio was less than 1, reflecting a longer plane on the left side. Of those individuals showing a reversal of this pattern, however, most were female. If a reversal is assumed to reflect greater bilaterality of function, the findings with human subjects are consistent with the other data reviewed so far. Females seem to be less lateralized.

Sex differences in brain asymmetry have also been reported for a species of white rat.[7] Marian Diamond and her colleagues found that male rats showed significantly thicker right hemispheres at all ages except very old. Female rats, in contrast, showed somewhat thicker left hemispheres, although the differences for females were not significant statistically.

Asymmetries in subcortical structures were also observed in this series of studies. Measurements of the hippocampus, discussed in Chapter 7 as playing an important role in memory, show laterality effects as well. The male rat has large, significant differences favoring the right hippocampus early in life: these differences decrease considerably with age. The female rat shows the reverse asymmetry; the left hippocampus is thicker than the right, with the differences reaching statistical significance only at 21 and 90 days of age.

Other data have shown the effect of sex hormones on the development of the corpus callosum in rats. The size of the corpus callosum is larger in the male rat than in the female rat. If testosterone is administered to newly born female rats, the corpus callosum becomes larger. Male fetuses exposed to an antiandrogen (a drug that interferes with testosterone), on the other hand, have a smaller corpus callosum.[8]

Does the corpus callosum show sexual differentiation in humans? A recent study of brain scans from 146 healthy subjects by neuroanatomist Laura Allen and neuroendocrinologist Roger Gorski of UCLA showed a dramatic sex difference in the shape of the corpus callosum.[9] Although there were no significant differences in overall size of the corpus callosum as a function of sex, the splenium (the last one-fifth of the corpus callosum) was more bulbous shaped in females and more tubular in males. It is not known whether this difference is related to a sex difference in the number or relative distributions of axons. If it were, it might, at least in part, underlie sex differences in cerebral lateralization.

We must reemphasize, however, that the link between anatomical asymmetries and functional asymmetries is, at present, an untested assumption. That link must be firmly established before anatomical data can be used to infer function.

...

Cerebral Blood Flow

A review of research on sex differences in spatial ability concluded that large differences favoring males are found consistently only on measures of mental-rotation ability.[10] Some recent research using cerebral blood flow has looked at sex differences during a mental rotation task.[11] (See Figure 4.8.)

Women scored significantly lower than men in terms of both accuracy and the number of items completed, but both men and women showed greater right-hemisphere activation during the task, a result suggesting no sex differences. However, when the regional pattern of increases within the right hemisphere was analyzed, it was found that males showed much greater increases in the right frontal lobe, whereas females showed greater increases in the temporal-parietal region (Figure 8.2).

Whether this difference in regional activation within the right hemisphere is somehow related to poorer female performance is not known. However, in another study condition involving a linguistic task (identification of words containing a "br" sound from among a tape-recorded series containing many words with similar sounds such as "pr"), males and females also showed a similar difference in the regional activation pattern seen in the left hemisphere, despite the fact that the two groups performed the task equally well. Males showed greater posterior frontal flow increases in the left hemisphere, whereas females showed greater increases in the left temporal lobes.

Overall, the most apparent sex difference in these studies was that males demonstrated greater asymmetries in frontal lobe activity while performing the two entirely different tasks. These findings suggest that other reported sex differences in lateralization may specifically stem from sex differences in the organization or utilization of the frontal regions of each hemisphere.

There is recent neuropsychological data that also supports the presence of sex differences in left and right frontal lobe organization. A model of hemispheric lateralization that we describe in greater detail in Chapter 12 proposed that hemispheric differences in frontal organization revolve around "set shifting" (for the right hemisphere) and maintaining "set constancy" (for the left hemisphere). That is, the right frontal lobe plays a major role in the ability to alter strategy or approach with tasks, whereas the left frontal lobe is involved in the ability to carry through with an approach.

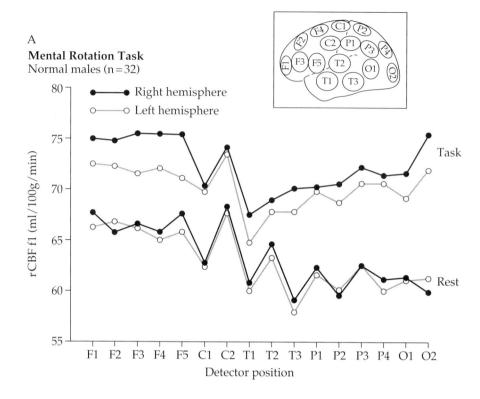

A
Mental Rotation Task
Normal males (n=32)

B
Mental Rotation Task
Normal females (n=29)

FIGURE 8.2 (*Left*)   Sex differences in frontal blood flow during a mental rotation task. Graphs plot cerebral blood flow at 16 locations in each hemisphere during rest and while performing mental rotation operations on complex cube arrays. The inset shows approximate detector positions. F, frontal; C, central; T, temporal; P. parietal; O, occipital. Note how coupled left and right flow is across equivalent regions of the two hemispheres at rest. During the rotation task, however, asymmetries in blood flow appear, with many regions showing greater increase in the right hemisphere. Although both genders show greater right hemisphere activation during this visuospatial task, sex differences appear in the regional pattern of blood flow. Males (A) show much greater frontal lobe asymmetries in flow (detectors F1–F5) than do females (B).

Initial studies to test this model used male patients with frontal lobe lesions and indeed found the expected side-of-lesion on a test designed to measure "shifting" versus "constancy" tendencies.[12] Furthermore, when both male and female frontal lobe patients were recently studied with similar tests, females did not show the predicted effects. This result supports the idea of the existence of a sex difference in left and right frontal lobe organization.[13]

·········

EVIDENCE FROM TESTS INVOLVING LATERALIZED PRESENTATION

···

Auditory and Visual Studies

Many researchers doing traditional behavioral studies of laterality looked for sex differences. Several verbal dichotic listening studies have reported that males have a greater right-ear advantage than do females. M. P. Bryden, a psychologist who has conducted numerous dichotic-listening studies to assess brain asymmetry, has combined the data from several of his studies that use dichotically presented digit pairs to look for possible sex differences.[14] Of the 98 subjects he tested, 73.6 percent of the males (11 left-handers and 42 right-handers) showed a right-ear advantage, and 62.2 percent of the females (3 left-handers and 42 right-handers) showed right-ear superiority. Sex differences in ear asymmetries have also been found in studies that use spoken syllables as dichotic stimuli.

Not all attempts to look for sex differences in verbal dichotic-listening performance have found them, however. Overall, about half of the verbal dichotic-listening studies that look for sex differences do not find them; the remaining half report greater lateralization for males.

Much less attention has been paid to possible sex differences in the processing of nonverbal auditory stimuli. Two studies that have measured ear asymmetry for melodies and familiar sounds reported a significant left-ear advantage for women and a small, statistically insignificant left-ear advantage for men.[15] These findings suggest that lateralization for certain nonverbal auditory stimuli may be greater in women than in men, in contrast with the trend found in studies using verbal stimuli.

Visual-field studies have also been employed to address the possibility of sex differences in brain organization. For the most part, the results show greater lateralization in males when tasks involve the processing of words, and there is also a weak trend toward greater lateralization in males when subjects are asked to indicate the location of a dot or to judge the number of dots represented in a display. A number of other visual-field studies, however, have failed to find sex differences.[16]

…

Studying Sex Differences in Children

Significant sex differences in the lateralization of spatial functions have been found in children. Standard behavioral techniques for studying the right hemisphere's role in spatial processing proved difficult for young children. Thus, Sandra Witelson devised a test of tactual perception that could be used over a wide range of ages.[17]

The test, known as the dichaptic stimulation test, requires that the subject simultaneously feel two different objects held out of view, one in each hand. After holding the meaningless shapes for 10 seconds, the subject chooses the two shapes from among a group of six that are displayed visually. The data are then scored for the number of objects correctly selected by each hand. Figure 8.3 shows this test.

Witelson tested 200 strongly right-handed children ages 6 to 13. The results showed a significant interaction of hand and sex. The left-hand scores of the boys were significantly better than their right-hand scores, but there was no difference between hands for the girls. A dichotic digits test administered to the same subjects did not show any sex difference in the proportion of children showing a right- or a left-ear advantage.

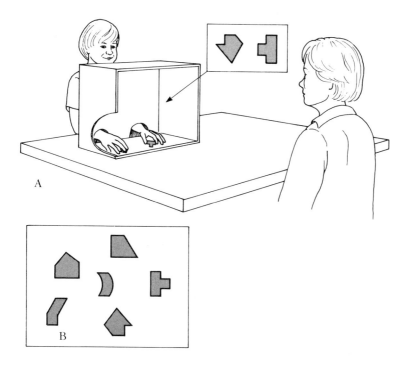

FIGURE 8.3   Dichaptic stimulation test. The subject is given two objects with meaningless shapes, such as those shown in the inset. Without being able to see the objects, he or she simultaneously feels both of them, one with each hand, for 10 seconds. B. The subject is asked to identify the two shapes from among a group of six displayed visually.

The results of the Witelson study suggest that sex differences in lateralization of spatial abilities may have their origins quite early in life. In a later section, we consider mechanisms that may underlie these differences.

·········

ARE SEX DIFFERENCES IN LATERALITY REAL?

The failure of many studies to find reliable sex differences have led some investigators to question the reality of sex differences in laterality in the first place. Some have argued that this area of research is plagued by the type I error.

Type I is the name given to the kind of error made when an investigator concludes that the differences observed in a study are real when in fact they are due to chance. Investigators are much more willing to report differences between groups (and journal editors are much more eager to accept such studies) than they are to publish negative or "no-difference" results. Critics have suggested that journals contain only the tip of the sex-differences-in-laterality-research iceberg and that the majority of studies with negative results are never published.

Those who believe that sex differences in laterality are real counter this argument with one that challenges the sensitivity of studies that fail to find evidence of sex differences. They note the tremendous variability in lateralization within a given sex and point out that this variability makes it quite difficult to detect real, but small, differences between the sexes. Small studies with 10 or 15 subjects per group (the size of many studies) will especially suffer from this problem.

Are there sex differences in the distribution of verbal and spatial functions between the hemispheres? Much of the data reviewed in the preceding sections suggest that there are. A variety of evidence suggests that males tend to be more lateralized for verbal and spatial abilities, whereas women show greater bilateral representation for both types of functions. But what about type I error? Are there studies (some of which we do not know about because they are unpublished) that fail to find these purported sex differences?

Our review of the lateralization literature in general has given us a healthy respect for the type I error and the scientific chaos it can create. The frequency as well as the consistency of reports of sex differences in cerebral organization, however, lead us to accept their reality, at least as a working hypothesis. The strength of the case, in our opinion, rests on the diversity of methodologies (clinical studies, behavioral work, neuro-imaging) that point to the same conclusion: Females are less lateralized than males.

A review of the studies that do not support this conclusion shows that most studies report no differences between the sexes. It is the rare study that reports sex differences in the direction of greater lateraliza-tion in females. This consistency suggests that there are true differences that are small in magnitude and easily masked by individual variability or other factors that may not be controlled.

·········

THE ORIGIN OF SEX DIFFERENCES

If we assume that sex differences in laterality are real, then we must ask what mechanisms might be responsible for them. Noting that females generally gain physical maturity at an earlier age than males, Deborah Waber proposed that sex differences of the sort reviewed here are attributable not to sex per se, but, rather, to differences in the rates at which males and females develop.[18]

Waber tested her hypothesis by comparing early and late maturers of both sexes on a series of verbal and spatial tests. Late maturers scored better on spatial tasks, and early maturers scored better on verbal tasks. Further analysis showed that only the spatial scores were related to maturational rate. Differences due to sex alone were not significant.

Waber concluded that the hormonal changes responsible for the timing of puberty are also responsible for sex differences in cognitive abilities. Although her idea is interesting, it has difficulty accounting for sex differences in tasks such as mental rotation that occur well before puberty. Data have also shown that the association between spatial ability and age at puberty is quite small.

Jerre Levy has suggested an evolutionary basis for sex differences.[19] She argued that males have been the hunters and leaders of migrations throughout hominid evolution and that those with good visuospatial skills enjoyed a selective advantage. At the same time, females were likely to have had selective pressures for skills involved in child rearing, such as use of language as a tool for communication, development of social sensitivity, and facility with nonverbal communication.

Levy proposed that greater bilateralization of function may facilitate the skills needed by females, because those skills appear to require a blending of the specializations of the hemispheres that may be best achieved by their representation within each hemisphere. In contrast, Levy's cognitive crowding hypothesis presented in Chapter 5 suggested that stricter separation of function would be necessary to ensure the high level of visuospatial skills in males that was needed for hunting. (Recall that the cognitive crowding hypothesis holds that if two or more cognitive abilities are primarily controlled by the same hemisphere, they compete for available neural tissue. Verbal skills are presumed to displace spatial skills when they share the same "neural space.")

...

Hormones and Cognitive Function

In Chapter 5 we discussed a theory by Geschwind and Galaburda that proposed that high levels of prenatal testosterone slow neuronal growth in the left hemisphere, allowing relatively greater development in the right hemisphere. Because males are usually exposed to higher levels of testosterone during prenatal development (from their own developing testes as well as smaller amounts from the mother), this theory is offered to explain, among other things, the greater incidence of left-handedness in males. The theory can also be applied more generally, however, to overall differences in brain organization between males and females.

There is a great deal of evidence pointing to the profound effect of sex hormones on mammalian development, both physical and behavioral, although much remains to be learned about their effects on brain organization and cognitive functioning in humans. As background for the discussion to follow, we should note that sex hormones are secreted by the testes in males, by the ovaries in females, and by the adrenal glands in both males and females. Both males and females produce the hormones found in both sexes, with the relative concentrations of these hormones varying by sex and life-cycle stage. Females have greater concentrations of female hormones, estrogen and progesterone, whereas males show greater concentrations of male hormones, the androgens (testosterone is an androgen).

Early in life the action of sex hormones establishes sexual differentiation; if the testes of a genetically male organism do not produce androgens or if the hormones cannot act on the developing tissue, the organism will develop as a female. Sex hormones also organize gender-specific behaviors early in life. If a rodent with functional male genitals is deprived of androgens right after birth, it will show enhanced female sexual behavior and reduced male sexual behavior as an adult. The reverse is also found; if androgens are administered to a female directly after birth, her behavior as an adult is more characteristic of a male. These effects are well established.[20]

Studies relating prenatal hormones and cognitive behavior in humans, however, have been relatively recent and few in number. Nevertheless, the results are intriguing. June Reinisch and Stephanie Sanders looked at the relationship between prenatal sex hormones and cognitive function in ten male subjects whose mothers had taken diethylstilbestrol (DES) while pregnant.[21]* A control group consisted of ten male siblings who were not exposed to DES. The Witelson Dichaptic Shapes Test was administered to both groups. Correct matches in the DES-exposed group were evenly distributed between left and right hands, a pattern typical of females, whereas the control group showed the male pattern of higher scores with the nonpreferred hand. The authors had

---

* DES, a synthetic form of estrogen, was commonly used in the 1950s as a treatment to prevent miscarriage. It subsequently has been shown to be ineffective and to be the probable cause of a rare form of genital cancer found in the female offspring of women who took DES while pregnant.

predicted this outcome, because DES is known to have a feminizing effect on the male fetus.

The Wechsler Intelligence Scales were also administered. The DES-exposed group scored lower than their nonexposed brothers on the spatial component of the test, which included measuring the time to find the missing parts of a picture and complete a jigsaw puzzle. Although overall performance and IQ did not differ between the groups, the researchers believed that exposure to DES in utero changes, very subtly, the way men approach spatial tasks.

Studies of children with a genetic disorder known as congenital adrenal hyperplasia (CAH) have also provided evidence bearing on the cognitive effects of hormones present early in life.[22] In CAH the adrenal glands produce abnormally high quantities of androgens, beginning in the third month of fetal life. Researchers have found that girls affected by CAH performed better than unaffected girls in tests of spatial manipulation, spatial rotation, and a task that involved finding a simple figure hidden within a more complex one, all tasks usually performed better by males. No differences between groups were found on other perceptual or verbal tasks, nor were any effects of exposure found for males with CAH.

Other studies have looked at the effect of hormone levels on performance in adults. A study by Valerie Shute looked at the relationship between the level of androgens in blood taken from males and females.[23] Even though all subjects had androgen levels within the normal range for their sex, Shute found that females with relatively high androgen levels performed better on spatial tests than females with lower androgen levels. For males, relatively low androgen levels were associated with better performance. A study measuring testosterone in saliva produced similar results. High-testosterone women performed better than low-testosterone women, but low-testosterone men were superior to high-testosterone men. The investigators suggested that there may be some optimum level of androgen for spatial ability, perhaps in the low male range.

The research we have just reviewed paints an intriguing picture of the effects of hormones on cognitive abilities. But what about the effects of hormonal fluctuations within an individual? Are cognitive abilities sensitive to those as well?

Research by Elizabeth Hamson and Doreen Kimura has shown that the performance of women on certain tasks changes throughout the menstrual cycle.[24] Hamson and Kimura chose tasks that typically show the largest male-female differences, such as speed of articulation and spatial tests. They found that women performed significantly better at midcycle (when estrogen and progesterone are at their highest levels) than during menstruation (when hormones are low) on speed of reciting a tongue twister, verbal fluency, and a manual dexterity task. Performance on spatial tasks, however, was better during the low-hormone part of the cycle. A control group of nonmenstruating women receiving hormone replacement therapy showed the same pattern of performance, whereas a control group of those not receiving replacement therapy did not show the variation.

These results have been confirmed by subsequent studies. More recently, Kimura has reported observing seasonal fluctuations in spatial ability in men, with improved performance in the spring when testosterone levels are lower.[25] Taken together, the findings on the effects of prenatal and postnatal hormones on cognitive functions are striking. It is clear that an eventual understanding of their meaning will be critical to a full explanation of sex differences in cognition and the differential involvement of the two hemispheres.

...

Mathematical Talent:
Sex, Handedness, and Immune Disorders

Mathematical talent is one of the newest areas to attract the interest of neuropsychologists looking at possible biological bases for cognition. It has been defined as a high level of mathematical reasoning ability demonstrated at an early age. One of the most striking characteristics of the mathematically highly talented is that they are much more frequently male than female.

Using the mathematics section of the College Board's Scholastic Aptitude Test (SAT-M) to measure mathematical talent, Camilla Benbow and Julian Stanley have analyzed data from 40,000 intellectually talented seventh graders, with males and females equally represented. The results showed that the ratio of boys to girls scoring 500 on the SAT-M was 2.l; increasing to 4.1 for students scoring 600; and to 12.9 for those scoring 700.[26*]

The authors concluded that there are many more mathematically talented boys than girls, especially at the higher levels. Further studies have shown that these differences could not be attributed entirely to socialization or environmental factors.

---

* A score of 600 on the SAT-M falls in the seventy-eighth percentile for twelfth-grade males, and a score of 700 falls in the ninety-fifth percentile.

In seeking an understanding of these sex differences, Benbow has looked at handedness as a variable. She limited her subject sample to students who had scored at least 700 on the SAT-M or at least 630 on the verbal portion of the SAT before age 13 (the top 1 in 10,000 in their respective abilities for this age group). She found frequency of left-handedness, as measured by a questionnaire, to be twice the figure found in the general population. She also noted that about 50 percent of these extremely precocious students were either left-handed, mixed-handed, or were right-handed with left-handed family members. Benbow proposed that this evidence supports the idea that bilateralization, rather than greater specialization of the hemispheres, is associated with extreme mathematical or verbal ability. To account for the surprising similarity of findings for extreme verbal and mathematical ability, Benbow suggested that verbal reasoning, what is measured by the SAT verbal test, may be more under the influence of right hemisphere processing than language production or syntax.[27]

The incidence of allergies was also very high in this population; over 50 percent of the extremely precocious students had allergies, twice the frequency found in the general population. Benbow related both the allergy data and the handedness data to the Geschwind and Galaburda idea that higher testosterone levels in utero slows the development of the left hemisphere while simultaneously affecting immune development.[28]

Although much more work remains to be done before the bases of mathematical talent are understood, the data we have presented add yet another piece to the sex-differences-in-cognition puzzle.

....

THE SIGNIFICANCE OF SEX DIFFERENCES

From a theoretical standpoint, the significance of sex differences in brain organization is considerable. If sex differences are real, what is (or was) their adaptive advantage? How does brain organization relate to patterns of higher mental function? Do sex differences in child-rearing practices affect brain asymmetries? These are a few of the many important questions that remain unanswered.

Particularly interesting is the issue of how ability is related to extent of lateralization. Does greater lateralization for a given function imply superior performance for that function? Is the spatial ability of males better than that of females because males seem to rely more on one hemisphere to process spatial information? There is, of course, no logical reason to expect that greater lateralization necessarily leads to superior ability. In fact, we have to assume the opposite to explain the superior verbal ability of females. According to behavioral tests and clinical data, women appear to be less lateralized for language functions, yet as a group they are superior to men in language skills. And, as we have just seen, mathematical talent may be related to greater bilateralization of function as well.

There may be a relationship between lateralization and ability that is different for different tasks. If this is the case, it would be fascinating to know why the brain organizes itself so differently for the optimal functioning of different abilities. At this point, we can only speculate about the relationship of lateralization and ability. For example, assume that complex visuospatial capability preceded the evolution of language in humans (which is a reasonable assumption). One can then postulate that in men only the left hemisphere became involved in language, leaving visuospatial functions intact in the right, whereas in women language was established in both hemispheres, crowding visuospatial capability. If this in fact occurred, "more lateralized" would be better for visuospatial function, whereas "less lateralized" would be better for language.

Although most investigators would probably agree that theoretical questions of this sort are significant, undoubtedly there would be less agreement concerning the practical meaning of sex differences in brain organization and their possible correlates in cognitive function. Sex differences in higher mental functions are typically on the order of one-fourth of a standard deviation. In other words, there is a great deal of overlap in the distribution of ability across men and women. Some women have better spatial abilities than most men, whereas some men have better verbal skills than most women.

Awareness of the extent of the overlap in ability tends to temper any suggestion that sex be used as a major criterion, by itself, for determining career options and educational opportunities. The need for curricula and programs better geared to the abilities of specific groups is clear. It is perhaps wiser, however, to determine the composition of those groups through individual testing than to determine it solely on the basis of gender.

NINE

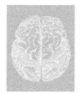

PHYLOGENY AND ONTOGENY: The Evolution and Development of Asymmetry

If one dates the beginning of the study of hemispheric asymmetry to coincide with Broca's observations, the field of laterality is now approximately 130 years old. For much of this time, investigators have viewed the lateralized brain as the end point of an evolutionary and developmental progression—human beings, but not other animals; older children and adults, but not infants—were believed to possess lateralized brains. In the last 25 years, however, new evidence has called into question these assumptions and has substantially increased our understanding of brain lateralization and its significance.

The study of the evolution of a trait or characteristic across different species is known as phylogeny. Ontogeny, in contrast, is the study of development within an organism over time. In this chapter we shall look at evidence bearing on the phylogeny of asymmetry. We shall see if animals other than humans show asymmetries that might be related to those found in humans. At the core of questions about asymmetries in animals are the assumptions that laterality is a true biological trait that can be studied in much the same way as other biological phenomena, such as color vision and digestion, and that precursors of human laterality will be found by studying other species.

Research demonstrating the existence of hemispheric asymmetries in animals would have important implications for our understanding of the origin and significance of asymmetry in humans. Some investigators have argued that brain asymmetry is intimately related to higher linguistic abilities. The presence of hemispheric differences in nonlinguistic animals would suggest that this view is not correct. The asymmetries found may then provide clues to the actual evolutionary basis for brain asymmetry. Conversely, convincing evidence pointing to the absence of asymmetries, even in the closest evolutionary relatives of human beings, would argue that brain asymmetry is unique to *Homo sapiens* and may be fundamentally related to language ability.

After studying laterality in animals, we shall turn to the ontogeny of asymmetry and ask whether the asymmetry we find in humans is present and complete at birth or whether it develops over time. The presence of at least some asymmetry at or near birth would be strong support for a biological basis, because there would be little or no opportunity for learning or experience to play a role so early in life. Evidence bearing on the development of asymmetry in an individual and the conditions under which it can be modified might also contribute in important ways to our understanding of language disorders and other problems that have been linked to the division of function between the hemispheres.

·········

WHICH PAW DOES YOUR DOG SHAKE HANDS WITH?

The most obvious sign of lateralization in humans is handedness. Thus, investigators have looked for paw or limb preferences in animals as evidence of brain lateralization, and they have found that many species do show such preferences.[1] Cats typically use one paw in tasks that involve reaching for an object; mice show consistent preferences in a task in which they must use one paw at a time to reach for food.

Although the pattern of limb preference in a given animal bears some resemblance to hand preference shown by human beings, there is an important difference. Approximately 50 percent of cats, monkeys, and mice show a preference for the right paw, and 50 percent show a preference for the left paw. This result is strikingly different from the breakdown found in human beings—90 percent right-hand preference, 10 percent left-hand preference.

The 50-50 split in animals has led some investigators to propose that paw preferences are the result of chance factors. According to this hypothesis, the limb first used by an animal is determined by chance. The additional dexterity gained as a result of the experience increases the probability that the same limb will be used again. Some support for such a mechanism has come from geneticist Robert Collins's work with paw preference in mice, which was discussed briefly in Chapter 5 when we considered the factors that determine handedness.

If a trait is under genetic control, it should be possible to select for it. That is, if individuals with the trait are selectively mated, each successive generation should show a higher incidence of the trait. If the trait is determined by chance, however, no such increase across generations should occur.

Collins began by mating mice that shared the same paw preference. In the next generation, he mated those offspring who showed the same paw preference as the parents. After repeating this selective inbreeding three times, Collins looked at the proportion of left-pawed and right-pawed offspring in the last generation. He found a 50-50 split, the same proportion he had started with in generation 1.[2]

·········

HAND PREFERENCE IN PRIMATES

Until recently, most reviews of paw preference in animals reported that monkeys showed a pattern of limb preference similar to that of cats or mice, that is, individual animals would show a preference for the use of one limb, but that overall there was no population preference for one limb over the other. This result proved particularly troublesome for an evolutionary view of asymmetry, because one would expect to find such evidence in the closest evolutionary relatives of humans.

Peter McNeilage, Michael Studdert-Kennedy, and Bjorn Lindblom have reopened this issue.[3] They argued that inconclusive findings about hand preference in nonhuman primates result from the use of inappropriate tasks as well as the use of animals too young to demonstrate a consistent preference. Taking these factors into account, the authors reexamined existing data and reported evidence of a left-hand specialization for visually guided movement (i.e., reaching) and a right-hand specialization for manipulation and bimanual coordination. They concluded that

> both the left and right hand preference patterns observed in nonhuman primates may be precursors of human specialization. However, monkeys and humans would seem to be separated by an evolutionary progression in which the importance of the ability to operate on the environment (including the use of bimanual coordination and the consequent right-hand preference) has so increased that the right hand now normally preempts the left, even for visually guided movement.[4]

Their analysis has generated a great deal of controversy. At the same time, it has stimulated increased interest in primate hand usage.

Joel Fagot and Jacques Vauclair suggested yet another approach to primate hand usage.[5] They noted that humans show stronger hand preferences for highly skilled tasks. The act of picking up an object shows less lateralization than tool use, for example.[6] With this in mind, they distinguished between high level tasks that require finely tuned motor actions resulting from spatial or temporal complexity and/or cognitive complexity (e.g., controlling the movement of a cursor on a computer screen with a joystick) and low level tasks that involve gross movements or familiar, highly practiced activities or both (e.g., reaching for food).

Fagot and Vauclair predicted that high level, but not low level, tasks are most likely to show a lateral preference. Their analysis of a large number of studies was generally consistent with their prediction.[7]

In drawing their final conclusions, Fagot and Vauclair differentiated between handedness (the preference that may be shown by an individual animal for the use of one hand in a low level task) and manual specialization (the preference for one hand shown by a group of animals in a high level task). It is the latter, they suggested, that holds the most promise in helping us understand the evolution of lateralization in humans.

·········

DAMAGE TO ONE HEMISPHERE:
Are the effects asymmetrical?

Many studies have focused on the kinds of deficits in behavior that follow surgical lesions in specific brain structures. In general, deficits following lesions on one side only (unilateral lesions) are less serious than those that follow bilateral brain damage, regardless of which side the lesion is on.

In monkeys, for example, studies have shown that visual discriminations involving color, shape, and orientation are disturbed equally by lesions in a particular region of the left or the right hemisphere and that the deficits are independent of the monkey's limb preferences.[8] Deficits in the discrimination of complex sequences of auditory stimuli after damage to the auditory region also have been shown to be independent of the side of the lesion.[9] More recently, however, it has been shown that the side of a temporal lobe lesion significantly affects the ability of macaque monkeys to discriminate species-specific vocalizations, that is, vocalizations made by members of their own species.[10]

What differentiates studies that have found lesion effects from those that have not? One factor that is likely to be of critical importance is the nature of the stimuli and the task to be performed. Some studies have employed stimuli that would probably not show an asymmetry in humans. Why should one be expected in primates? To fairly test the hypothesis of hemispheric specialization in primates, tasks are needed that are sufficiently complex to tap the brain asymmetries that may exist in these animals.

·········

SPLIT-BRAIN RESEARCH WITH ANIMALS

In Chapter 2 we considered at some length what has been learned about brain asymmetry from split-brain studies with human beings. In principle, split-brain research is an ideal way to test for hemispheric specialization in animals. Cutting the fiber bands that connect the two hemispheres allows the investigator to study separately the abilities of each half of the same brain. Except for possible hemispheric differences, which are the object of the research in the first place, both hemispheres

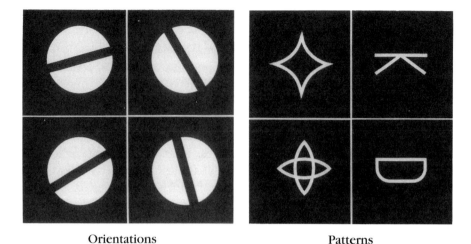

Orientations   Patterns

are genetically identical and have been exposed to the same environmental influences.

In contrast to research with human patients, limited by necessity to persons with epilepsy (generally of long standing), animal studies may be done with healthy animals with two intact hemispheres. Interpretation of any differences that might be found is therefore much more clear-cut. In addition, split-brain research avoids the problem of inferring the function of specific regions of the brain from the effects of lesions in those areas. Lastly, in lesion studies, investigators must have some idea in advance about which parts of the brain control specific functions. In split-brain work, it is not necessary to localize a function to a specific region; the performance of the whole hemisphere is studied.

What are the results of studies that use monkeys and cats and investigate the relative abilities of the two hemispheres to learn and perform different types of problems? Results from tests of simple pattern discrimination suggest that the two hemispheres possess similar learning capabilities.[11] A few studies have reported quantitative differences between the hemispheres in learning and performance. However, there are no consistent differences favoring one hemisphere in these studies.[12] The absence of consistency within a study suggests that the differences found may be a consequence of asymmetrical damage resulting from the surgical procedure.

Like the lesion work, however, most of the tasks used to study asymmetries in split-brain animals are simple and bear little resemblance to the stimuli and tasks that reveal asymmetries in humans. An exception are the several studies by Charles Hamilton that have tested the surgi-

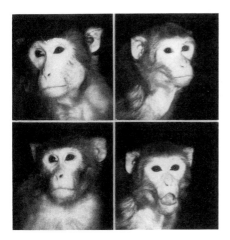

Faces

FIGURE 9.1   Representative   stimuli for three types of discriminations used by Hamilton.

cally separated hemispheres of rhesus monkeys with stimuli similar to those that show evidence of asymmetry in humans.[13]

Hamilton and his colleagues chose stimuli that were similar to those known to elicit lateralized processing in humans, including lines in different orientations and facial expression and identity (using monkey faces). Geometrical patterns not expected to show lateralized differences were used as control stimuli. Examples are shown in Figure 9.1. Because the monkeys had a complete section of the cerebral commissures and the optic chiasm, it was possible to present stimuli to one hemisphere by presenting it to the ipsilateral eye. The monkeys were taught to discriminate between the members of pairs of stimuli by pressing the screen after seeing one member of each pair and refraining from pressing after seeing the other. The number of trials needed for each animal to reach a criterion of 90 percent was measured.

As expected, the geometrical patterns did not show any evidence of asymmetry and were learned equally well by both hemispheres. In addition, there was no systematic relationship between sex, hand preference, or hemisphere retracted during surgery. These control tasks demonstrated that Hamilton had been successful in eliminating some of the biasing factors that may have affected other studies, and they provided further evidence that the two hemispheres of the monkey brain are equally capable of learning a simple pattern discrimination. Spatial discriminations, however, were processed significantly better by the left hemisphere. Discriminations of monkey faces, in contrast, were processed better by the right hemisphere.

How are we to interpret these findings? We join Hamilton in believing that the differences he observed indeed reflect complementary hemispheric specialization. Evidence in support of this comes from the geometrical control patterns, which show no evidence of lateralization. Moreover, an analysis of the data from the 25 monkeys who learned both the orientation and facial-discrimination tasks showed convincing support for complementary specialization; of those 25 animals, 16 discriminated oriented lines better with the left hemisphere and faces better with the right hemisphere. This result shows that possible unrecognized asymmetries in surgical or testing procedures did not produce an asymmetry artifactually. Hamilton would be the first to agree, however, that additional work is necessary to help us understand the nature of hemispheric asymmetry in monkeys and how it may be similar to, as well as different from, human asymmetry.[14]

·········

ANATOMICAL ASYMMETRIES IN ANIMALS

Anatomical studies have suggested that in the temporal lobe region of some nonhuman primates there may be structural asymmetries between the hemispheres similar to the asymmetries found in human brains. One study found asymmetries favoring the left hemisphere in humans and, to a lesser extent, in chimpanzees, but no significant differences between sides in the rhesus brain.[15]

Another study examining the brains of a variety of monkeys and apes produced a similar conclusion. Sixteen of 28 great apes (orangutans, chimpanzees, and gorillas) showed an asymmetry favoring the left hemisphere. One showed the opposite. In contrast, only 3 cases among 41 monkeys and lesser apes (gibbons) showed a sizable asymmetry.[16] Skull size, rather than brain size, has been studied by another investigator. In this study examining skull length in three species of gorilla, only the mountain gorilla showed evidence of gross asymmetry. The other species did not.[17]

It is tempting to speculate that these asymmetries are related to the ability of the apes, particularly chimpanzees, to learn language. Chimpanzees have shown an ability to learn words, some grammar, and even some abstract concepts through the use of sign language or the manipulation of plastic symbols. Some investigators have suggested the anatomical asymmetries in the great apes are a reflection of their having reached a "prelinguistic" evolutionary stage in which their thought patterns are similar to those of humans but much more primitive.

Evidence for anatomical asymmetries in the brain has not been limited to primates, however. For almost 20 years, Marian Diamond and her colleagues studied how the cerebral cortex in the rat could be altered by environmental experience. They had pooled the data from the two hemispheres, assuming they would be similar; but renewed interest in hemispheric differences led Diamond to begin to examine the hemispheres separately, thereby revealing an intriguing pattern of asymmetries that differed as a function of sex of the animal. We reviewed these data in Chapter 8.[18]

Of course, it is still important to keep in mind that we do not yet have evidence linking anatomical asymmetries in animals to actual asymmetries in function, such as those for speech and language in human beings. In fact, there is little convincing evidence of a link between anatomical asymmetries and functional asymmetries in human beings. It is possible that asymmetries in the brain of primates and rats are not related to behavioral asymmetries, just as it is possible that the asymmetries in the human brain may be unrelated to behavioral differences. Underlying much of the interest in anatomical asymmetries, however, is the as yet unproven assumption that such a relationship will ultimately be established.

·········

PHARMACOLOGICAL ASYMMETRIES

Further evidence suggesting that the rat may be a useful animal in which to study brain asymmetries comes from the work of Stanley Glick and his colleagues at the Mt. Sinai School of Medicine.[19] They found that rats rotate or move in circles at night, and that individual rats show a preference in the direction in which they run. Some prefer to run to the left, and others consistently prefer to run to the right. This preference seems to be established very early—the direction in which newborn rats turn their tails predicts their turning preferences later in life.

Glick has shown that a rat's characteristic turning preference is related to a chemical imbalance in the region of the brain called the nigrostriatal pathway, an area that helps regulate movement. They found that the concentration of dopamine, a chemical transmitter released by the neurons in the nigrostriatal pathway that is responsible for circling behavior, is higher by about 15 percent in the side of the brain opposite the direction of the animal's turning preference. Thus, animals with a higher concentration of dopamine in the left side of the brain prefer to turn right, and those with a higher concentration on the right prefer to turn left.

Studies with humans have also revealed asymmetries in the concentration of neurotransmitters in the brain. In reanalyzing data collected by others, Glick and colleagues found higher concentrations of some chemicals in the left hemisphere, and higher concentrations of others in the right hemisphere. A particularly intriguing finding was the observation that dopamine concentrations were higher in the left side of the brain. Because most of the patients whose brains were studied at postmortem may be assumed to have been right-handed, this finding suggests that dopamine concentration apparently is higher on the side contralateral to the preferred hand, a finding consistent with the rat data they obtained.

This work suggests that studies in the rat may reveal functions and mechanisms of brain asymmetry that apply to humans as well. Although research to test this began only recently, Ernst Mach considered the possibility more than a century ago:

> The idea that the distinction between right and left depends upon an asymmetry, and possibly in the last resort upon a chemical difference, is one which has been present to me from my earliest years. . . Human beings and animals that have lost their direction move, almost without exception, nearly in a circle . . . we have here a teleological device to help parents to find their hungry young again when they have been lost.[20]

·········

BEHAVIORAL TESTS

In many respects the search for asymmetries in animals has followed a progression similar to that of laterality research with human beings. A major difference between the human and animal research, however, lies in the role played by behavioral studies. Behavioral work forms a large part of the literature on human laterality, but, with the exception of research on paw preference, until recently few studies have used behavioral approaches to hemispheric differences in animals.

In one such study Japanese macaque monkeys were taught to discriminate two different types of vocalizations made by members of their own species. The sounds were prerecorded and presented to the left or the right ear in a random sequence. The investigators found that all five of the monkeys tested performed more accurately when the sounds were presented to the right ear. Only one of five monkeys of other species showed ear asymmetry when presented with the Japanese macaque vocalizations.[21] If we assume that sounds presented to the right ear are preferentially delivered to the left hemisphere, these results suggest a hemispheric asymmetry in Japanese macaques for the processing of vocalizations produced by members of their own species.

William Hopkins and colleagues have taken a different approach in their study of language-trained chimpanzees.[22] Their subjects were a small number of chimpanzees who have received language training with geometrical visual symbols over the past 12-18 years. The task required them to hold down a response button until a response cue occurred. On each trial, a geometrical symbol, in some cases meaningful and in some cases nonmeaningful but familiar, was presented as a warning stimulus in either the left or the right visual field. The warning stimulus was expected to prime the hemisphere to which it was presented, resulting in greater readiness to respond. Results showed a right-visual-field advantage in priming for the meaningful symbols. Hopkins concluded that

> the data suggest that the manner in which these chimpanzees perceive symbols that have acquired functional meaning may be similar to that observed in human subjects in the processing of words. Further research using traditional lateralized recognition and memory paradigms should help to determine the relations between these simple priming effects and other higher cortical processes.[23]

· · · · · · · · ·

AVIAN ASYMMETRIES:
What the bird's brain can tell us

Up to this point, our review of asymmetries in animals has been confined to studies using mammals, particularly the nonhuman primates. There is some evidence to suggest the existence of asymmetries in these species, but the evidence is far from clear-cut. Given this background, it is especially interesting to note that researchers working at Rockefeller University have discovered a striking asymmetry between the halves of the brain in an unexpected source—songbirds. To appreciate their findings, we must make a brief digression to consider how bird song is produced.

The vocal system of birds essentially consists of a set of bellows that act on an air-driven structure called the syrinx. The position and tension of tissue folds and membranes in the syrinx determine the frequency and amplitude of the sounds produced. The syrinx is divided into a left half and a right half, which are controlled independently by the left and the right hypoglossus nerves, respectively.* Song birds typically develop song during the first year of life. They require auditory feedback both to acquire and to maintain normal song.

Fernando Nottebohm and his colleagues demonstrated that sectioning the left hypoglossus in adult chaffinches and canaries results in a dramatic change in song. Most of the song components disappear and are replaced either by silence or by poorly modulated sounds. Sectioning of the right hypoglossus, in contrast, has minimal effects on song; for the most part, song remains intact.[24]

Further investigation has shown that the right hypoglossus may come to control song to various degrees, depending on the age at which the left hypoglossus is cut. Canaries with the left hypoglossus cut within two weeks after hatching develop song of normal complexity that is completely controlled by the right hypoglossus. Birds operated on as adults also show some plasticity in that they can learn new song under control of the right hypoglossus; the end result, however, is less accomplished than that produced by intact canaries and canaries with damage occurring earlier in life.

The asymmetries in control of bird song appear to extend to the highest vocal-control stations in the brain. Results show that lesions of the left hemisphere produce a song almost completely lacking in structure, without any of the components that were present preoperatively. In contrast, the song in right-lesioned birds retains its structure, although some components are lost. With time, canaries with damaged left hemispheres recover their ability to sing; the right hypoglossus assumes control as it did when the left hypoglossus was cut. Again, however, the resulting song is less accomplished than that found in normal birds.

At first glance, the similarities between asymmetry in bird song and in human language are striking. Several factors, however, suggest caution in interpreting these findings. First, Nottebohm and colleagues were unable to find any gross asymmetry between the left and right sides of the higher-vocal control stations in the canary brain. Thus, the functional differences in the canary appear in the absence of any observable anatomical differences. Second, the evolutionary significance of left hypoglossal dominance in birds remains uncertain. It clearly is not a condition for vocal learning, because even prolific vocalizers such

---

* Notice that control of the syrinx is same-sided, or ipsilateral, in contrast with the crossed, or contralateral, control we have come to expect.

as parrots do not show hypoglossal dominance. Finally, some recent physiological data have suggested that song production may actually be bilaterally controlled in the brain and that peripheral asymmetries can explain earlier findings.[25]

These points, as well as the remoteness of the evolutionary relationship between birds and humans, caution against uncritical interpretations of the song bird evidence. It does, however, remain intriguing, especially in light of very recent work in Nottebohm's laboratory pointing to hemispheric differences in avian song discrimination.

Zebra finches were given unilateral lesions that disrupted auditory input to either the left or the right hemisphere of the song-control system. When taught to discriminate between pairs of bird songs, right-lesioned birds did better than left-lesioned ones at discriminating between the song of a cage mate and their own. Left-lesioned birds did better in a task requiring discrimination between two versions of an unfamiliar song differing only in the harmonic structure of one part of the song. The investigators concluded that the two hemispheres of song birds perceive and process song produced by their own species differently, a phenomenon analogous to hemispheric asymmetry in humans.[26]

·········

THEORETICAL IMPLICATIONS
OF ANIMAL ASYMMETRIES

Comparative research with nonhuman species may help to answer two fundamental questions about brain lateralization: Why are there asymmetries in the first place? Why are such asymmetries generally consistent in their direction—that is, why is speech usually represented in the left and not the right hemisphere?

The evidence we have reviewed points to the existence of anatomical, pharmacological, and/or behavioral asymmetries in a wide range of animals. Much work remains to be done, however, to firmly establish the existence of these asymmetries and to determine what their relationship might be to the asymmetries found in human beings. Norman Geschwind, one of the researchers primarily responsible for current interest in the biological foundations of laterality, has speculated on some of the more far reaching implications of animal asymmetry research.

Geschwind argued that the widespread belief that humans have certain completely distinctive characteristics, such as language and high levels of artistic and musical abilities, would be discredited as more is learned about asymmetries in animals.[27] He was particularly interested in the recent scientific debate as to whether chimps could be taught "true" language. Chimpanzees had been specially trained to communicate with sign language, but there is much controversy over whether this represented language in the same sense as spoken language used by humans.

Geschwind proposed a hypothetical experiment to help resolve the issue. If the chimpanzee's language abilities were impaired by a left-side lesion in the region of the brain comparable to the human language centers and if a bilateral lesion in other locations did not disrupt performance, the results would be consistent with the idea that chimpanzee "language" and human language were similar in mechanism. If the chimpanzee's abilities were impaired as a result of the bilateral lesions in areas not homologous to human language centers, however, and were not impaired with the left-side lesion, he argued, this would be evidence against the linguistic nature of the chimpanzee's performance.*

The fact that asymmetries are found in animals that do not seem to possess linguistic abilities does not weaken the argument, Geschwind claimed. He postulated that perhaps there is a forerunner of language that does not involve communication among individuals but is still useful to the individual animal. Geschwind stated:

> It is clearly conceivable that such an internal method of coding might have appeared very early in evolution and could have been used by individual non-human animals. The ability to communicate, although of great interest, might be a later "technical" development that enabled transmission of the code from one individual to another, but the essential step in the development of the internal code might have occurred much earlier.[28]

Although these ideas are speculative, they are representative of the problems that neuroscientists wishing to understand lateralization are starting to confront. By extending the search for asymmetries beyond human beings, researchers have begun the process of discovering the

---

We agree with Geschwind that a "positive" outcome to this hypothetical study would be powerful indirect evidence for the linguistic nature of the chimpanzee's performance. However, we believe the failure to demonstrate hemispheric asymmetry in chimpanzees of the same sort found in humans would not necessarily rule out the possibility that chimpanzee language was linguistic in the same manner as human language.

answers. In the next sections of this chapter, we shall turn to another issue critical to an understanding of lateralization—the ontogeny, or development, of asymmetry in humans.

·········

THE DEVELOPMENT OF ASYMMETRY

At birth, the brain of a human infant is one-fourth the weight of an adult brain. By the time a child is two years old, the brain will have more than tripled its mass and come close to its full size. Accompanying this dramatic change in physical size are equally dramatic changes in the child's capabilities. By the age of two years, the average child has begun to talk and to show the beginnings of many of the higher mental functions that characterize human beings.

In the sections that follow, we shall discuss how and at what point the basic differences between the left brain and the right brain found in adults fit into this picture of physical and functional change in childhood. Do these asymmetries emerge over time as the child develops, or are they present at birth or even before? What roles do genetic and environmental factors play in the establishment of asymmetry? Can the pattern of asymmetry be changed and, if so, what are the limiting factors?

These fundamental questions relating to the ontogeny of asymmetry are the focus of research efforts that use many different methodologies. The answers have the potential for contributing in important ways to our understanding of language disorders, both in children and in adults. They may also help investigators better understand other problems that have been linked to the division of functions between the hemispheres.

·········

BRAIN INJURY IN CHILDHOOD: Laterality and plasticity

The person perhaps most responsible for current interest in the development of lateralization is Eric Lenneberg, a psychologist at Cornell University. In the mid-1960s, Lenneberg reviewed a variety of evidence and concluded that lateralization of function in the brain develops over time but is complete by puberty.[29] His research also indicated that puberty marks a crucial turning point in the ability to learn new languages, without signs of a foreign accent, through mere exposure. Lenneberg believed it was not merely coincidence that both lateralization and language-learning ability appear fixed at puberty. He saw one as the biological basis of the other.

In drawing his conclusions about the time course of lateralization, Lenneberg relied heavily on clinical data collected by the neurologist L. S. Basser.[30] Basser reported that about half of a group of 72 children with brain injury occurring before the age of two years began to speak at the usual time, whereas the other half showed some delay. The results were the same for children with damage to the left or the right hemisphere, outcomes suggesting that hemispheric asymmetry for language is not well established by the age of two years. Results from a group of children with injuries occurring between the onset of speech and the age of 20 years, however, showed the emergence of hemispheric differences. In this group, injury to the left side resulted in speech disturbances in 85 percent of the cases, but injury to the right side produced disturbances in only 45 percent of the cases.

Despite these differential left-right effects, this pattern of impairment is still different from that found in right-handed teenagers and adults who sustain brain injury. Here, aphasia very rarely follows damage to the right hemisphere but occurs even more often after damage to the left half of the brain. On the basis of this evidence, Lenneberg concluded that lateralization begins at the time of language acquisition but is not complete until puberty.

...

Lateralization by Puberty Reconsidered

Lenneberg's interpretation of these data has not gone unchallenged. A careful reexamination of Basser's findings has shown that each of the cases where damage to the right hemisphere resulted in speech disturbances involved injury occurring before the age of five years. In the sole case where right-hemisphere injury occurred after that age, no speech loss was noted. Thus, Basser's findings are consistent with the hypothesis that lateralization is complete by the age of five years rather than by puberty. They do not, however, provide an adequate number of patients to test the hypothesis that lateralization is completed later.[31]

Marcel Kinsbourne argued that the data are consistent with the hypothesis that lateralization is complete at birth, not by the age of five years or at puberty. He has reviewed the neurological records in Basser's cases and argued that most of the cases in which right-hemisphere damage in infancy resulted in aphasia were really cases of injury to the left as well as the right hemisphere.[32] If this is so, the early childhood data look no different from adult data in terms of the incidence of aphasia after damage to the left or the right side of the brain.

In 1978 Bryan Woods and Hans Lucas Teuber reported 65 cases of children with unilateral hemispheric injury occurring after the onset of speech.[33] They found that 25 of the 34 children with left-hemisphere lesions were initially aphasic, whereas only 4 of the 31 children with right-hemisphere lesions (including two left-handers) were aphasic. In reviewing earlier literature, the authors concluded that there had been a striking change in the incidence of aphasia after right-hemisphere injury in children, with a sharp drop seen in studies begun after 1941.

They attributed this difference over time in part to the use of antibiotics, which resulted in the virtual elimination of aphasia and hemiplegia in children as a consequence of complications from scarlet fever and other diseases. Studies had shown that these infections, if severe and untreated, could produce localized brain lesions as well as diffuse damage to both hemispheres. A child who showed both left hemiplegia and aphasia after such an infection probably would have been classified as a right-hemisphere case, when, in fact, the left hemisphere was most likely also affected. The investigators concluded that the incidence of aphasia after right-hemisphere lesions in children had been greatly overestimated and that the data as a whole supported the idea that the pattern of language functions seen in adults is essentially complete soon after birth.

Thus, clinical evidence suggests that hemispheric specialization for language is present at birth and does not develop over time. This conclusion, however, does not question in any way what we know about the ability of the right hemisphere to take over language functions after very early lesions of the left hemisphere. We know that there are dramatic differences in recovery from aphasia in children and in adults, and we shall consider the theoretical implications of this finding later in this chapter.

·········

HEMISPHERECTOMY IN INFANCY:
Removing half a brain

Occasionally, it is medically necessary to remove most of one cerebral hemisphere. We discussed in Chapter 6 some of the consequences of hemispherectomy in adults. The operation is also done early in infancy when extensive damage to one hemisphere threatens to impair the function of the undamaged side as well.

Reports of several dozen hemispherectomy cases have appeared in the literature and serve as a source of information on the development of hemispheric asymmetry of function. The consequences of the operation are a function of the age of the patient at the time of the surgery and of which hemisphere is removed. As we discussed, adult patients with the right hemisphere removed typically show little or no language impairment, but the removal of the left hemisphere generally results in marked aphasia that improves only slightly with time. Similar lateralized effects occur in children. The severity of impairment is directly related and the prognosis for recovery of language is inversely related to the age of the child at the time of surgery.[34]

Several reports have noted that if surgery is performed early enough in infancy, no signs of lateralized deficits in higher mental functions remain in adulthood. This finding suggests that the remaining hemisphere, whether it is the left or the right, is able to take over for the hemisphere that is removed and to perform those functions that ordinarily would be lateralized to the other half of the brain.

It is possible to draw at least two different theoretical conclusions from these data. One is that no shift of functions has taken place in early hemispherectomy cases because lateralization of function is not present in early infancy. A second interpretation is that hemispheric differences are present early in infancy, but the young brain has a tremendous ability to reorganize itself in the face of damage to specific regions.

Some recent, in-depth studies of the abilities of patients with left and right hemispherectomies suggest that of the two possibilities, the latter "plasticity" explanation is more likely to be correct. Maureen Dennis and Harry Whitaker tested early hemispherectomy patients on various language tests and found very subtle signs of lateralized effects.[35] Standard measures of verbal intelligence do not seem to differentiate between early left and early right hemispherectomy. This failure to find a difference does not mean, however, that other tests might not reveal one.

Dennis and Whitaker studied three nine- to ten-year-olds who had undergone hemispherectomy by the age of five months. One was a right-hemispherectomy patient; the other two had had the left hemisphere removed. Results showed that both discrimination and articulation of the sounds of speech were normal in all three children. The three were also equally good at producing and discriminating words. Important differences between the hemispheres, however, appeared in tests of the patients' abilities to deal with syntax—the rules for combining words into grammatically correct sentences. For example, each child was asked to judge the acceptability of the following sentences:

1. I paid the money by the man.
2. I was paid the money to the lady.
3. I was paid the money by the boy.

The right-hemispherectomy patient correctly indicated that sentences 1 and 2 are grammatically incorrect and that sentence 3 is acceptable. The two left-hemispherectomy patients did not make these distinctions.

The researchers concluded that the right hemisphere in the left-hemispherectomy cases does not accurately comprehend the meaning of passive sentences. Other tests led them to conclude that the right-hemisphere defect is an organizational, analytical, and syntactical problem rather than one rooted in the conceptual or semantic aspects of language. The results suggest that there are limits to the plasticity of the infant brain and, what is more important for our purposes, that the asymmetries between the hemispheres are present very early in life.

Dennis and Whitaker's conclusions, however, have been criticized as premature, considering the evidence presented in support of them. Dorothy Bishop noted problems with the statistical analysis used, as well as with the absence of appropriate control groups against which to compare patients' performances.[36] She noted that later studies showed that the sole right-hemispherectomy patient studied by Dennis and Whitaker did better than most other right-hemispherectomy patients in a variety of linguistic tasks and that it is unsound to use one patient as the sole standard against which to evaluate the linguistic abilities of the left-hemispherectomy patients. Bishop argued for caution in accepting Dennis and Whitaker's conclusions until stronger data are presented.

It may well be the case that data definitively showing the limits of plasticity eventually will be provided. These limits, however, whatever they might be, would not detract from the very important role plasticity plays in much of the dramatic recovery from aphasia that is found after left-hemisphere damage in children. The ability of a brain to readjust its function relatively quickly makes it hard to distinguish between a system in which lateralization does not exist or exists only in rudimentary form and one in which lateralization is extensive but rapid compensation for unilateral damage is possible. Only through the use of very sensitive tests designed to measure subtle differences in performance can we begin to tease apart these alternatives.

·········

THE SEARCH FOR THE BEGINNINGS
OF LATERALIZATION

Clinical evidence dealing with the effects of early brain damage on language functions has played a central role in shaping current thinking about the development of asymmetry. Several other sources of evidence bearing on this issue are also available, and we shall now consider them.

...

Anatomical Asymmetries in Infants

Other evidence to support the idea that brain asymmetry has its origin early in life comes from anatomical studies in fetuses and infants. In the largest study, 207 brains were measured. Ages ranged from 10 to 44 weeks after conception. A longer left temporal plane was present in 54 percent of the brains; the relationship was reversed in 18 percent of the cases. In 28 percent no significant difference in the sizes of the two temporal planes was observed.[37]

In another large study of 100 brains, comparable results were found. The mean age in this study was 48 weeks, including the gestational period. The left temporal plane was 77 percent larger, for the average case, than the right temporal plane. There were 12 infants with the right side larger than the left side and 32 with approximately equal measurements on the left and the right.[38]

Once again, however, there is a major difficulty in interpreting such anatomical studies. We do not know the precise nature of the relationship between anatomical asymmetry and functional asymmetry. Is the former the structural basis of the latter? If so, are functional differences between the hemispheres operative whenever we find anatomical differences? Only when additional information is available to help answer these questions will we be able to interpret the asymmetry data with confidence. Until then, the evidence will remain suggestive and intriguing but by no means a complete answer to the issue of whether lateralization of function is present at birth.

...

Head-Turning in Infants

Newborns are very limited in their range of behaviors, a condition leaving little opportunity to observe any lateral preferences such as hand usage. However, infants do turn their heads to the left and the right, and thus the frequency of left-side turns and right-side turns becomes a measure of potential interest. Several studies have shown that infants just a few days old show a marked preference for right-side head turns.[39] Although the meaning of this preference has not been firmly established, there is some preliminary suggestion that it may be related to hand preference later in life.

One group of investigators has reported a statistically significant correlation between direction of head-turning in infancy and lateral preference at the age of seven years, although the correlation is not large.[40] There are at least two possible explanations for this relationship. The first holds that head-turning preference in infancy affects the subsequent development of hand preference. For example, those infants who prefer to turn their heads to the right would see their right hands more often than their left hands. This circumstance might result in better eye-hand coordination with the right hand, thereby leading to a preference for the right hand in visually guided reaching. A second possibility is that both head-turning preference and later hand preference are related because they are determined by the same set of brain mechanisms.

...

Evoked Potentials in Infants

Because electrophysiological recording techniques do not require a deliberate response of any sort from the subject, they are ideally suited to the study of hemispheric asymmetries in infants. Psychologist Dennis Molfese was one of the first investigators to find evidence of asymmetries in the electrical recordings of the left brain and the right brain in neonates. In one study, he and his collaborators presented speech sounds, such as "ba," to infants ranging in age from one week to ten months while they recorded evoked potential (EP) activity from both hemispheres.[41]

Molfese found responses of greater amplitude, presumably reflecting greater involvement in the processing of the sounds, on the left side in nine of the ten infants tested. The effect held for the youngest infants as well as for the older ones. The one infant showing a reversal was eight months of age. When Molfese presented the infants with certain nonspeech sounds, such as a noise burst or a piano chord, the opposite results were obtained: All ten infants showed EPs of greater amplitude in the right hemisphere. These findings are exciting because they suggest that although a newborn may not "understand" what is being presented, the brain is already equipped with specialized centers that will be responsible for processing the sounds at deeper levels later in life.

Wada and Davis have taken another approach to the study of EP asymmetries in infants. "If fundamental asymmetry of the neurocircuit exists before the development of language and speech function," they noted, "then we ought to be able to disclose such a difference without using verbal stimuli."[42] Wada and Davis recorded the EP to clicks and flashes of light and measured the coherence (similarity of the forms) of the EP in the temporal and occipital regions of the brain in infants.

In earlier work with adult patients tested with sodium amobarbital, they had observed that coherence was largest for clicks in the speech-dominant hemisphere and for flashes in the non-speech-dominant hemisphere. Similar results were found in their study of 50 infants ranging in age from one day to five weeks. Findings indicated that the forms of the occipital and temporal responses to clicks were more similar within the left half of the brain than within the right half; the similarity shifted toward the right hemisphere when flashes were presented. The investigators argued that their findings reflect the specialization of the two hemispheres for processing different kinds of information and that this specialization is present at birth.

...

Dichotic Listening in the Crib

Many dichotic-listening studies have sought to determine the earliest age at which the right-ear advantage may be found. This technique, discussed at length in Chapter 3, involves the presentation of two different speech messages simultaneously, one to each ear. Subjects are typically asked to report what was heard, a procedure that obviously places a lower limit on the age of the children who can be tested. The standard dichotic listening test has been used with children as young as three years old, however, and a right-ear superiority has been found.[43]

Ingenious methods have been devised to take the dichotic technique to the crib to determine whether infants show a right-ear advantage. In one study, infants averaging 50 days of age first learned to suck on a nipple in order to receive dichotic presentations of a pair of words. Each time infants sucked with a previously specified force, the same words were presented to them. This procedure continued until the infants habituated to the dichotic pair, as evidenced by a sustained reduction in the sucking rate. At this point, either the left-ear stimulus or the right-ear stimulus was changed, and the investigator monitored the infants for changes in sucking rate. The results showed that the infants noticed a change in either ear (the sucking rate increased), but a change in the right ear produced a larger increase in sucking.[44]

Because infants typically increase their rate of sucking when a novel stimulus is presented, the results with the dichotic speech stimuli suggest that the difference between old and new stimuli is easier to detect in the right ear—a right-ear advantage. When nonspeech stimuli were used, there was a greater increase in sucking rate following left-ear change. This finding is further evidence that the "ear difference" in the dichotic task reflects brain asymmetry.

Although this modification of the dichotic paradigm is ingenious and encouraging to those who believe lateralization of function is present at birth, other investigators have had difficulty replicating the findings. One study repeated the work with speech stimuli modifying the procedures slightly to prevent inadvertent experimenter bias.* That study failed to obtain evidence of differences in the sucking rate in response to stimuli changed in either ear.[45] Further work is needed to determine whether ear asymmetries can be found in newborns.

·········

DOES LATERALIZATION CHANGE OVER TIME?

The fact that the effects of unilateral brain damage occurring early in life contrast with the effects of later damage certainly suggests that important changes in the brain occur with time. Language impairments

---

* Experimenter bias is a potential problem in all behavioral research. In the study just discussed, the experimenter was not "blind" to the order of stimulus conditions; that is, the investigator knew which ear received a change in sound stimuli on a particular trial and may have inadvertently influenced the infant to respond in the predicted direction. In the attempted replication of this work, the experimenter present in the room with the infant had no knowledge of the particular condition being tested at any given time.

after damage to the left hemisphere generally are less severe and of shorter duration the younger the individual at the time of the injury. Does this imply that lateralization becomes more extensive or complete with age? Not necessarily. Another interpretation of these brain-damage findings is that the plasticity of the brain decreases with age; that is, as the individual grows older, the right hemisphere loses the ability to take over the control of language.

To answer the question of whether lateralization itself changes with age, we must obtain measures of lateralization in subjects of different ages and compare the degree of asymmetry present in each age group. This approach has been used most extensively in investigations of dichotic listening.

The pattern of findings, unfortunately, is not consistent. For example, one large study using 30 children at each of five ages (5, 7, 9, 11, and 13 years) in a dichotic consonant-vowel task found a right-ear advantage across all age groups, with the magnitude of the ear asymmetry similar at all age levels.[46]

In contrast, another study using 24 subjects in each of five age groups (6, 7, 10, 12, and 14 years) found an increase in the magnitude of the ear asymmetry over this age range. The right-ear advantage was significantly different from zero in the 12- and 14-year-old groups only.[47] In a review paper dealing with the issue of developmental change, the authors tallied four dichotic-listening studies showing an increase in asymmetry over this time period and five showing either a mild decrease or a plateau after three to five years of age.[48]

Other measures have also been used to address the question of change in lateralization with age. Molfese's study of EPs to speech and nonspeech stimuli mentioned earlier in this chapter also involved children between 4 and 11 years of age and adults 23 to 29 years old.[49] Analyses showed that the asymmetry in the size of the EP to the non-speech stimuli was proportionately greater in the infants than in the children and adults. The speech stimuli resulted in a comparable asymmetry in the infants and children, whereas both groups showed greater asymmetry in response to these stimuli than did the adults. The authors suggested that the EP asymmetry may decline with age because of the maturation of the cerebral commissures that connect the hemispheres. To support their argument, they cited anatomical studies showing that the corpus callosum is incompletely developed at birth.

We noted earlier that anatomical asymmetries have been found in infant brains. One study used both infant and adult brains measured in a manner permitting comparison of the degree of asymmetry in the two groups. By expressing the size of the right temporal plane as a percentage of the size of the left temporal plane, a measure independent of absolute size is derived. The investigators could then directly compare the infant and adult series. The average R/L ratio was 67 percent for infants and 55 percent for adults, a result indicating a greater degree of asymmetry in the adults.[50] These findings suggest that the asymmetry in the size of the temporal plane in the two hemispheres increases with age.

Given the variability in outcome of studies using different methodologies, as well as the variability found in studies using the same measure of lateralization, it is clearly premature to draw conclusions regarding change in asymmetry with age. Further research using more refined measures of lateralization should provide the answers. It would also be valuable to investigate hemispheric asymmetries over the entire life span to see if the aging process differentially affects the hemispheres. Very little work has been done in this area.

·········

THE ROLE OF THE CORPUS CALLOSUM IN DEVELOPMENT

The brain of most mammals, including humans, is largely underdeveloped at birth and undergoes a major portion of its structural and functional maturation during infancy and early childhood. In addition to its obvious growth, the brain undergoes dramatic changes at the microscopic level. The connections between neurons multiply tremendously in the first few years and are thought to continue changing throughout a person's lifetime. In addition, insulating fatty layers called myelin are laid down around nerve fibers, thereby making them more efficient conductors of electrical impulses.

The corpus callosum is present at birth but appears disproportionately small in cross section when the brain of a newborn is compared with the brain of an adult. Figure 9.2 shows the growth of the cerebral commissures during three stages of human development.

Sandra Witelson has been particularly interested in the changes in the corpus callosum that take place between birth and adulthood.[51] She has analyzed all of the studies bearing on the development of the corpus callosum and has found that the most rapid growth of the corpus callosum takes place during fetal development. Between birth and the age of two years, the corpus callosum continues to grow at a rapid rate, although somewhat more slowly than during fetal development. There is a paucity of data on callosal size between ages 2 and 18 years, but

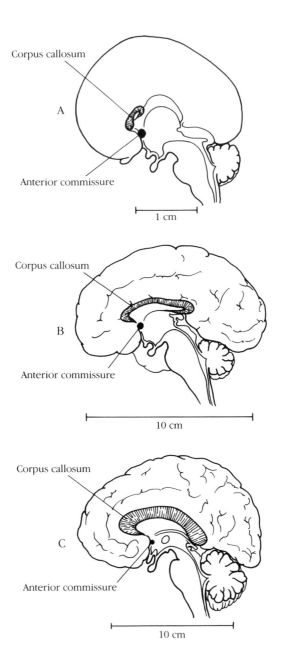

FIGURE 9.2 The corpus callosum and anterior commissure at three stages of human development. A. Fetus (16 weeks). B. Neonate (40 weeks). C. Adult. [From Trevarthen, "Cerebral Embryology and the Split Brain," Fig. XI-7, pp. 228–229 in *Hemisphere Disconnection and Cerebral Function*, ed. M. Kinsbourne and L. Smith, Springfield, Ill.: Charles C. Thomas, 1974.]

Witelson noted that if the callosum were to continue growing at the same rate as it grew in infancy, the adult callosum would be 300 percent bigger than it is.

Witelson suggested two possibilities regarding the development of the corpus callosum between ages 2 and 18 years. The first is that the corpus callosum continues to grow at the same rate it grew in infancy, reaching adult size at three to four years of age. The second is that there is a significant decrease in the rate of callosal growth between ages 2 and 18 years, with very slow growth occurring until the adult size is reached. Although there are no data on callosal size between these ages to answer this question directly, Witelson favored the second hypothesis, citing other changes in the brain (e.g., myelinization of the corpus callosum and brain size itself) that follow a time course in which rapid development between birth and the age of two years is followed by much slower growth until adult development is reached.

Witelson saw implications of this pattern of brain growth and cortical development and cited cognitive and "neurocognitive" events fitting this time frame. She noted, for example, that brain damage occurring during the first year of life differs in its effects from damage sustained after one year. Specifically, damage before one year is associated with lower overall IQ scores and with lower nonverbal—relative to verbal—abilities. After one year of age, damage has less effect on overall IQ, with the pattern of deficits linked to the locus of the damage. Hand preference in normal children also shows signs of stabilization by the age of one year. Perhaps, Witelson suggested, callosal growth represents cortical changes and, accordingly, cognitive changes.

...

Agenesis of the Corpus Callosum

What would happen if the cerebral commissures were severed at birth? What role do the commissures play in lateralization and in the normal development of cognitive functions? Although there are no cases of split-brain surgery performed in infants, cases of a congenital absence, or agenesis, of the corpus callosum provide a unique opportunity to look at these questions.

The earliest work on callosal agenesis focused on how language is organized in the brain. If the corpus callosum plays an important role in the development of hemispheric asymmetry, perhaps by inhibiting simultaneous activation in related areas in the other half of the brain, then one might expect to find language functions bilaterally represented in acallosal subjects. This did not prove to be the case. Most subjects with callosal agenesis show a clear hand preference and small, but reliable, asymmetries in dichotic listening and visual half-field tests, as well as left-hemisphere speech as determined by the Wada test.[52]

Until relatively recently, cases of callosal agenesis came to the attention of investigators as a result of other neurological abnormalities, often accompanied by impaired mental function. The introduction of noninvasive procedures such at CT scans and magnetic resonance imaging (discussed in Chapter 4), however, has led to the detection of additional cases without gross neurological dysfunction in the normal to near-normal IQ range.

In one recent study of acallosal subjects, they did not show any cognitive deficits that could be specifically attributed to callosal agenesis when compared to IQ-matched subjects with an intact corpus callosum.[53] For example, acallosal subjects had verbal and performance IQ scores that were comparable to each other, with no suggestion of the kind of imbalance between verbal and performance scores that can accompany brain damage. Acallosal subjects did show deficits, however, compared with IQ-matched controls on tasks measuring dexterity in using one hand and bimanual coordination.

Christine Temple has conducted intensive studies of a small number of normal-IQ acallosal children to ask whether a finer grained analysis of cognitive development using specialized tests might reveal specific cognitive impairments.[54] Her initial results showed that these children display deficits in tasks involving the production and recognition of rhyme. Examples of the tasks include a fluency task in which the subjects are asked to generate in one minute as many words as possible that rhyme with a given word (e.g., fear, ring, nine) and a recognition task in which each word from the rhyme fluency task is paired with four other words (e.g., fear-beer; fear-feel; fear-four; fear-hen). Pairs are spoken aloud in a random sequence and subjects are asked to judge whether each pair rhymes.

Deficits in these tasks were surprising because the subjects show no gross impairments; their speech is clear and well formed and their overall language skills are normal. Yet, as Temple noted, "on rhyming tasks which require more explicit decomposition, analysis, and synthesis of speech-related material, there are significant deficits in performance."[55] Subsequent work showed that although overall reading level in these children is normal, they are impaired in the ability to pronounce aloud nonwords (letter strings that conform to the orthographic rules of language, e.g., gip, sutter). Normal young children are better at reading words than nonwords, but the difference declines with age as they become increasingly familiar with the rules of English. For acallosal children, the difficulty in reading nonwords aloud persists.

Temple found that acallosal children could read irregular words like *yacht* yet have difficulty with a nonword like *gip*. She suggested that phonological (speech sound) reading is impaired in these children, whereas lexical (whole word) reading is normal. Subsequent tests showed that the impairment extended to simple speech sound discriminations in which subjects had to judge whether pairs of words spoken aloud were identical (e.g., tub-tug). Temple concluded that while overall language development may be normal in children with callosal agenesis, there is a consistent deficit in phonological processing.

Might certain aspects of spatial cognition be similarly impaired in these children, despite generally normal performance? Using a variety of visuospatial tasks, Temple found that all of the acallosal subjects were deficient in certain kinds of visuoconstructional skills that require the coordination of a series of movements, for example, putting pieces of a puzzle together to form an abstract pattern. Temple concluded that

> the results therefore implicate a number of selective cognitive domains in which the corpus callosum may play a critical role in normal performance. The results also indicate that acallosal subjects provide useful evidence about the nature of the modular subcomponents of cognitive skill which may develop in relative independence of each other.[56]

Much more work remains to be done with larger samples of subjects to see if the deficits observed by Temple can be generalized to acallosal children more broadly. The apparent normality, for the most part, of individuals with callosal agenesis points to the ways in which noncallosal commissural pathways can compensate for the absence of the callosum. The existence of highly selective deficits, however, may help our understanding of the nature of lateralization and the role played by the corpus callosum in the development of cognitive functions.

·········

THE ROLES OF NATURE AND NURTURE IN THE ESTABLISHMENT OF ASYMMETRIES

···

Nature

Much of the evidence reviewed in this chapter suggests that hemispheric asymmetries in some form are present at or near birth. The earlier the age at which asymmetries are detected, the more confident we may be

that they are part of the biological makeup of the organism and independent of experience.*

Several genetic models have been proposed to account for hemispheric asymmetries. Chapter 5 contained a brief review of this topic in
the context of our discussion of handedness.

More recently, some investigators have begun to consider other
ways, not genetic in the strict sense, in which patterns of lateralization
may be inherited. Research has shown that cytoplasm, the fluid contained in all cells, including the maternal egg, can transmit certain traits
from parent to offspring in some species. Such "cytoplasmic inheritance" has been proposed as a possible basis for the transmission of
asymmetry from parent to offspring in human beings.

Michael Corballis and Michael Morgan proposed that there is an
underlying cytoplasmic gradient operating during embryonic development that favors the left side of the body.[57] This gradient, they claimed,
is responsible for physiological asymmetries in humans and animals,
which, in turn, are responsible for the functional asymmetries we see.
According to this view, the left-sided control of song in certain birds,
the enlargement of the left temporal plane of the brain in chimpanzees,
orangutans, and humans (discussed earlier in this chapter and in Chapter 4), and the leftward displacement of the heart in vertebrates, are all
examples of consequences of this developmental gradient. Both right-
handedness and left-cerebral control of speech in humans are seen as
further manifestations of this gradient.

Why are some people left-handed, and why do some have speech
represented in the right or, perhaps, both hemispheres? Corballis and
Morgan suggested that the hypothesized gradient is absent in some
individuals and that in these cases, environmental factors play a major
role in determining which pattern a given individual will show.

Corballis and Morgan's ideas are intriguing ones and are an attempt
to place human hand preference and hemispheric asymmetry in a
broader biological context. A gradient favoring faster development on
the left side is a fundamental one shared by many species, they argued,
and handedness and speech lateralization are simply a species-specific
consequence of that gradient. Critics of their views, however, point to
other examples, in both humans and other animals, in which the right
side of the body appears to be favored.[58]

---

*Asymmetries occurring later may also be part of an organism's biological makeup.
Genetic factors may determine the emergence of asymmetries in later stages of
development.*

···

Nurture

What can be said about the role of experience or environmental factors in determining hemispheric asymmetries? At one extreme, we have seen that early damage to one hemisphere of the brain can result in a dramatic reorganization of lateralized functions. The fact that persons with the left hemisphere removed in infancy develop language skills in the right hemisphere is but one piece of evidence pointing to the tremendous plasticity of the brain. The compensation for early removal of one hemisphere, however, is not total. Sensitive tests reveal language deficits, a result suggesting that the basic blueprint for asymmetry is present very early in life and that its traces remain despite damage-induced reorganization. In our earlier discussions of left-handedness, we noted that some investigators believe all left-handedness (and presumably all right-hemisphere or bilateral control of speech) is a result of brain injury, however subtle. Other evidence, however, has suggested that the quality and quantity of exposure to language itself may affect the development of lateralization.

···

Exposure to Language

Some evidence pointing to early environment as a factor in asymmetry is based on the study of Genie, an adolescent girl who endured 11½ years of extreme social and experiential deprivation. Genie was discovered at the age of 13½, after having spent most of her life in almost complete isolation, during which time she was punished for making any noise whatsoever. Two years after she was found, she was reported to have made slow but steady progress in language learning. This fact is of considerable significance for the theoretical issue of whether a first language may be acquired after puberty.

Of particular interest to us here, however, is Genie's performance on two special dichotic-listening tests. One was composed of familiar words, the other of familiar environmental sounds. Genie was able to identify correctly each of these stimuli when she was tested one ear at a time. When the words were presented dichotically, however, Genie showed an extreme left-ear advantage instead of the moderate right-ear advantage that is generally found in right-handed subjects. Her left ear performed perfectly, whereas the performance of her right ear was at chance level. For the environmental sounds, Genie showed a small left-ear advantage, in keeping with the prediction that such sounds are processed more efficiently in the right hemisphere.[59]

These findings suggest that the processing of both language and nonlanguage stimuli took place in Genie's right hemisphere. The investigators who worked with her have argued that her left hemisphere may have begun language acquisition before her confinement but through disuse was no longer able to fulfill its original function. As Genie began to learn language a second time, the right hemisphere assumed control because its functions presumably had been exercised (by visuospatial processes) in spite of her confinement.

The problem with a single-subject study such as this is that there is no way of knowing the pattern of asymmetry that would have developed in Genie's brain had she had a normal childhood. Perhaps she would have shown right-hemisphere specialization for language and nonlanguage stimuli anyway. Nevertheless, the results are intriguing, especially in light of work looking at hemispheric asymmetry in the congenitally deaf.

Helen Neville of the Salk Institute has studied hemispheric asymmetry in profoundly deaf individuals born to deaf parents.[60] All had learned American Sign Language (ASL) from their parents at the normal age for language acquisition, but none had acquired speech. When asked to write single words presented in the left or right visual field, normally hearing control subjects showed a right-visual-field advantage. The deaf subjects, however, performed similarly to stimuli in both fields. When deaf subjects were presented with lateralized images of a person signing, however, and asked to repeat a sign, all responded more accurately to right-visual-field presentations.

Neville concluded that experience with language presented auditorily is not necessary for specialization of the left hemisphere and that critical to the maintenance of the specialization of the left hemisphere is the acquisition of competence in the grammar of language. American Sign Language is not sound based, but it is highly grammatical.

Neville's findings fit nicely with data on the effects of stroke-induced damage to the left or right hemisphere in six profoundly deaf persons, all of whom had used ASL as their primary mode of communication. Left-lesioned patients were able to process visuospatial relations well but showed severe "aphasia" in the use of ASL. In contrast, the right-lesioned patients were severely impaired in visuospatial relations but were unimpaired linguistically. The authors concluded that hearing and speech are not necessary for hemispheric specialization and that congenitally deaf signers show separate specialization for sign-based language processing and nonlanguage spatial processing, despite the spatial-manipulative aspects of ASL.[61]

...

The Bilingual Brain

Does the experience of acquiring two languages change the pattern of brain organization? This question is currently the subject of considerable controversy. A number of studies have concluded that the left hemisphere is dominant for processing both the native language and the nonnative language. Other studies, however, have reported weaker left lateralization for language among bilinguals; still others have reported differential hemispheric asymmetry for language. A review by Loraine Obler and her colleagues has attempted to bring order out of the seeming chaos of findings by identifying some factors that may account for the differences among studies.[62] These factors include the level of proficiency in the two languages, age at second-language acquisition, and the way in which the second language is acquired.

Michel Paradis has argued that such efforts to account for differences among studies in terms of increasingly specific subgroups of bilingual subjects is not productive, and that there really is no good evidence that bilingual subjects, of any variety, show lateralization patterns that differ from those of monolingual subjects.[63] He noted in particular that clinical data do not provide any evidence for reduced asymmetry in bilingual subjects for either or both languages. Crossed aphasia, in which damage to the hemisphere ipsilateral to the preferred hand produces aphasia, is not significantly higher in bilingual subjects than in monolingual subjects. The results from Wada testing show a similar picture—both languages are disrupted only by left-hemisphere administration of the drug.

Not everyone, however, agrees with Paradis's conclusion that it may be time for neuropsychologists to move on to more productive research.[64] The field remains highly controversial and will continue to be until we have good explanations for the diversity of findings.

....

SOME THEORETICAL ISSUES

Although investigators are far from having definite answers to the questions about the development of asymmetry, a pattern of findings is emerging. Of great theoretical significance are the observations suggesting that hemispheric differences are present at birth. In apparent conflict with the lateralization-at-birth view is clinical evidence showing that the effects of very early unilateral brain damage do not vary as a function of the side of injury. The latter data, however, are compatible with the lateralization-at-birth position if we take into account the plasticity that allows the young brain to compensate for the effects of damage. In this context, we pointed to the importance of tests that are very sensitive to subtle impairment and could perhaps differentiate between the results of damage-induced reorganization and the absence of lateralization in the first place (presuming damage-induced reorganization is in some way less than optimal).

Research investigating the time course of lateralization and the factors that affect it is difficult for several reasons. First, our measures of laterality are far from perfect. Does failing to find differences between the hemispheres mean such differences do not exist? Can we be sure that we have not simply failed to set up conditions that would allow us to detect a real difference?

A related issue is that many tests apparently are sensitive to factors other than brain lateralization. In Chapter 3, we discussed how differences in the way a task is approached can dramatically affect the type of asymmetry observed in behavioral tests. Perhaps differences found in hemispheric asymmetry as a function of age reflect different strategies rather than differences in lateralization per se.

A second major problem in studying factors involved in lateralization is related to the difficulty of answering nature-nurture questions with human beings in general. We are severely limited in the kinds of environmental effects that can be studied, and genetic models frequently cannot be adequately tested.

The state of affairs is a challenging one for which there are no simple solutions. As more and more investigators appreciate the significance of developmental issues and the care with which they have to be investigated, we can expect progress toward some answers.

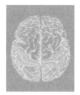

ASYMMETRY'S ROLE IN DEVELOPMENTAL DISABILITIES AND PSYCHIATRIC ILLNESS

Research in the area of hemispheric differences has had an impact on many fields involved in the investigation of human function and dysfunction. In Chapters 1, 6, and 7 we discussed the clinical symptoms of injury to the right and left hemispheres. In this chapter we shall consider other disabilities and abnormalities in human behavior that have been related to the division of function between the hemispheres. Although not the consequence of any obvious physical damage, these disabilities may in fact arise from subtle problems in either the left or the right side of the brain.

Is stuttering the result of competition for control of speech by the two hemispheres in a less than normally lateralized individual? Does incomplete lateralization predispose a child to reading problems, despite otherwise normal intelligence? Why does psychiatric depression seem to respond better to right-hemisphere shock treatment than to left-hemisphere shock treatment? These are a few of the questions investigators have pursued in an attempt to determine the roles of the left brain and the right brain in pathological processes.

Evidence dealing with right-hemisphere involvement in emotion plays a role in current thinking about certain psychiatric disorders and hemispheric differences. We shall briefly review experiments with neurologically normal subjects that bear on this topic and add to the data on hemispheric differences relating to emotion discussed in Chapter 7.

There are at least two ways in which pathological processes can be related to hemispheric asymmetry of function. The pathology can be directly related to dysfunction in one of the hemispheres, that is, to dysfunction of one or more of the hemisphere's specialized abilities. Alternatively, the pathology can be associated with patterns of hemispheric asymmetry that differ from normal. Both kinds of dysfunction have been claimed to play a role in pathology.

·········

READING DISABILITY:
A failure of dominance?

One of the first investigators to propose a link between lateralization and reading disability was Samuel T. Orton, a physician who had worked during the early decades of this century with children suffering from reading and writing problems. Orton noticed that these children sometimes wrote in mirror form, reversing the orientation of individual letters as well as their sequence within a word. For example, the word *cat* might be written "ɪɒɔ" as it would appear if one viewed in a mirror. Similarly, these children often reversed letter sequences in reading, so that *saw* was read as *was*.

Orton observed that children who made mirror-image reversals in reading and writing also tended to have unstable handedness preferences. He interpreted this finding as a sign of incomplete cerebral dominance. This association of reading disability and incomplete cerebral dominance led him to propose that the two were related.

Because the two sides of the brain are symmetrical about the midline, information about the visual world, he suggested, is represented in mirror-image form on each side. Orton argued that information represented in the dominant hemisphere was oriented correctly, whereas information in the nondominant hemisphere was in mirror-image form (see Figure 10.1). In the absence of sufficiently developed cerebral dominance, the two representations would cause confusion in reading and writing. Orton used the term *strephosymbolia* to describe the resulting condition.[1]

Orton's term for this type of reading and writing difficulty is no longer used, and his ideas of how representations are laid down in mirror-image fashion in each hemisphere have been shown to be incorrect. Nevertheless, the basic notion that reading disability may be linked to hemispheric asymmetry is still under active investigation. The development of new behavioral tools to study hemispheric asymmetry has made it possible to test more directly the idea that reading disability is

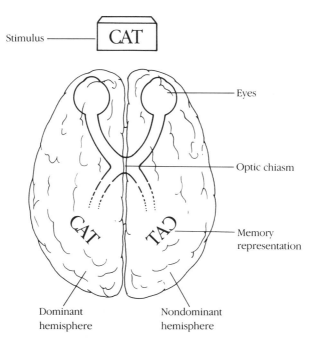

FIGURE 10.1   Schematic representation of Orton's theory. Orton assumed that a visual stimulus is represented in opposite orientations in the two hemispheres. [From Corballis, "The Left-Right Problem in Psychology," *Canadian Psychologist* 15 (1974).]

linked to atypical brain asymmetry. It turns out that Orton may have been right, but for the wrong reasons.

Dyslexia is the term currently used to refer to a marked impairment in the development of reading skill compared with that expected on the basis of intelligence level and education.[2] It is common in school-age children, affecting anywhere from 2 to 8 percent of them, and in most cases appears to be a language deficit rather than a visual-perceptual problem.

In general, dyslexia is considered to involve decoding—the ability to read words accurately—rather than reading comprehension per se. The context present in written material can often help dyslexic individuals decode specific words they would have difficulty reading in isolation. Over time, many dyslexic children improve and no longer show obvious signs of reading impairment. However, neuropsychological tests frequently reveal subtle deficits that remain in phonological coding—the ability to recognize individual phonemes, or speech sounds, in words and to apply the phonological, or sound-symbol, rules of English. For example, the ability to read nonwords, which requires application of the rules of phonology, may be impaired even though there is no problem reading familiar words. Spelling may also be impaired. Recent data suggest a strong genetic component to dyslexia. Approximately 35-40 percent of boys with a dyslexic parent show dyslexia themselves; the figure is 17-18 percent for girls. Thus, having an affected parent increases the probability a boy will have dyslexia 5- to 7-fold; girls show a 10- to 12-fold increase in risk.[3]

...

Behavioral Studies with Normal and Impaired Readers

What is the evidence bearing on possible brain mechanisms underlying dyslexia? A large number of behavioral studies have been conducted to explore lateralization of function in children with reading disability by comparing normal and poor readers on tasks that consistently show a lateral asymmetry in normal children and adults. These include dichotic-listening and tachistoscopic studies and the tactile dichaptic task discussed in Chapter 8.

A review of this literature by M. P. Bryden identified 51 such studies.[4] Of these, 30 claimed to show that poor readers are less lateralized than good readers. No difference between groups was found in 14 studies, and 7 studies reported that poor readers show greater lateralization. Looked at as a whole, there were significantly more studies showing weaker lateralization in poor readers than there were studies showing greater lateralization. The same pattern of results was found for the three different techniques used to measure lateralization. Of the 35 dichotic-listening studies, 20 showed less lateralization in poor readers, and 5 showed greater lateralization; 10 showed no difference between groups. Of the visual-field studies, 8 of 14 showed weaker lateralization in poor readers, 2 showed more lateralization, and 4 showed no difference. Evidence for weaker lateralization in poor readers was found in both dichaptic studies reported.

Our discussion of behavioral tests in Chapter 3 identified several factors, such as attentional strategies, that may affect the outcome of dichotic and other tests, independent of hemispheric asymmetry. While acknowledging the need to better control for these factors that can cause variations from study to study, Bryden concluded his review with the suggestion that "there is at least some fire in the smoke of reading ability and laterality. Although almost all possible results have been obtained at one time or another, the general pattern that appears is that poor readers are less lateralized for receptive language than are good readers."[5]

...

Structural and Functional Asymmetries from Anatomical and Imaging Studies

Anatomical evidence pointing to a relationship between brain asymmetry and dyslexia has been reported and provides a promising basis for further exploration of differences in lateralization between dyslexic and normal readers. Albert Galaburda and colleagues performed autopsies on the brains of seven dyslexic persons, most of whom died from accidents. Their study of four dyslexic men showed unusual symmetry in the planum temporale.[6] In Chapter 4, in contrast, we presented evidence showing that the planum is larger on the left side of the brain in 65-75 percent of the general population. Microscopically, the four brains also showed a large number of neural anomalies—dysplasias and ectopias, in the left perisylvian area. These neural anomalies are believed to occur during the second trimester of fetal development when neurons migrate in the developing brain to reach their ultimate location. Another study of three female brains also showed highly symmetrical plana and displaced neurons.[7] The symmetry is not due to a decrease in the size of the left planum, but to an increase in the size of the right planum.

Neuroanatomic imaging methods are also being used to examine cerebral asymmetries. They offer the obvious advantage over autopsy studies of permitting testing of greater numbers of subjects, who can also be tested behaviorally.

Both computerized tomography (CT) and magnetic resonance imaging (MRI) work has recently been undertaken with dyslexic subjects, particularly in the measurement of posterior hemispheric asymmetries. Studies of normal persons show that the left occipitoparietal lobe is generally larger than the right. In studies of dyslexic subjects, both increased symmetry and reversal of normal asymmetry have been reported.[8] In some studies, increased symmetry is due to increases on the right, although others have reported decreases on the left. One study has reported an increase in the area of the posterior corpus callosum, possibly reflecting an increase in the number of fibers connecting with an enlarged right planum.[9]

Functional neuroimaging studies, using positron emission tomography (PET) and regional cerebral blood flow techniques, are also beginning to appear. These studies present control and dyslexic subjects with a simple, language-based task (for example, when presented with word pairs, identify those that rhyme) while activation in different regions is compared with a baseline resting state. Early results suggest different patterns of activation for dyslexic subjects, although it is too soon to identify consistent patterns across tasks, studies, and methods.[10] Particularly exciting are studies that are planned to relate MRI data on temporal lobe asymmetries and corpus callosum structure to patterns of activation measured with PET.

...

Evaluating the Evidence

Overall, the data just presented are highly suggestive of a relationship between brain lateralization and reading disability, although differences among subjects and tasks probably play an important role in the outcome of such studies. Even if this relationship were to be reliably established, however, we could not be sure that the extent or type of brain lateralization determines reading abilities.

Orton assumed that weak cerebral dominance caused reading disability. One could easily argue, however, that some third factor is responsible for the relationship observed and that there is no direct causal link between lateralization and reading skill.

For now, it is important to keep two points in mind when considering the relationship between lateralization and reading ability. First, most subjects who show little evidence of asymmetry (or even reversed asymmetry) on measures of lateralization do not show evidence of reading problems. Second, many subjects with reading problems have normal lateralization, as measured by these tests. Thus, reduced lateralization is neither a necessary nor a sufficient condition for reading problems. Reading difficulties are a complex class of problems to which many different factors may contribute. Similarly, brain lateralization may be but one aspect of a complex of brain functions that provide the neurological substrate for reading.

·········

STUTTERING:
The case for competition for control of speech

Most people have probably heard the claim that it is unwise for parents to force a child showing a natural preference for the left hand to use the right hand. It has been argued that such attempts have potentially serious consequences for the child's overall adjustment, including increasing the chances that the child will stutter.

Samuel Orton played an important role in establishing this idea. Orton believed that in some cases stuttering is the result of competition between the hemispheres for the control of speech. In individuals with well-established cerebral dominance, the left hemisphere assumed control, whereas those with poorly established dominance were at risk for stuttering. Forcing children to switch hands against their natural preference could disrupt the establishment of dominance and result in a stuttering problem. In his own practice with stutterers, Orton observed that children allowed to use their naturally preferred hand after having been forced to use the right hand would stop stuttering.

Stuttering is defined as a disruption in the fluency of verbal expression characterized by involuntary audible or silent repetitions or prolongations in the production of sounds and syllables. It is estimated that about 1 percent of the population stutters to some degree.

What evidence links hemispheric organization to stuttering? One piece of evidence sometimes mentioned is the purported higher incidence of left-handedness and ambilaterality among stutterers than in the general population. Other studies, however, have challenged the figures showing a higher incidence of left-handedness among stutterers.[11]

Some evidence addressing this question more directly has come from dichotic-listening studies. One of the first such studies showed that 55 percent of adult stutterers had a left-ear advantage in a dichotic task, whereas only 25 percent of normal subjects showed a left-ear advantage.[12] Later studies, however, have been unable to replicate these findings with either adults or children.[13]

Another interesting approach has involved stutterers who underwent sodium amobarbital testing for an unrelated neurological problem.[14] In one study, all four patients—three left-handers and one right-hander—showed speech impairment following injection on either side. This result contrasts with the typical sodium amobarbital finding, in which transient aphasia follows injection on one side (usually the left) but not on the other. Moreover, in each case, stuttering was reported to have stopped after the surgical removal, for medical reasons, of one of the presumed speech centers. This finding is perhaps the strongest evidence linking stuttering to the bilateral distribution of speech.

An attempt to replicate the sodium amobarbital work, however, failed to obtain similar results.[15] The subjects in this study were four right-handers, only one of whom showed any evidence of bilateral representation of speech. The fact that even one of the right-handers showed bilateral speech is important, however, for it is extremely rare in normal right-handers. The sodium amobarbital data can thus be viewed as a partial, but certainly not total, confirmation of the idea that stutterers have speech bilaterally represented in the brain.

One might argue, on the basis of the Wada test, that tests sensitive to the lateralization of speech production, rather than speech perception, are best suited to the search for possible differences between stutterers and normal control subjects. In another effort to study lateralization of speech production, Harvey Sussman and Peter MacNeilage have developed a task called pursuit auditory tracking in which a subject hears two tones simultaneously: a target tone in one ear and a cursor tone in the other ear. The subject's task is to track the frequency of the randomly varying target tone with the cursor tone, which the subject can vary through movements of the jaw.

Sussman and MacNeilage found that normal subjects tracked more accurately when the cursor was presented to the right ear and the target to the left ear than when the tones were presented in the reverse arrangement.[16] In contrast, when a group of 28 stutterers was tested, no laterality effects were found.[17] The investigators concluded that these findings were consistent with the hypothesis that stutterers have bilateral control of speech production.

Regional cerebral blood flow has also been used in a limited way to study stuttering. In one study, two stutterers showed reduced blood flow to Broca's area while reading aloud compared with the blood flow in the homologous area of the right hemisphere. When the same task was performed while the subjects received haloperidol, a drug that reduces stuttering in some persons, greater blood flow was found in the left hemisphere.[18]

In a more recent study measuring regional cerebral blood flow in resting subjects, 20 adult stutterers were tested and compared with nonstuttering control subjects. Blood flow was measured in several locations. Overall, stutterers showed reduced regional cerebral blood flow compared to that of normal subjects at all locations measured. For three of those locations, the stutterers showed asymmetry patterns that differed significantly from those of the controls: relatively greater right-side flow compared to left.[19] The authors concluded that stuttering is a neurogenic disorder involving recognized cortical regions of speech and motor control.

Overall, the case for the role of brain asymmetry in stuttering is not as strong as that for its role in reading disability. First, far fewer studies have looked for such a relationship in stutterers. Second, stuttering is now viewed as a disorder with many possible causes, only one of which may be related to brain organization. Differences in subject populations could be a major factor in failures to replicate results, and until we are able to identify specific subgroups, the replication problem will persist.

What of the claim that forcing a child to switch hands increases the likelihood that the child will stutter? At this point, no conclusive evidence even links stuttering and brain lateralization, let alone the notion that switching hand usage at an early age has important consequences for the distribution of language functions between the hemispheres.

·········

AUTISM

Autism is one of the most puzzling of all behavioral abnormalities in children. The classic symptoms of autism include inability to use speech to communicate in a normal way, stereotyped and obsessive movements, and deficient social interaction. The first signs of autism are sometimes noticed when the child is an infant. Such children may be unresponsive to parental handling and do not seem to react to their environment. Other autistic children may develop normally well into the toddler stage, when regression of their sociability, language, and play takes place.

Autism varies widely in severity and prognosis. Intelligent, highly functioning autistic adults may function well enough to live independently and be employed in a sheltered environment. Those with more severe impairment may require lifelong care by their families, in a group home, or in an institution. In most cases, the behavioral deficits associated with autism remain detectable for the life of the individual.[20]

Until relatively recently, autism was seen primarily as a disorder having psychodynamic origins. Faulty patterns of interaction established by the parents were believed to be the basis of the disorder, and attention was focused on the characteristics of the parents of autistic children.

Current approaches to autism focus on its origins in brain dysfunction. Although the nature of that dysfunction is far from clear, several investigators have suggested that the disorder may differentially involve the left hemisphere. One source of evidence that these investigators point to comes from the behavior of autistic children. A salient characteristic of autism is the failure of these children to acquire language normally. Intelligence per se does not seem to be a factor, because even severely retarded (but not autistic) children learn to speak without special training.

Even though autistic children have depressed language skills, they sometimes show considerable artistic or musical ability or extraordinary memory abilities in selected areas. It is not uncommon to find autistic children who are able to tell the weekdays on which a particular date falls over several centuries. The ability to perform elaborate mental arithmetic problems has also been reported. A case history of an autistic girl with extraordinary drawing ability has been documented.[21] At the age of $3\frac{1}{2}$, Nadia was producing lifelike drawings with considerable detail (see Figure 10.2). Like the skills that characterize other autistic children, Nadia's performance was quick and almost without conscious effort. It has been suggested that the nature of these special abilities is a reflection of the contributions of the right hemisphere. Nadia's drawing skills diminished as therapy continued; however, it is impossible to tell whether the change was a consequence of the therapy or would have resulted naturally as she matured.

A limited amount of other evidence is consistent with the hypothesis that abnormal patterns of hemispheric asymmetry are involved in autism. A recent review of the literature that combined the findings of a number of studies on handedness in autistic children reported that 52 percent did not have an established hand preference or were left-handed.[22] Autistic children who had an established hand preference performed better on a variety of cognitive tasks than did children with mixed handedness. These figures point, albeit indirectly, to differences in hemispheric asymmetry between normal and autistic children. They do not, of course, provide any information about the reasons for the

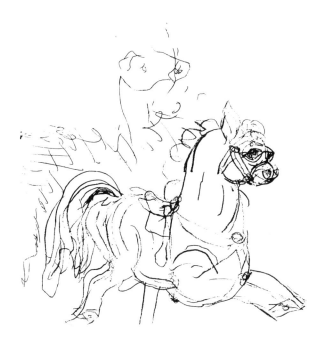

FIGURE 10.2   Horses were among Nadia's favorite subjects. She drew this merry-go-round horse before she was four years old. [From Selfe, *Nadia: A Case of Extraordinary Drawing Ability in an Autistic Child* (New York: Academic Press, 1977).]

differences; early brain damage and genetic factors are both possibilities.

A variety of tests to measure lateralization have been used with autistic subjects. Studies looking at ear preference have typically reported a left-ear advantage or no ear preference for autistic subjects, although the results are not compelling.[23]

A more convincing picture emerges from studies of electrical activity in the brain. A study comparing EEG activity in autistic subjects with age- and handedness-matched normal controls looked at performance in several verbal and spatial tasks.[24] Data were analyzed in terms of the ratio of alpha activity recorded from the right hemisphere to alpha activity in the left hemisphere (R/L ratio). As alpha activity is reduced when a hemisphere is engaged in a task, higher ratios indicate relatively greater left-hemisphere activation, whereas lower ratios indicate relatively greater right-hemisphere involvement. Results showed that the autistic and control groups did not differ significantly in the pattern of hemispheric activation during the spatial tasks, but the autistic subjects showed greater right-hemisphere activity in the linguistic tasks. Seven out of 10 autistic subjects and 3 out of 10 control subjects showed right-hemisphere dominance during the verbal tasks.

A subsequent study with autistic subjects recorded cortical auditory evoked potentials from the left and right hemispheres. Eleven out of 17 subjects showed evidence of right-hemisphere specialization for speech, with right-hemisphere specialization associated with poorer language ability and greater degree of asymmetry.[25]

Because these results supported the hypothesis that inferior language ability in autism is associated with right-hemisphere involvement in language, the investigators postulated that subgroups of autistic children could be distinguished on the basis of their degree of reliance on the left hemisphere for language. One subgroup with severe left-hemisphere dysfunction would rely on the right hemisphere for language, a reliance leading to poor language ability. A second subgroup with a lesser degree of left-hemisphere impairment presumably would still rely on the left hemisphere for language and would show better language functions.

The small number of cases available for study has limited anatomical studies of the brain in autism. New neuroimaging techniques, however, have made it possible to look for both structural and functional abnormalities in vivo. Both CT and MRI studies, however, do not reveal any abnormalities in the cerebral hemispheres or subcortical structures of autistic persons. No statistically significant abnormal frontal or posterior brain asymmetries have been found.[26]

Studies focusing on the cerebellum, however, have found reductions in cerebellar size. Autopsy findings are consistent with the neuroimaging data and have shown Purkinje neuron loss. All such abnormalities appear to be bilateral and symmetric.[27] Functional neuroimaging studies have been few in number and inconsistent to date.[28] Although the cerebellum appears at first to be unlikely as an anatomical correlate of autism, a disorder of higher cognitive functions, recent evidence suggests that an intact cerebellum is important for normal cognitive functions.[29]

What can be concluded about the role of atypical hemispheric asymmetry of function in autism? A review of this topic written before the neuroimaging data became available called for considerable caution in reaching conclusions.[30] Delays in language development, rather than deficits as such, characterize much of autistic speech, the reviewers argued, making the case for left-hemisphere dysfunction weaker. Moreover, they maintained that this type of analysis ignores the deficits of autistic children in the areas of prosody, the social use of language, and the ability to read emotional expression in language. To the extent these functions are lateralized in normal adults, it is the right hemisphere, and not the left, that is involved.

In drawing conclusions from their review, the authors argued that the hypothesis of left-hemisphere dysfunction can be useful if it is pursued on an individual-by-individual basis, rather than looking at entire groups. Although the hypothesis may be useful in some cases, they believed that the neurological deficits in autism may be more variable and more pervasive than what is assumed by the left-hemisphere dysfunction hypothesis.

The newest data from neuroimaging studies suggest additional reasons for caution. We now have evidence suggesting the involvement of the cerebellum in autism, thus complicating the picture further. It is clear that autistic symptoms vary greatly from individual to individual—perhaps there are different forms of autism, with different etiologies or causes. Further research using the tools of modern cognitive neuropsychology should lead to a better understanding of this disorder and to better classifications or discriminations among those grouped together under the label *autistic*.

·········

HEMISPHERIC ASYMMETRY AND PSYCHIATRIC ILLNESS

Within the last 15 years, investigators have begun to explore the possibility that certain psychiatric disorders, particularly schizophrenia and depression, may involve the hemispheres asymmetrically. These ideas mesh well with general notions about the functions of the left and right hemispheres. The thought disorders and verbal hallucinations that are frequently symptoms of schizophrenia fit with the view of the left hemisphere as the analytic, language half of the brain. The mood disorders characteristic of affective illness are consistent with the conceptualization of the right hemisphere as the one controlling nonverbal functions.

···

Observations from the Clinic

One of the first attempts to link psychopathology with a model of hemispheric specialization was made by the psychiatrist Pierre Flor-Henry about 25 years ago.[31] Flor-Henry compared 50 cases of temporal lobe epilepsy that also showed psychotic symptoms with 50 cases without psychotic symptoms. When both groups were subdivided on the basis of location of the epileptic focus, he found that a left-hemisphere focus was more common in schizophrenia and a right-hemisphere focus was more common in affective psychoses.

Although this work has been criticized as weak statistically, other studies have produced results pointing in the same general direction. A large-scale review of the literature on schizophrenialike psychoses and central nervous system disturbance, for example, reported that delusions and catatonic symptoms were most strongly associated with left cerebral lesions, especially temporal lobe lesions.[32]

Of course, most psychoses are not associated with brain damage occurring in adulthood and are believed to be neurodevelopmental in origin. Perhaps, it is argued, dysfunction of lateralized regional brain systems, or abnormal modes of integration between the hemispheres, may characterize such disorders.

Additional clinical evidence comes from findings on unilateral electroconvulsive shock (ECS), used occasionally in the treatment of depression, in which current is delivered through electrodes placed on the scalp. Although the conventional treatment generally has been bilateral, numerous reports have suggested that posttreatment confusion and memory loss frequently accompanying ECS can be reduced by using electrodes placed on only one side of the head. Of three carefully conducted studies comparing the therapeutic effect of left, right, or bilateral ECS, two found the left-hemisphere-only condition to be less effective in relieving depression than the right-hemisphere-only treatment. One study found no difference.[33] The general picture that emerges is one in which depression responds more effectively to right-hemisphere ECS than to left-hemisphere ECS, suggesting an asymmetry in hemispheric involvement in depression.

...

Behavioral, Electrophysiological, and Neuroimaging Studies

A variety of behavioral and electrophysiological techniques have been used to explore the role of brain organization in mental illness. John Gruzelier and his colleagues studied the skin conductance of both schizophrenic and depressed patients in response to repeated auditory stimuli.[34] When a subject is alert and presented with a novel stimulus, the resistance of the skin on the arm to mild electric current decreases. This is one of several peripheral physiological changes that take place when a person is alerted to something new or different.

Among the schizophrenic subjects, most showed little, if any, conductance response in the left hand. In contrast, the response amplitudes of depressed patients were smaller for the right hand than for the left. Because these orienting responses are believed to be controlled by the ipsilateral hemisphere, Gruzelier argued that a left-hemisphere disorder and a right-hemisphere disorder are implicated by his findings in schizophrenia and depression, respectively.

Evidence from postmortem examinations shows a significant increase in the size of the corpus callosum in chronic schizophrenic individuals. Graham Beaumont and Stuart Dimond speculated that the increase reflects compensation for defective interhemispheric communication.[35] To test this hypothesis, they used a tachistoscopic task in which subjects were asked to respond "same" or "different" to pairs of stimuli presented simultaneously. The largest differences between schizophrenic patients and control subjects were found when each of the two stimuli in a pair was presented to separate hemispheres.

Smaller differences were observed when the two stimuli were presented to the same hemisphere. Beaumont and Dimond argued that the difficulty encountered by schizophrenic patients in the task involving both hemispheres is the result of a defect in communication between the two sides. A review of findings with schizophrenic patients generally supported this conclusion.[36]

Recently, psychiatrist Wayne Drevets and colleagues have identified specific brain regions involved in severe depression.[37] Using PET techniques, Drevets measured blood flow in 13 adults suffering from depression at the time of testing and 10 others previously diagnosed as suffering from depression but showing no signs at the time of testing. In all patients, one or more close blood relatives also suffered from depression. Subjects with no history of depression served as controls.

The investigators found markedly increased blood flow (a result indicating increased brain-cell activity) in the left side of the amygdala (a subcortical structure involved in the modulation of emotion) of all depressed subjects. Increases in blood flow were also found in the left prefrontal cortex of all patients currently depressed but not in those in remission. Drevets proposed that elevated blood flow in the left prefrontal cortex indicates that a depressive episode is in progress and that the left prefrontal cortex may process the constant negative thoughts that characterize depression. These data thus implicate special left-sided involvement in severe depression.

...

Theoretical Considerations

Two main models of hemispheric involvement in psychosis have been proposed as a result of work in this area. One is the hemispheric dysfunction hypothesis, in which a given hemisphere is believed to be deficient, possibly in very subtle ways. The psychosis would follow from this deficiency. The second model is the functional hemispheric imbalance hypothesis, in which normal interhemispheric functions mediated by the corpus callosum are thought to be impaired.[38]

It is clearly premature to argue strongly for one model over the other in any form of psychopathology. In fact, although much of the evidence in this area points to some involvement of brain lateralization in psychopathology, each piece alone is not particularly compelling. Like reading disability and stuttering, mental disorders probably have a number of different causes, many of which produce the same overall symptomatology. Perhaps brain asymmetry is involved in some forms of schizophrenia and affective illness but not in all. Careful classification of patients and new technologies to measure brain activity should be particularly valuable in addressing the possible role of brain lateralization in psychopathology.

....

THE ROLES OF THE LEFT BRAIN
AND THE RIGHT BRAIN IN PATHOLOGY

The pathologies considered in this chapter are diverse, ranging from stuttering to schizophrenia. In each case a lateralized abnormality of some sort is believed to exist but has not been unequivocally demonstrated. Before attempts are made to apply research findings to the treatment of persons with problems like those just considered, we must be sure that the findings are firmly established.

We have repeatedly noted the importance of recognizing that many dysfunctions probably have more than one cause. To assume that similar symptoms always result from the same cause is to grossly oversimplify the intricacies of human brain-behavior relationships. Lateralized dysfunction may be involved in some, but not all, forms of a disorder. It is also important to remember that lateralized dysfunction may not be sufficient by itself to result in a particular problem; other factors may have to operate at the same time before a deficit will occur. We have noted that a full range of patterns of lateralization are observed in normal persons, an observation suggesting that particular patterns of lateralization per se are not sufficient causes for certain deficits.

ELEVEN

HEMISPHERICITY, EDUCATION, AND ALTERED STATES

The rapidly growing body of knowledge dealing with the nature of hemispheric asymmetry has led quite naturally to speculation about the consequences of asymmetry for everyday behavior. Does the specialization seen in the hemispheres of normal individuals correspond to distinct modes of thought? Do some people rely more on the left side of the brain, others more on the right? Are there cultural differences in hemisphericity? Do the educational systems of Western Civilization emphasize so-called left-brain thinking and perhaps neglect the potential of the right brain? These are some of the popular issues raised by the discoveries discussed in earlier chapters. In this chapter we shall consider several such issues.

·········

TWO BRAINS, TWO COGNITIVE STYLES?

We have seen evidence that, after the surgical division of the two hemispheres, learning and memory can continue separately in the left brain and the right brain. Each half of the brain of a split-brain patient is able to sense, perceive, and perhaps even conceptualize independently of the other. Furthermore, in virtually every approach to the study of hemispheric processes, including approaches using normal individuals, findings support the existence of hemispheric differences. In earlier chapters we discussed the difficulty in characterizing the differences. Some investigators talked of a verbal-nonverbal distinction. Others argued that the halves of the brain differ in terms of how they deal with information in general.

Since the first split-brain operations, a progression of labels have been used to describe the processes of the left brain and the right brain. The most widely cited characteristics may be divided into five main groups, which form a kind of hierarchy. Each designation usually includes and goes beyond the characteristics above it:

Left Hemisphere	*Right Hemisphere*
Verbal	Nonverbal, visuospatial
Sequential, temporal, digital	Simultaneous, spatial, analogical
Logical, analytical	Gestalt, synthetic
Rational	Intuitive
Western thought	Eastern thought

The descriptions near the top of the list seem to be based on experimental evidence; the other designations appear more speculative. The verbal-nonverbal distinction, for example, was the earliest to emerge from split-brain studies and behavioral research with normal subjects. The sequential-simultaneous distinction reflects a current, although not universally accepted, theoretical model holding that the left hemisphere tends to deal with rapid changes in time and to analyze stimuli in terms of details and features, whereas the right hemisphere deals with simultaneous relationships and with the more global properties of patterns. In this model, the left hemisphere is something like a digital computer, the right like an analog computer.

Many investigators speculating on these issues have attempted to go beyond these distinctions. A popularly accepted view of the differences between the hemispheres is that the left brain operates in a logical, analytical manner and the right brain works in a Gestalt, synthetic fashion.

Once one starts using such labels to describe the operations of the hemispheres, several questions come to mind. Are they just convenient descriptions of how the hemispheres deal with information? Or do they imply that the hemispheres differ in their styles of thinking? Is it possible to view the specialized functions of the left brain and the right brain as distinct modes of thought?

Historically, philosophers and students of the mind have shown a tendency to divide intellectual faculties into two types. For example, consider the following quotation from a Yogic philosopher who wrote, in 1910:

> The intellect is an organ composed of several groups of functions, divisible into two important classes, the functions and faculties of the right hand, the functions and faculties of the left. The faculties of the right hand are comprehensive, creative, and synthetic; the faculties of the left hand critical and analytic . . . The left limits itself to ascertained truth, the right grasps that which is still elusive or unascertained. Both are essential to the completeness of the human reason. These important functions of the machine have all to be raised to their highest and finest working-power, if the education of the child is not to be imperfect and one sided.[1]

Many Western thinkers have also talked of mental organization as if it were divided into two parts. Rational versus intuitive, explicit versus implicit, analytical versus synthetic, abstract versus concrete, objective versus subjective are some examples of these dichotomies.

Why so many two-part divisions? Do they label truly distinct and separate qualities, or do they just describe the extremes of a set of continuous behaviors? In other words, are we dealing with all-or-none differences, or are there gradations in between? Some have insisted on the former view because, they claim, it conforms best to a neuroanatomical reality—the existence of a left brain and a right brain capable of operating independently. Another view is that the formulation of dichotomies or opposites is just a convenient way of viewing complex situations.

Psychologist Robert Ornstein has argued that Western men and women have been using only half of their brains and, hence, only half of their mental capacity.[2] He noted that the emphasis on language and logical thinking in Western societies has ensured that the left hemisphere is well exercised. He went on to argue that the functions of the right hemisphere are a neglected part of human abilities and intellect in the West and that such functions are more developed in the cultures, mysticism, and religions of the East. In short, Ornstein identified the left hemisphere with the thought of the technological, rational West and the right hemisphere with the thought of the intuitive, mystical East. Many outlandish claims and misinterpretations have followed in the wake of Ornstein's position. For example, some have equated the left hemisphere with the evils of modern society.[3]

As we have seen, ideas about the nature of hemispheric differences are diverse. They have evolved from verbal-nonverbal distinctions to ever more abstract notions of the relationship between mental function and the hemispheres. In this process, ideas concerning hemispheric differences have moved further and further away from basic research findings. Some have found this progression disconcerting because the distinction between fact and speculation is often blurred. The term *dichotomania* has been coined to refer to the avalanche of popular literature fostered by the most speculative notions. One investigator has noted:

> It is becoming a familiar sight. Staring directly at the reader—frequently from a magazine cover—is an artist's rendition of the two halves of the brain. Surprinted athwart the left cerebral hemisphere (probably in stark blacks and grays) are such words as "logical," "analytical," and "Western rationality." More luridly etched across the right hemisphere (in rich orange or royal purple) are "intuitive," "artistic," or "Eastern consciousness." Regrettably, the picture says more about a current popular science vogue than it does about the brain.[4]

·········

HEMISPHERICITY

The idea that the two hemispheres are specialized for different modes of thought has led to the concept of hemisphericity—the idea that a given individual relies more on one mode or hemisphere than on the other. This differential utilization is presumed to be reflected in the individual's "cognitive style"—the person's preferences and approach to problem-solving. A tendency to use verbal or analytical approaches to problems is seen as evidence of left-side hemisphericity, whereas those who favor holistic or spatial ways of dealing with information are seen as right-hemisphere people.

Hemisphericity has been claimed by different sources to extend not only to perception but to all kinds of intellectual and personality dimensions. Several years ago, a cartoon appeared in a well-known magazine showing a very fancy country club with a little sign outside reading, "Left Hemisphere People Only." The idea that differences among people may be related to differences in the degree to which they use their two hemispheres is a very appealing one that has captured the fancy of the popular media. Culture and occupation are two areas that have been studied experimentally.

...

The Role of Culture and Occupation

Some attempts by anthropologists to characterize the cognitive processes of different cultures and subcultures seem similar to many notions about the left brain and the right brain. One school of thought suggests that there are qualitatively distinct intersocietal, interclass, and interindividual ways of thinking. Most anthropologists, however, insist that "average" human minds function in the same way, regardless of cultural differences. Some have suggested that there is an inconsistency in simultaneously asserting that the human mind functions the same way everywhere and that fundamental ways of thinking differ radically with cultural background.[5]

One way out of the dilemma is to say that every human brain is capable of more than one kind of logical process and that cultural differences exist with respect to the processes used to deal with various situations. The idea that two different structures within the brain are capable of qualitatively distinct logical processes appealed to investigators interested in resolving the "culture-cognition" paradox.

Can differences in cognitive style between cultures be accounted for on the basis of differences in left- versus right-hemisphere usage? One study compared the performance of 1220 persons of varied backgrounds, including Hopi Indians, urban blacks, and rural and urban whites, on two tests considered reasonably selective in the hemispheric performance they tap. One test, the Street Gestalt Completion Test, is believed to involve primarily processing in the right hemisphere (see Figure 11.1). The other test, the Similarities Subtest of the Wechsler Adult Intelligence Scale, is thought to involve processing primarily in the left hemisphere. A sample question in the latter test is, "How are a screwdriver and a hammer alike?"

The investigators estimated the relative "right- versus left-hemisphere mode of thought" in each subject group by constructing a ratio

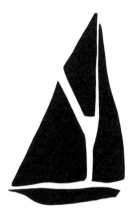 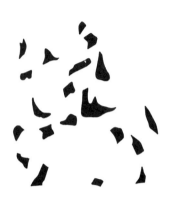

FIGURE 11.1   Examples from the Street Gestalt Completion Test. What do these figures depict?

of the average Street Gestalt/Similarities scores for each group. High ratios (larger numerator) were interpreted as signifying more right-hemisphere thought; lower ratios (larger denominator) were believed to signify greater left-hemisphere thinking. The results showed rural Hopi Indians to have the highest ratio, followed by urban black women, urban black men, rural whites, and urban whites. The investigators concluded that Hopis and blacks rely relatively more on their right hemispheres in thinking than do the other groups.[6]

A critique published soon after this research appeared argued convincingly that the reported cultural differences were a restatement of cultural differences on verbal IQ tests rather than evidence for greater right-hemisphere thinking among often disadvantaged groups. The authors pointed out that no appreciable differences exist between the groups on the Street Gestalt ("right-hemisphere") Test and that the groups differ only on the verbal Similarities Subtest. If one is to interpret the findings in hemispheric terms, they concluded, the only thing that can be said is that "the right hemisphere appears to develop similar levels of ability in radically different cultural groups whereas development of the left hemisphere is depressed by lack of educational opportunity."[7]

Another problem with this and many studies that claim to show patterns in the use of the two sides of the brain is the questionable nature of the measures employed. Although tests such as the Similarities Test certainly seem verbal rather than spatial, it is by no means certain that they are just testing the abilities of the left hemisphere. The situation is even more questionable with many of the standardized nonverbal tests. Many so-called tests of spatial ability have been shown to involve a large and sometimes essential verbal component. At the present time, there are no confirmed right-hemisphere-only or left-hemisphere-only tests.

Of course, these criticisms do not rule out the possibility that in certain situations there are cultural differences in hemispheric involvement. In Chapter 3 we considered the importance of the subject's strategy in determining the outcome of laterality studies. If specific groups consistently use different strategies in a wide variety of tasks, we would expect to find some evidence of those differences in laterality studies. Studies looking specifically for these effects, however, require the use of tests that are sensitive to small differences in hemispheric utilization.

A limited number of studies employing dichotic listening and EEG measures of asymmetry have suggested that this is an area worthy of further exploration. However, the evidence is scanty, and often conflicting. Much more work is needed to determine whether cultural differences in hemispheric utilization are real and, if so, to what they are attributable.

Similar questions regarding hemisphericity can be asked about people in different occupations. For example, do artists make greater use of the right hemisphere than lawyers do? Here, too, a limited number of studies have provided suggestive, supportive findings.[8] However, effects suggesting differential hemispheric involvement as a function of occupation are generally weak and have failed to be replicated in some studies. Differences in the sensitivity of the tests used, as well as variability in the subject populations tested, no doubt contribute to these problems. Further work is needed before a strong statement for or against the notion of occupational hemisphericity can be justified.

It is also important to remember that findings suggesting the possibility of differential hemispheric utilization as a function of occupation do not necessarily support the idea that hemispheric organization per se is different for different groups. Studies supporting the notion of hemisphericity are consistent with the view that the pattern of activation of the hemispheres may vary among groups as a function of occupation but that the underlying asymmetric brain organization is comparable.

...

Can Hemisphericity Be Measured with Questionnaires?

A number of people have developed paper-and-pencil tests that claim to assess hemisphericity. They have asserted that by completing one of these tests and having it scored (frequently for a substantial fee) an individual can determine his or her preferred hemisphere. In turn, they have promised, this will be useful information when selecting a career or a spouse, or when making any other choice where hemispheric compatibility seems desirable.

Managers, in particular, are often targeted as potential users of such questionnaires, with claims that the knowledge gleaned from the results can be used for enhancing the productivity of employees as well as for individual and organizational problem-solving. A whole industry has developed around consultants who provide corporate training seminars that promise new marketing and sales directions as well as greater employee performance and satisfaction, all based on the concept of "hemisphericity."[9] Figure 11.2 nicely illustrates this point.

One hemisphericity questionnaire that has undergone the scrutiny of persons other than its developers is "Your Style of Learning and Thinking."[10] Developed for research purposes by educational psychologist E. P. Torrance and colleagues, the questionnaire has 36 items with three alternative responses per item: one indicating left-hemisphere specialization (for example, not good at remembering faces—inhibited in expression of feelings and emotions), one indicating right-hemisphere specialization (for example, not good at remembering names—able to express feelings and emotions freely), and one signifying an "integrative" style (for example, equally good at remembering names and faces—controlled in expression of feelings and emotions).[11]

A careful look at the questionnaire shows that the scores correlate highly with tests designed to measure creativity. This is not surprising in view of the logic underlying such tests. As the "nonverbal" hemisphere, the right hemisphere is seen as responsible for intuition which, in turn, is seen as a core characteristic underlying creativity. According to this line of reasoning, a test measuring creativity would reflect the degree of right-hemisphere involvement, and hence, hemisphericity.

A similar approach has been taken by Ned Herrmann, developer of the "Herrmann Brain Dominance Instrument (HBDI)."[12] According to his

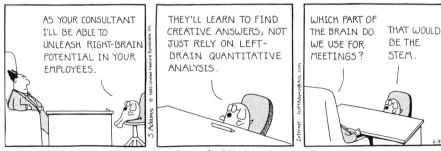

DILBERT reprinted by permission of UFS, Inc.

advertising literature, the HBDI is an "extensive, computer-analyzed, scientifically developed questionnaire that is the word standard for identifying brain dominance." Going beyond a simple left-right dichotomy, Herrmann describes four types of mental preference—analytical/logical, organized/detailed, interpersonal/expressive, and imaginative/conceptual—and promises that understanding these preferences will lead to valuable insights and performance improvements for both executives and employees.

In evaluating the claims that have been made about questionnaires and hemisphericity, we need to separate the possible usefulness of the results from statements that have been made about the questionnaires themselves. Corporate executives may indeed find practical value in the applications that are proposed; they are in the best position to determine whether a particular technique results in greater productivity or enhanced employee satisfaction. What we wish to focus on here is the more basic claim that the questionnaires measure hemisphericity.

A major problem with these claims is that there is little in the way of scientific evidence linking creativity to the right hemisphere, let alone evidence tying degrees of creativity to the degree of right-hemisphere utilization. Before the idea of hemisphericity can be fairly evaluated, we will need good measures of differential hemispheric activity. There are a number of possible candidates for such a measure—ear asymmetries in dichotic listening, evoked potential measures, regional cerebral blood flow—but each currently has problems that limit its usefulness as a measure of hemispheric activity in a particular individual. Such measures, and perhaps others, may ultimately prove useful in testing the notion that each of us relies more on one hemisphere than on the other, but we cannot do so at present. Hemisphericity thus remains an interesting but untested hypothesis.

·········

ALTERED STATES

In the preceding section we explored the possibility of differential hemispheric involvement in different groups of subjects—namely, the idea that certain characteristics of individuals are predictive of the degree to which the two hemispheres will be brought into play in a particular task. In this section, we consider a related idea—that differences in a given individual's mental state will be associated with differences in hemispheric activity. Thus, although the first approach deals with differences between subjects, the second considers differences within a subject at different times. The hypnotic trance and dreaming are two altered states that have received the most attention from the standpoint of hemispheric differences.

...

Dreaming and the Hemispheres

The association between hemispheric activation and dreaming found its origin in occasional reports that patients with brain damage in the posterior region of the right hemisphere no longer had dreams.[13] The right-hemisphere effect fit nicely with the idea that dreams are frequently nonlogical and involve visual images and emotional ideas. Because data depended on the patients' reports, however, the results could be explained in terms of the inability of the patients to remember the dreams that they actually had, rather than in terms of lack of dreams per se. A direct test of the notion that it is the right hemisphere only that is involved in dreaming came from an investigation with split-brain patients discussed in Chapter 2. As the patients slept, their EEGs were monitored for occurrence of dream activity. When awakened at that point, patients were able to report their dreams, thereby indicating that the left hemisphere had access to dream content.[14]

The nature of dreams in split-brain patients has been studied by Klaus Hoppe, a psychoanalyst. Hoppe analyzed the dreams of 12 split-brain patients and reported that "patients after commissurotomy reveal a paucity of dreams, fantasies, and symbols. Their dreams lack the characteristics of dream work; their fantasies are unimaginative, utilitarian, and tied to reality; their symbolization is concretistic, discursive, and rigid."[15]

This description suggests that the left hemisphere lacks access to imagery and fantasy, functions presumably localized in the disconnected right hemisphere. It should be remembered, however, that these patients had epilepsy of long standing, and it would be important to determine how much of these results could be attributed to hemispheric disconnection and how much to other factors.

...

Hypnosis and Hypnotizability

The possibility of differential hemispheric involvement during hypnotic trance first received attention in studies of hypnotic susceptibility. Subjects differ widely in how easily they can be hypnotized, and investigators have tried to determine what factors are involved. The abilities to concentrate and to be absorbed by a novel are two of the factors that positively correlate with hypnotizability. The similarity between these abilities and what is thought to be characteristic of the right hemisphere led naturally to the hypothesis that hypnotic susceptibility correlates with right-hemisphere activation.

Some evidence consistent with this idea has come from a study of lateral eye movements.[16] In these studies, greater hypnotizability was found in subjects showing a preference for leftward eye movements. Eye movements, as discussed in Chapter 3, have been a controversial indicator of hemispheric activity.

Another study looking at the neuropsychological correlates of hypnotizability measured EEG during the performance of a variety of tasks, including spatial orientation, tonal memory, verbal categorization, and mental arithmetic. It was expected that the first two tasks would suppress alpha activity more in the right hemisphere, whereas the second two tasks would suppress alpha activity more in the left hemisphere. The results showed that subjects classified as highly hypnotizable showed a greater shift of cortical activation between the cerebral hemispheres appropriate to the tasks than low-hypnotizable subjects, although most subjects in both groups showed a shift in the appropriate direction. In contrast to the eye-movement data pointing to greater right-hemisphere involvement in highly hypnotizable subjects, these data suggest greater task specific hemispheric involvement in such subjects.[17]

The relationship between handedness and degree of hypnotizability has also been examined.[18] Half of all the right-handed subjects were in the medium hypnotizability category, whereas left-handed subjects were overrepresented in the low- and high-hypnotizability groups. These findings are intriguing because of the relationship between handedness and hemispheric asymmetry, although their meaning remains unclear.

A more direct approach to hypnosis and hemispheric activity has involved looking at hemispheric involvement during hypnosis itself. In one study, subjects listened to dichotically presented speech before, during, and after a hypnotic trance. The right-ear advantage obtained before and after the trance was significantly reduced during the trance, because of improvement in the left-ear scores.[19] These results suggest that hypnosis may involve differential activation of the hemispheres. More research needs to be done, however, before any firm link can be drawn between hypnosis—or any other altered state—and hemispheric asymmetry.

·········

EDUCATION AND THE HEMISPHERES

Does an elementary school program restricted to reading, writing, and arithmetic educate mainly one hemisphere and leave half of an individual's potential unschooled? Is the entire educational system biased against developing right-hemisphere talents?

Joseph Bogen, one of the pioneers of the commissurotomy procedure, has been an especially avid proponent of developing what he calls "appositional thinking" in school.[20] The word *propositional* was adopted by neurologist John Hughlings Jackson in the nineteenth century to describe the left hemisphere's dominance for speaking, writing, calculation, and related tasks. In contrast, Bogen coined *appositional* to refer to the information processing of the right hemisphere in well-lateralized right-handers.

In Bogen's view, society has overemphasized propositionality at the expense of appositionality. Intelligence tests, for example, are aimed at propositional left-hemisphere abilities. Their use is justified by the claim that they predict success in a society that most often measures success monetarily and in terms of productivity. Bogen argued that such measures are very narrow and do not take into account artistic creativity and other right-hemisphere skills that are not easily quantifiable.

The idea that half—more precisely, the right half—of our mental capability is neglected has been appearing with increasing frequency in educational journals, self-help manuals, and a variety of other publications. Articles usually include a background summary of some of the data on laterality along with the author's personal interpretation of what the data mean. Some end with advice about "boosting right-hemisphere thinking" or "training the right hemisphere."

The major business of the left hemisphere, these articles often claim, is the logical representation of reality and communication with the external world. Thinking, reading, writing, counting, and worrying about time are also usually attributed to the left hemisphere. The business of the right hemisphere, in contrast, is said to be understanding patterns and complex relationships that cannot be precisely defined and may not be logical. The qualities of the right hemisphere, an author will state, are essential for creative insight but tend to be inadequately developed.

One writer's statement is representative of a common interpretation of why the right side of the brain is neglected:

> Because we operate in such a sequential-seeming world and because the logical thought of the left hemisphere is so honored in our culture, we gradually damp out, devalue, and disregard the input of our right hemispheres. It's not that we stop using it altogether; it just becomes less and less available to us because of established patterns.[21]

Classroom teachers at all levels have been exhorted to encourage greater right-brain involvement in their students. This has ranged from recommending "show and tell" as an activity that stimulates both sides of the brain, to the use of drawings and graphs to augment "left-brain" text, to spending more time listening to music and looking at art, to the greater use of television as a "right brained input system."[22]

With the possible exception of more television watching, there is little that is controversial about these suggestions. Most primary grade teachers already employ these approaches and find value in them. The problem, as we see it, is the attempt to justify these and other more controversial approaches with claims about what is known about the two hemispheres of the brain.

Our educational systems may be deficient and may limit a broad spectrum of human capabilities. We question, however, the division of styles of thinking along hemispheric lines. It may very well be that in certain stages the formation of new ideas involves intuitive processes independent of analytic reasoning or verbal argument. Preliminary schemes ordering new data or reordering preexisting knowledge could possibly arise from even aimless wanderings of the mind during which a connection is seen between a present and a past event or a remote analogy is established. But are these right-hemisphere functions? We do not think it is as simple as that, and there is certainly no conclusive evidence to that effect. Our educational system may miss training or developing half of the brain, but it probably does so by missing out on the talents of both hemispheres.

...

From Theory to Practice: Learning to Draw

The ideas concerning education and the hemispheres considered up to this point have been very general. In this section, we shall consider two approaches that are much more specific in their recommendations.

Betty Edwards, a California art teacher, has presented her method of teaching people to draw in a book entitled *Drawing on the Right Side of the Brain*.[23] Her basic premise is straightforward: Under ordinary conditions, it is the right hemisphere of the brain that has the ability to draw. When left alone, the right hemisphere will produce very respectable drawings, even in untrained adults. The catch is that for most of us, the right brain is not given the opportunity to display its talents. The verbal, analytical, left hemisphere (lacking in artistic ability) becomes involved and interferes. The natural tendency to label and analyze a picture or a scene before drawing it, in Edwards's view, is the source of this interference.

Edwards's method of instruction is designed to reduce the amount of left-hemisphere involvement in the drawing process. One of her first exercises involves having students copy a fairly detailed pencil drawing of a person—with the picture held upside down. The reasoning is simple. Held upside down, the picture is no longer easily recognizable. In fact, it is difficult to label any part of it. Thus, Edwards proposed, the upside-down copying task is one in which the right hemisphere may proceed without interference from the left. According to Edwards, most adults will be pleasantly surprised when they finish their drawings and rotate them 180 degrees.

There are several stages in Edwards's method, and we cannot do it justice here. Briefly, however, it involves creating conditions to minimize the likelihood of left-hemisphere involvement. As part of this process, she has suggested that the student verbally reassure the left hemisphere that it is not being abandoned and that a new technique is being tried out only temporarily.

Does Edwards's method work? We know of no research that addresses this question, but her book is filled with before-and-after drawings produced by her adult students. The differences are striking. If they are truly representative, then Edwards's method works, and we do not wish to quarrel with success. We do note, however, that at this point there is no way of knowing whether her methods work for the reasons she indicated.

As a general rule, there is no evidence that just one hemisphere is involved in a given cognitive task, including language, which is known to be well lateralized. During language tasks, for example, blood flow is greater to the left hemisphere, but it also increases to a lesser extent in the right hemisphere. There is no reason to believe that this is not also the case for drawing or that the left hemisphere interferes with the right hemisphere as it engages in drawing.

Although split-brain research has shown that the left hemisphere is inferior to the right in ability to draw certain figures, other data show that both hemispheres contribute to drawing, but in different ways. Patients with damage to the parietal lobe show impairments in drawing, regardless of the side of injury; the nature of the impairment, however, varies as a function of side. The left hemisphere appears to be more involved in identification of details and internal elements, whereas the right hemisphere is more involved in orientation, location, and dimensionality.[24]

This analysis of the contribution of the two hemispheres suggests, in fact, an alternative interpretation for Edwards's finding. Rather than producing right hemisphere involvement in drawing by inverting a picture, inversion may result in greater reliance on left-hemisphere skills by encouraging the individual to break the picture up into smaller parts to be copied feature for feature, line for line. As further support for this interpretation, psychologist Lauren Harris noted that upright faces are more likely to be recognized when presented in the left visual field (and hence to the right hemisphere), whereas inverted faces are better recognized when they are presented to the right visual field (left hemisphere).[25] This finding is consistent with the idea that the left hemisphere is better at the analytic, feature-by-feature approach that is required when a face is no longer recognizable as a face.

It will remain for future research to demonstrate why Edwards's method works. For now, the value of the method is independent of its hypothesized mechanism. The value is not increased because of the neuropsychological rationale offered to explain the method, nor does the rationale receive any support because of the method's success.

...

Hemispheric "Therapy"

The idea that atypical patterns of hemispheric asymmetry may be present in certain disorders such as reading disability and stuttering (see Chapter 10) led naturally to the development of educational programs described to be therapeutic. Glen Doman, a physical therapist, and Carl Delacato, an educational psychologist, have developed and promoted an educational program specifically designed for retarded and handicapped children.[26]

The program is known as "patterning" and is based on the assumption that normal cortical dominance develops through a series of stages. The program is individualized for each child and is based on the "level of neurological organization" the child has reached without skipping any developmental stages. Children who are not yet walking are required to spend most of their day on the floor, with crawling emphasized. A team of therapists, parents, and volunteers take turns manipulating the head and limbs of a child who is unable to make the necessary movements alone. Other techniques used in particular children include restricting the use of one arm, occluding one eye, and prohibiting singing and listening to music. The rationale is to develop total cortical dominance extending not only to language but to a dominant eye, hand, and foot.

Although the Doman and Delacato method is still in use, it has been severely criticized on many grounds.[27] First, many of the assumptions they make are known to be false. For example, hemispheric asymmetry, as seen in Chapter 9, most likely is present at birth and does not develop over time. Moreover, occluding the left eye and restricting musical activities are unlikely to result in development of a dominant left hemisphere. Critics also point out that the methods have been promoted in such a way that parents cannot refuse treatment without calling into question their adequacy as parents, and unsubstantiated claims of success have been made, extending even to claims of making normal children superior.[28]

It may well be the case that the "patterning" treatment does have some residual benefits. It is totally unclear at this point, however, whether those benefits are specific to the treatment. After all, any "close supervision, repeated testing, structured environment, and a favorable atmosphere also may produce substantial benefits in IQ and social functioning."[29]

·········

SCIENCE, CULTURE, AND THE CORPUS CALLOSUM

After accepting the distinction that the left hemisphere is analytic and the right intuitive, astronomer-biologist Carl Sagan has gone on to speculate about how the two modes have interacted to generate the accomplishments of our civilization. In his book *The Dragons of Eden*, Sagan described the right hemisphere as a pattern recognizer that finds patterns, sometimes real and sometimes imagined, in the behavior of people as well as in natural events. The right hemisphere has a suspicious emotional tone, for it sees conspiracies where they do not exist as well as where they do. It needs the left hemisphere to analyze critically the patterns it generates in order to test their reality:

> There is no way to tell whether the patterns extracted by the right hemisphere are real or imagined without subjecting them to left-hemisphere scrutiny. On the other hand, mere critical thinking, without creative and intuitive insights, without the search for new patterns, is

sterile and doomed. To solve complex problems in changing circumstances requires the activity of both cerebral hemispheres: the path to the future lies through the corpus callosum.[30]

Sagan went on to suggest that intuitive thinking does well in situations where we have had previous personal or evolutionary experience. "But in new areas—such as the nature of celestial objects close up—intuitive reasoning must be diffident in its claims and willing to accommodate to the insights that rational thinking wrests from Nature."[31] Sagan described science as paranoid thinking applied to nature, a search for natural conspiracies, for connections in data:

> Our objective is to abstract patterns from Nature (right-hemisphere thinking), but many proposed patterns do not in fact correspond to the data. Thus all proposed patterns must be subjected to the sieve of critical analysis (left-hemisphere thinking). The search for patterns without critical analysis, and rigid skepticism without a search for patterns, are the antipodes of incomplete science. The effective pursuit of knowledge requires both functions.[32]

He concluded that the most significant creative activities of a culture—legal and ethical systems, art and music, science and technology—are the result of collaborative work by the left and right hemispheres. We completely agree. Sagan also suggested, "We might say that human culture is the function of the corpus callosum."[33] This may be true, not so much because the corpus callosum interconnects "analytic" with "intuitive" thinking, but because every structure in the brain plays a role in human behavior, and human culture is a function of human behavior.

TWELVE

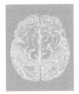

CONCLUDING HYPOTHESES AND SPECULATIONS

A great deal more has been said about the left brain and the right brain than we have reported in the preceding chapters. Speculation concerning the implications of hemispheric asymmetry has followed closely behind discoveries with split-brain patients and other investigations into the functioning of the halves of the brain. This is not surprising, for great indeed is the temptation to account for observations about our own minds and the varieties of human experience in light of discoveries about the brain.

Much speculation has touched on the nature of consciousness. What does laterality research have to offer the age-old question about the relationship between mind and body (or between mind and brain)?

Does it provide any experimental evidence for Freud's concept of the "unconscious"? Does each hemisphere in a split-brain patient possess a consciousness of its own?

In addition, researchers have posed and attempted to answer on a provisional basis a great many theoretical questions concerning the "how" and "why" of hemispheric specialization. Why is language localized in the left brain? What is the evolutionary reason for lateralization? Just how much of one hemisphere is different from the other? To what extent are the many observed asymmetries a consequence of hemispheric differences in language capacity rather than a sign of some other processing differences? Does the verbal left hemisphere truly dominate behavior? Is it instrumental in creating a feeling of mental unity?

The issues are diverse, and discourse about even one topic may operate at several levels. For example, consciousness is an especially confusing topic because the term means different things to different investigators. One calls consciousness a style of thinking or a way of viewing the world. Another may use the term to mean "self-awareness." Yet another may mean all the information of which one is aware at a given moment. Despite these and other problems, in this chapter we shall survey some of the complex and controversial ideas that have emerged as investigators have attempted to theorize about hemispheric differences as well as to extend the implications of left brain and right brain beyond the data.

·········

THE "WHY" AND "HOW"
OF HEMISPHERIC SPECIALIZATION

Although much has been said about what each hemisphere can and cannot do, there is still little understanding of the reasons for hemispheric specialization in the first place. There is also little knowledge about the physiological mechanisms that may underlie these fundamental differences. Dealing with these "why" and "how" issues should help answer the "what" of specialization, a question that has preoccupied us throughout much of this book. It is not clear which question is more important or should be answered first. Insight into any one helps reformulate ideas about the other two. An ultimate understanding of hemispheric specialization undoubtedly will arise from the interaction of successively better answers to all three questions.

In earlier chapters, we mentioned different investigators' speculations concerning the evolution and the mechanisms of hemispheric asymmetry. We now try to bring these speculations together as well as to consider some more recent hypotheses about the nature of hemispheric specialization and callosal function.

...

Is Dominance Based on Motoric Skills?
An Evolutionary Perspective

Why is the hemisphere that controls speech also the one that usually controls a person's dominant hand? Is it a coincidence, or is there a profound relationship that should tell us something about what is involved in both speech and manipulative skills?

Doreen Kimura and her colleagues have obtained evidence that the left hemisphere may be essential for certain types of hand movement.[1] Patients with damage to the left hemisphere but without paralysis of the right side may have difficulty copying a sequence of hand movements and complex finger positions with either the left or the right hand. Kimura suggested that this finding bears a relationship to reports in the clinical literature of deaf-mutes who sustained left-hemisphere damage in addition to their earlier speech and hearing disabilities. These individuals used hand-movement communication, but after damage to the left hemisphere, they displayed disturbances of these movements similar to the disruption of speech suffered by normal speakers who sustain such damage.

Kimura has also studied the gestural hand movements of a group of normal subjects, including individuals with right-hemisphere speech dominance, as determined by dichotic-listening tests. When speech is controlled by the left hemisphere, as it is in most people, the right hand makes more of the free hand movements; conversely, when speech is controlled by the right hemisphere, the left hand makes more of those movements.

Kimura and others have proposed that left-hemisphere specialization for speech is a consequence not so much of an asymmetric evolution of symbolic functions as of the evolution of certain motor skills "that happen to lend themselves readily to communication."[2] In other words, the left hemisphere evolved language, not because it gradually became more symbolic or analytic per se, but because it became well adapted for some categories of motor activity.

It is possible that the evolutionary advantages offered by the development of a hand skilled at manipulation also happened to be a most useful foundation on which to build a communication system, one that at first was gestural and utilized the right hand but later came to utilize the vocal musculature. As a result, the left hemisphere came to possess a virtual monopoly on control of the motor systems involved in linguistic expression, whether by speech or writing.

Although the differences are considerably less striking than in the case of expression, the left hemisphere also appears to be somewhat superior to the right in its comprehension ability. Researchers at the Haskins Laboratories have shown that the left hemisphere is better at decoding the extremely rapid transitions in frequency that are part of certain speech sounds. Using the dichotic-listening technique, they found that right-handed subjects show a right-ear advantage for consonant–vowel syllables such as "ba," "da," and "ga." These differ only in terms of the rapid frequency changes taking place in the first 50 milliseconds or so of the syllable, so the left hemisphere appears to have an advantage in processing this quickly changing information.[3]

Some evidence directly implicating the left hemisphere in the processing of this information comes from a study in which the duration of this information was increased by using computersynthesized speech. In one set of syllables, the frequency changes occurred within the first 40 milliseconds of the stimulus, and in the second set, the information was extended synthetically to 80 milliseconds. Overall identification was not affected by this process, and a significant right-ear advantage for both types of syllables was found when they were presented dichotically. The magnitude of the right-ear advantage, however, was significantly reduced when the stimulus information was extended from 40 to 80 milliseconds. Subjects produced fewer correct right-ear responses and more correct left-ear responses with the 80-millisecond set than they did with the 40-millisecond set.[4]

But is the left-hemisphere advantage simply one of being able to track rapid frequency changes in speech? There is reason to believe that more is involved. Investigators at Haskins have discovered that the rapid frequency changes that signal *b* in the syllable "ba" are different from those that signal *b* in "be" or "bo." Similarly, the acoustic configuration of other consonants also changes as a function of the vowel in the syllable.[5] Figure 12.1 shows the nature of these changes for *d*.

What do all the different *b*'s or *d*'s have in common that allow our perceptual systems to hear them as identical sounds? Haskins researchers noted that they are similar in terms of the way they are

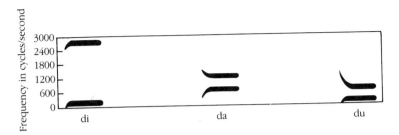

FIGURE 12.1   Idealized spectrogram of sound frequencies produced in voicing "di," "da," and "du." Each sound consists of air vibration concentrated mainly within two frequency ranges, called the first and second formants. Recognizing these sounds involves perceiving the rapid change at the beginning of the formant. Even this early part of the formant changes as the vowel sound changes, despite the fact that all sounds start with *d*.

produced. The similarity in production, they argued, is responsible for the similarity in perception.

This idea—the motor theory of speech perception—holds that to perceive speech sounds, the human brain actually figures out what it would have had to do to produce them. Speech researchers have worked hard to explain what allows speech pronounced in so many different ways to be understood so readily. One quality that seems invariant across any particular sound is the way the throat, mouth, lips, and tongue are controlled in its production. The Haskins researchers proposed that in perceiving speech, a listener is in some manner figuring out how he or she would produce the same sounds. Although this theory is not universally accepted, it is of interest to our discussion, for it suggests that finely controlled motor sequences may be an inseparable part of our language communication system, in terms of both production and perception.

Several neuroimaging studies have provided some surprising support for the motor theory of speech perception. A cortical blood flow study using the xenon-inhalation method reported significant increases in Broca's area during a task in which normal volunteers had to identify words containing a "br" sound in a tape recorded series of words.[6] A recent PET study also reported increases in blood flow in Broca's area during a task in which subjects had to decide whether pairs of speech syllables ended in the same consonant or not.[7] The task in both studies involved only perception of speech sounds and not production of speech. The investigators in both studies speculated that their data suggest an active role for the speech production regions of the brain (including Broca's area) in aspects of speech perception.

What about the right hemisphere? Has it changed during the period in which the left hemisphere acquired its motor and communication skills? Abilities unique to the right hemisphere remain elusive and difficult to define, although spatial ability is strongly implicated. Just as the left hemisphere evolved language, a symbolic system surpassing any single sensory modality, perhaps areas in the right hemisphere evolved ways of representing abstractly the two- and three-dimensional relationships of the external world grasped through vision, touch, and movement. In addition to the spatial tasks considered in earlier chapters, the ability to visualize a complex route or to find a path through a maze seems to depend on the right hemisphere. Although it is usually characterized as more spatial than the left, it is probably more accurately described as more manipulospatial, that is, possessing the ability to manipulate spatial patterns and relationships.

We have just considered how verbal skills may have grown out of the fine-movement skills of the left hemisphere. Perhaps the spatial skills of the right hemisphere are due to another kind of motor skill—the ability to manipulate spatial relationships. Our ability to generate mental maps, rotate images, and conceptualize mechanical contraptions could very well be an abstract, internalized, right-brain counterpart to the motor skills of the left brain.

Are these right-hemisphere skills a result of evolutionary specialization that developed in a fashion complementary to those occurring in the left brain? Or are they more ancient abilities that were at one time bilaterally represented but were essentially displaced in the left by the emergence of language? As mentioned in Chapter 2, different investigators hold different views on this issue. Jerre Levy, for example, has argued that the cognitive processes used for language and for spatial-perceptual functions are incompatible and, therefore, had to develop in separate areas. By analyzing the tasks and questions most difficult for each hemisphere of split-brain patients, she inferred that the left and right modes of processing would mutually interfere if they existed within the same hemisphere.

These kinds of data yield insights into why lateralization took place, but they do not necessarily invalidate the idea that it was mainly the left hemisphere that changed. The issue is not readily decided. Its resolution may depend on much more complete knowledge of what is both common and different about the two hemispheres, as well as the neural mechanisms behind the similarities and differences. Even when we achieve this knowledge, however, it is likely that several equally plausible evolutionary schemes for hemispheric specialization will remain.

...

Evidence for a Linguistic Basis
for Left-Hemisphere Specialization

Another view of hemispheric asymmetry holds that the essence of left-hemisphere specialization is the ability of the left hemisphere to deal with the grammar and syntax of language, and that the left hemisphere is uniquely predisposed for the mediation of language. Researchers at the Scripps Institute have conducted a series of studies with experienced users of sign language, using both deaf and hearing subjects, that support this perspective rather than other approaches that assume that left-hemisphere specialization derives from either the left hemisphere's role in the motor control of speech or its role in the expression and comprehension of symbols more generally.[8]

They employed the dual-task interference paradigm introduced by Kinsbourne, which we discussed in Chapter 3. The procedure assesses the amount of interference in a finger-tapping task as a function of the nature of the concurrent task. Kinsbourne interpreted the interruption patterns as a measure of resource competition with a given hemisphere. In the first phase of the Scripps study, 16 right-handed hearing adults fluent in American Sign Language (ASL) had to repeat a list of one-handed signs while tapping a telegraph key as quickly as possible. This was also done while the subjects spoke English words instead of signing. Baseline tapping rates in the absence of a competing task were also measured.

Results showed that repetition of both words and signs caused a greater drop in right-handed tapping than in left-handed tapping, an outcome suggesting greater involvement of the left hemisphere. When the experiment was repeated with 48 right-handed hearing adults with no knowledge of ASL, participants repeated common words and two types of manual gestures—symbolic (e.g., waving goodbye) and arbitrary (without meaning). Only word repetition produced a disruption in right-handed tapping. Finally, 12 right-handed deaf adults fluent in ASL repeated a list of common signs, symbolic gestures, and arbitrary gestures. Only repetition of sign language resulted in fewer right-handed taps.

The finding that only linguistic tasks disrupt the right hand demonstrates, according to the investigators, that the left hemisphere is specialized for linguistic processing, as distinct from muscle movement or symbolic abilities involved in language. In Chapter 3 we noted that the dual-task interference paradigm is far from completely understood or widely accepted as a tool to measure hemispheric involvement. In addition, the tasks used to assess the possible role of motor and symbolic processing were clearly not comprehensive. However, the findings are intriguing and make a case that bears consideration.

....

THE NATURE OF HEMISPHERIC SPECIALIZATION AND CALLOSAL FUNCTION: Recent ideas

...

The Routine and the Novel

Learning and new-task performance clearly involve dealing with situations in terms of codes and organizational schemes already present in the brain, that is, dealing with "what is out there" in terms of an already established repertoire of ways of describing and organizing events. This repertoire of ways in which an individual brain organizes and understands consists of a whole continuum ranging from biologically fixed visual pattern identification cells to natural language, musical notation, and culturally determined rules of games. Neuropsychologists Elkhonen Goldberg and Louis Costa called these built-in organizational schemes "descriptive systems" and proposed that hemispheric differences in function are rooted in the extent to which an individual's descriptive systems are or are not applicable to ongoing events. They hypothesized that the left hemisphere is highly efficient at processing that takes advantage of well routinized codes, such as the motoric aspects of language production, and that the right hemisphere is crucial for situations for which no readily apparent code (descriptive system) is available, that is, more novel situations. The model also predicts a shift in the hemisphere involved in a particular task, depending on the extent to which the task becomes efficiently performed and routine.[9]

Their model is based partly on observation of the nature of tasks where discrepancies from expected hemisphere involvement seem to appear and partly on some neuroanatomical considerations. As discussed in earlier chapters, not all language-related functions are in the realm of the left hemisphere, nor are all visuospatial functions in the realm of the right hemisphere.*

"Classes of materials may differ in the degree of their relevance to existing descriptive systems, thus forming gradients of relative left–right hemispheric involvement in their processing," according to Goldberg.[10] As an example, he notes that the recognition of line drawings of meaningful objects seems to suffer predominantly after posterior left-hemisphere lesions, whereas the recognition of full photographlike pictures may suffer after either left- or right-hemisphere lesions. Furthermore, the impairment of line-drawing recognition is greater than that of full-picture recognition in left-hemisphere patients. This difference in the involvement of the two hemispheres in processing these two types of materials cannot be explained in terms of language codability—both are pictures of meaningful objects. It can be explained, however, from a perceptual point of view. Line drawings are the visual models of a whole set or class of real objects, whereas pictures are unique representations (or representations of unique objects). The data just described lead to an example of such a gradient for visual perception, ranging from line drawings of symbols to line drawings of meaningful objects, to detailed pictures of meaningful objects, to nonsense shapes, to human faces, with line-drawing interpretation being most left-hemisphere dependent and face recognition most right-hemisphere dependent[11] (see Figure 12.2).

Goldberg and Costa discussed evidence for differences in neuro-anatomical organization of the two hemispheres that may account for two fundamental distinctions in processing. They brought together data suggesting that areas devoted to sensory- and motor-specific functions are greater in the left hemisphere,[12] whereas the right hemisphere is characterized by greater areas of "associative" (higher level, integrative) cortex[13] (see Appendix for a brief discussion of sensory–motor versus associative cortical areas). Combining the data from a study that suggested there is more tissue in the right hemisphere[14] with a study suggesting an asymmetry in the ratio of gray to white matter in each hemisphere,[15] Goldberg and Costa proposed that there is relatively more white matter in the right hemisphere, a condition indicating greater numbers of connections between regions in that hemisphere. Thus, "it appears that there is relatively greater emphasis on inter-

---

It is more the repetitive aspects of language —syntax (grammar) and phonology (sound structure) — that most clearly depend on left-hemisphere function. The right hemisphere appears to have some role in semantics (meaning) and a great deal to do with the contextual aspects of language.

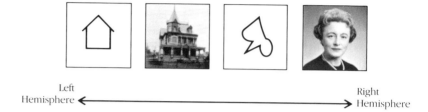

Left
Hemisphere ←——————————————————————→ Right Hemisphere

FIGURE 12.2   An example of visual stimuli that fall into a continuum in terms of left- versus right-hemisphere processing, as suggested by Goldberg et al.

regional integration inherent in the neuronal organization of the right hemisphere, and on intraregional integration in the left hemisphere." In Chapter 1 we mentioned a related conclusion by Josephine Semmes, who proposed that mental processes are distributed over larger regions of brain tissue in the right half of the brain than in the left half.[16]

Goldberg and Costa concluded that, as a result of these anatomical differences, the right hemisphere has a greater capacity for dealing with informational complexity and for processing many modes of representation within a single task, whereas the left hemisphere is superior at tasks requiring detailed fixation on a single, often repetitive, mode of representation or execution.

In summary, Goldberg and Costa argued against assigning fixed hemispheric specificities for particular materials or tasks and emphasized that "there is a gradient of relative hemispheric involvement in a wide range of cognitive processes, reflecting the degree of their routinization."

...

A Model of Callosal Function

In our discussions of models of hemispheric asymmetry of function up to this point, only minimal attention has been paid to the functions of the corpus callosum. In Chapter 2 we talked of the corpus callosum as a means of updating each hemisphere regarding information received by the other or perhaps suppressing one hemisphere while the other "takes over" some activity.

These hypothesized roles, however, lead to some paradoxical questions. As Jerre Levy has observed, if in fact the corpus callosum provides carbon copy-like information by transferring information from one hemisphere to the other, why have the corpus callosum, "if all you need to do is move your eyes around."[17] After all, most split-brain patients seem to do quite well after they recover from the operation. Conversely, if the corpus callosum only inhibits, allowing each hemisphere to function independently, why is it so complex, so intricate in its connections of so many regions of the brain? We need to develop a model that not only explains the need for its detailed connections, as the carbon copy model does, but also explains how these connections provide unique or truly useful information.

Psychologist Norman Cook considered four possible neurophysiological roles for the corpus callosum: two involving reduction of neural activity (inhibition) and two involving enhancement of neural activity (excitation) in the hemisphere opposite to the site of initial activity.[18] Either inhibition or excitation can operate at the global (diffuse) level, slowing down or activating the entire hemisphere, or at the regional level, doing so only in specific regions in a "point in one hemisphere" to a "point in the other hemisphere" manner (callosal fibers do connect corresponding regions of the two hemispheres in a point-to-point or "topographic" manner). Cook contended that neither the diffuse nor the topographic excitation model is sufficient—diffuse excitation would amount to using the callosum for purposes of arousing or alerting the other hemisphere, and topographic excitation would provide carbon copy information between hemispheres. In either case, the corpus callosum would tend to accentuate or duplicate what was already happening in the other hemisphere. Cook believed it must do more than that.

Cook similarly rejected the diffuse inhibition possibility, arguing that it is absurd to imagine so large a nerve fiber tract simply serving to shut down one hemisphere while the other is active. Besides, he argued, there is no electrophysiological or metabolic (e.g., blood-flow) evidence that there is any suppression of overall activity in one hemisphere as the other becomes more active. This elimination process left Cook with the topographic inhibitory model, which he discussed in terms of how it can serve to accentuate functional asymmetries.

To understand his model, we must first accept two assumptions, both of which have considerable support from experimental data. The first is that arousal and attentional mechanisms located deep in the brain tend to activate regions of both hemispheres symmetrically. The brain's main arousal system, the reticular activating formation, does in fact consist of subcortical groups of cell bodies and pathways that are not separated by cutting the callosum. As mentioned in Chapter 4, cerebral blood-flow data have also shown that when there are increases in metabolism, they tend to occur in regions of both hemispheres, even during speech production. The other assumption is that related aspects of some item in memory are represented in the brain anatomically near each other, or at least that access to these related aspects is provided by neighboring neurons.

Cook contended that topographic inhibition across the corpus callosum suppresses in one hemisphere exactly the same neuronal pattern of activity that originated in the other, but at the same time allows activity to develop in surrounding neurons representing complementary (e.g., contextual) aspects of the original information. Figure 12.3 illustrates how this might occur.

In most language-related activity it would be excitation in the left that inhibits equivalent neurons in the right and promotes surrounding context-associated processing. As an example, excitation of the cortical neurons that represent "cat" in the left hemisphere would inhibit "cat" in the right hemisphere while allowing excitation of peripheral cat-related neural assemblies ("kitten, lion, dog," etc.) in that hemisphere. If the ongoing language is, "The cat pounced on the mouse," then not only would individual words produce related contextual items in the right but also the meaning of the left hemisphere's sentence, as a whole, would generate right-hemispheric contextual meaning.

These complementary aspects of whatever item is being processed are the result of a "mirror-image negative relationship" between equi-

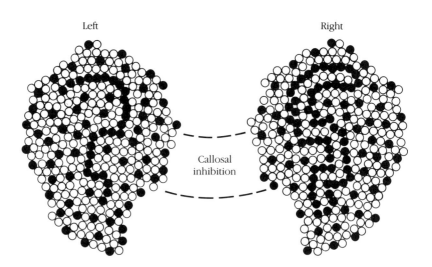

FIGURE 12.3   An example of topographic inhibition, mediated by the corpus callosum, creating a suppression of activity in the same grouping of cells of the right hemisphere that are active in the left. This is accompanied by increased activity in the immediately surrounding neurons in the right hemisphere that are thought to encode related or contextual information. Dark circles represent neurons or columns of neurons that are firing. [From Cook, "Callosal Inhibition: The Key to the Brain Code," Fig. 1, p. 102, in *Behavioral Science*, 1984.]

valent areas of the two hemispheres, created or at least accentuated by continuous topographic inhibition across the cerebral commissures. In the case of language, this implies that whatever the left hemisphere asserts explicitly, the right hemisphere connotes in a more generalized pattern with the explicit message omitted. Thus, by producing two distinctly different patterns of neural excitation within bilaterally identical regions (each of which was aroused by the general attentional system), "callosal homotopic inhibition allows the 'two brains' momentarily to hold different perspectives on the same information."[19]

Language-related examples are just one type of example of how this system works, according to Cook. The idea of complementary functions of equivalent areas extends to other functions including perception where, for example, perception of a visual figure versus its contextual background also operates in a similar manner. Cook's assumption that equivalent (homotopic) areas of the two hemispheres end up active for complementary aspects is supported by what is known about subtle language and cognitive deficits after right hemisphere injury—such as the deficits in context, metaphor, and humor discussed in Chapter 6.

...

Do the Hemispheres Make Use of Different Neural Circuits?

Psychologist S. H. Woodward has proposed a relationship between two different patterns of neuronal connectivity and the specialized functions of the two cerebral hemispheres. Bringing together some theoretical concepts of memory storage and some basic neurophysiological data, Woodward proposed that left-hemisphere processing relies primarily on tight connections between vertical columns of neurons, whereas right-hemisphere processing depends on weaker and longer horizontal connections.[20] Figure 12.4 illustrates the prominent horizontal and vertical dimensions evident in the major layers of cortical neurons and their interconnections. Both vertical and horizontal circuitry have been well studied by neurophysiologists, and there is no conclusive evidence that the connections actually differ in some way in the two hemispheres. What could differ, however, is which kind of circuitry is more utilized in each hemisphere.

Woodward reviewed several modern theories concerning ways to store information and noted the striking parallel between alternative models of memory storage and the kinds of processing horizontal and vertical neuronal connections can offer. Several theorists have examined

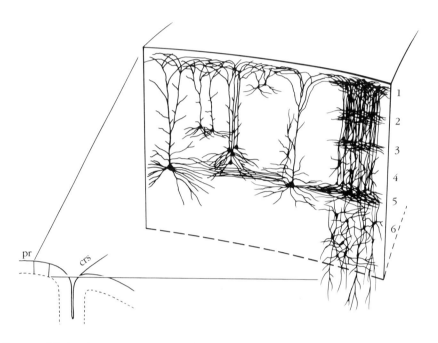

FIGURE 12.4   A cross section through a cortical gyrus illustrating the prominent horizontal and vertical dimensions of assemblies of cortical neurons and their interconnections. The interconnections are formed by both axons and dendrites, mostly from pyramidal cells. [Adapted from Scheibel, Davies, Lindsay, and Scheibel, "Basilar dendritic bundles of giant pyramidal cells," Fig. 1, p. 309, in *Experimental Neurology* 42, 307–319, 1974.]

ways of coding information while concentrating on the extent to which each way is accurate and efficient. Two theoretically different ways of storage that seem relatable to anatomical processes are "conjunctive encoding" and "coarse encoding."[21]

Conjunctive encoding uses a separate definite unit of memory or memory trace (for example, a connection between cells) to stand for every aspect and every important relationship (conjunction) between items. Such an encoding scheme is highly specific but quickly runs out of units. In coarse encoding each elementary unit of memory is broadly tuned, so properties or features specified by a unit overlap to various degrees with those specified by others. Any part or feature of, say, a visually presented item, is then represented by activity in a group of units within whose overlapping representational boundaries it falls.

Although efficient and quite flexible, coarse encoding system breaks down when it has to encode large numbers of highly similar, co-occurrent events.

In idealizing hemispheric differences along these lines, the left is presumed to be dominated by highly coupled, nonoverlapping connections between vertically arranged cell neighbors. Precision coding of small differences, like those needed for articulation or fine motor movements, would depend on this columnar organization. The right-hemisphere anatomy is presumed to be dominated by overlapping horizontal axonal connections, thought to involve greater distances and more cell groups, and to be weaker or less precise than the tight vertical columns of neurons in the left. The encoding potential of this kind of anatomy resembles that of coarse encoding and seems to be more applicable to encoding more diffuse, less repetitive information. The efficiency of coarse encoding increases as features of a stimulus are more dispersed and variable. "These characteristics appear to correspond closely to classical notions of the right hemisphere as excelling in the integration of spatially and temporally disparate features and the representation of stimulus 'wholes and continuities'"[22]

Because the vertical and horizontal anatomies do not appear to be lateralized, Woodward must account for hemispheric differences in physiological use rather than in anatomy itself. Neurophysiologists have shown that activities within a hemisphere tend to suppress or inhibit horizontal connections and that vertical circuitry tends to dominate local cortical patterns. (In fact, in Norman Cook's model of callosal function previously discussed, the surrounding contextual neurons are suppressed in the left hemisphere by inhibition created by initial processing of the stimulus material.)

If vertical cortical circuitry dominates the response to a stimulus, how does horizontal circuitry prevail in some situations? Woodward proposed that this happens through inhibitory signals carried over to the right hemisphere by the corpus callosum. He suggested that in the absence of hemispheric specialization, it is the vertical mode that prevails or is more primary, and that transcallosal input to the right hemisphere permits increasing utilization of horizontal, coarse coding-type storage and processing.

...

Comments on the Callosal Inhibition Models

It is interesting to note the similarities in the function of the corpus callosum postulated by Cook and by Woodward. In both cases the information transferred is mostly inhibitory in nature. In Cook's model the callosal signals suppress "identical patterns" of activity and foster activity in adjacent neurons thought to represent related or contextual information. In Woodward's model, callosal signals suppress vertical neuronal circuitry, thereby allowing the other kind of connections—horizontal—to be used to a greater degree. In both models callosal inhibition serves to suppress in the other hemisphere exactly the same pattern of activity started on one side of the brain and to foster some other kind of activity. In Cook's model, this other activity is highly related to the initial stimuli, so the hemispheres end up dealing with different aspects of the same information. In Woodward's model the callosal signals bias the way in which the right hemisphere deals with information in general.

·········

TWO BRAINS, TWO MINDS?

More than four centuries ago, the great French philosopher Rene Descartes concluded that the pineal gland, at the base of the brain, is the seat of consciousness. He based his conclusion on his belief in the unity of consciousness and on the fact that the pineal gland was the only brain part he could find that was not double in structure.

Assigning consciousness to part of the body seems an inconsistent twist in Descartes's thinking if one examines his writings on the relationship between body and mind. Although Descartes enjoyed mechanically analyzing some of the functions of living things and had great interest in human anatomy (see Figure 12.5), he felt there was something about human beings that could not be explained in these terms. He saw the human body as similar to the bodies of animals, but he questioned whether the human mind could be part of the same physical world. An analysis of one's own thought, he felt, cannot prove the existence of anything outside personal experience. Descartes concluded that an absolute distinction must be made between the mental and the physical.

The assertion that the mind is independent of the body came to be known as Cartesian dualism. Some modern skeptics have referred to it as the "ghost in the machine" idea. The philosophical issues revolving around the relationship between body and mind in general are referred to as the mind–body problem.

Within the past two and a half decades, work with split-brain patients has raised questions about the implications of split-brain surgery

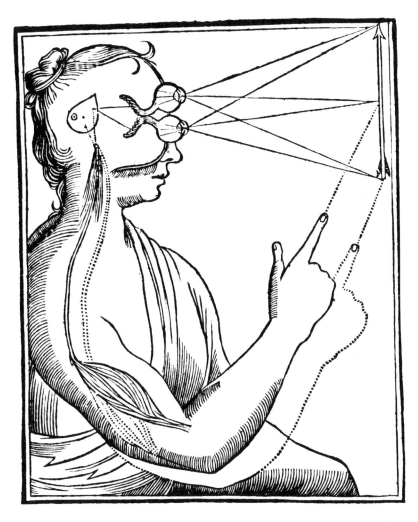

FIGURE 12.5   Descartes' diagram illustrating the interaction of mechanistic and mental processes in the pineal body. Light reflected from an object (an arrow) is imaged on the retinas of the eyes and conducted by the optic nerves to the brain. There, it is apprehended by the soul at the pear-shaped pineal body, which also initiates responsive movements. [Reprinted by permission of Sandford Publications, Oxford, England.]

for the mind–body problem. If the surgeon's knife accomplishes a separation of consciousness, then splitting the brain is splitting the mind. One is then forced, the argument goes, to accept the fact that mind is brain, or at least that mind arises from the workings of the brain.

Although one can argue with the premise that split consciousness implies mind is brain, most of the controversy in this areas focuses on whether such patients can actually be shown to possess two realms of consciousness, at least some of the time. In Chapter 2 this question was discussed on a theoretical level by Gustav Fechner and William McDougall. Fechner argued that the split-brain operation would result in a doubling of consciousness. McDougall argued that consciousness would remain unaffected by such a procedure.

Roger Sperry has argued that the results of split-brain research point to a doubling of consciousness in these patients:

> Everything we have seen so far indicates that the surgery has left these people with two separate minds, that is, two separate spheres of consciousness. What is experienced in the right hemisphere seems to lie entirely outside the realm of experience of the left hemisphere. This mental dimension has been demonstrated in regard to perception, cognition, volition, learning, and memory.[23]

For Sperry, the impression of mental unity in split-brain patients is an illusion, a consequence of the sharing by the two sides of the brain of the same position in space, the same sensory organs, and the same experiences in everyday situations outside the lab.

In contrast, Sir John Eccles (also a Nobel laureate, for his work in physiology) denied that there are two separate minds in a split-brain patient or that consciousness is in any way split by commissurotomy.[24] He claimed that the right hemisphere cannot truly think. He made a distinction between "mere consciousness," which humans share with animals, and the world of language, thought, and culture, which is uniquely human and essential to any idea of a mind.

In Eccles's opinion, everything that is truly human derives from the left hemisphere, where the speech center resides and where interactions between brain and mind occur. The split-brain patient who blushes or smiles when a pinup is flashed to her right hemisphere not only cannot report why she did so but truly does not know why she blushed. The right hemisphere cannot know because only the left hemisphere can have thoughts or knowledge.

Although such controversies are highly confounded by subjective definitions of consciousness, some attempts have been made to be more precise in using this term. One approach is to form an operational definition, which is a definition in terms of the procedures that may be used to measure a concept. Along these lines, Donald McKay, whose primary field is artificial intelligence, has noted that the split brain cannot be viewed as a split mind until it can be shown that each separated half has its own independent system for assigning values to events, setting goals, and establishing response priorities.

An experiment to address this point was conducted by Joseph LeDoux and Michael Gazzaniga with their unique commissurotomy patient, P.S. The study took advantage of the considerably greater than usual linguistic capabilities in P.S.'s right hemisphere which was able to express itself by arranging Scrabble letters with the left hand in response to questions. LeDoux and Gazzaniga's intention was to ask subjective questions of each hemisphere separately and to compare the results.

On each trial, P.S. was asked a question orally. The key word or words were replaced by the word "blank." The missing word or words were then visually presented in either the left visual field (to the right hemisphere) or in the right visual field (to the left hemisphere). The questions included, "Who (*are you*)?" "Would you spell the name of your favorite (*hobby*)?" "What is (*tomorrow*)?" The italicized items were the key words actually flashed in the respective visual field. When they were presented to the right hemisphere, P.S. was asked to spell out his answers using the Scrabble letters.

P.S. was also asked to rate how he felt about a particular word by pointing to a number from one (like very much) to 5 (dislike very much). Some of the words were chosen because of their personal significance to the patient. They included "Paul" (his name) and "Liz" (his girlfriend's name). A sample question is, "How much do you like ?" A word would then appear in either the left or the right visual field.

The results showed both that P.S.'s right hemisphere could answer the questions asked and that its answers and evaluations sometimes differed from those of the left hemisphere. For example, ratings by the right hemisphere were consistently closer to the "dislike" end of the scale in the word-rating test than were those by the left hemisphere. When asked the job he would pick, the right hemisphere spelled out "automobile race," in contrast to P.S.'s normal left-hemisphere verbal assertion that he wanted to be a draftsman.

Regarding the issue of double consciousness, the investigators stated:

> Each hemisphere in P.S. has a sense of self and each possesses its own system for subjectively evaluating current events, planning for further events, setting response priorities, and generating personal responses. Consequently, it becomes useful now to consider the practical and theoretical implications of the fact that double consciousness mechanisms can exist.[25]

Although P.S. is a special case because of the extent of verbal capabilities in both his hemispheres, the theoretical implications of demonstrating an apparent double consciousness in the same person extend beyond this one case. In addition to illustrating the older claim that splitting the brain can split the mind, LeDoux and Gazzaniga felt that their observations suggest "the nature and origin of those mental qualities unique to man." These, they feel, are dependent on an active language system:

> When this system is absent, as in the right hemisphere of most split brain patients, . . . the organism functions mainly at the perceptual motor level. Though certain cognitive skills can be demonstrated in such instances, the richness and characteristic flexibility of human behavior seems to be lacking in the absence of linguistic sophistication. . . Add a rich linguistic system to an isolated mass of non-verbal tissue as in the right hemisphere of P.S., and a human being with the capacity to value, aspire, and reflect on life experience emerges.[26]

The idea that consciousness is dependent on language or linguistic processes is not entirely new. Several philosophers and linguists have subscribed to so-called verbal access theories of consciousness. These theories have in common the concept that the brain events experienced as conscious are the events processed by the language system of the brain.

. . . .

CONSCIOUSNESS AND THE HEMISPHERES

. . .

The Origins of Consciousness: Verbal Access Theories

Until as recently as 3,000 years ago, members of the group *Homo sapiens* were virtually automatons, lacking both a concept of self-fulfillment and a sense of the brevity of life. They heard voices inside their heads and called them gods. These gods told them what to do and how to act. Their minds were divided into two parts: an executive part called "god" and a follower part called "man." When writing and more complex human activity started weakening the authority of the auditory hallucinations, this "bicameral mind" slowly broke down. The voices of the gods fell silent, and what we call consciousness was born.

This is the radical theory of Princeton psychologist Julian Jaynes. Jaynes proposed that the speech of the gods occurred in the right hemisphere and was heard by the auditory and speech centers of the left hemisphere by means of the cerebral commissures. Perhaps, he suggested, the pattern-recognition and spatial-processing mechanisms of the right hemisphere were communicating with the left hemisphere through primitive language.

Jaynes supported many of his contentions by reference to ancient literature and to history. He felt that the *Iliad,* for example, describes a people who are not conscious. They do not decide to fight, and they do not plan strategy or do anything else without the intervention of a god or some hallucination.

> These auditory and visual hallucinations, occurring whenever a novel situation arose, show us the structure of the bicameral mind. Achilles, like all bicameral people, had a split mind. One part, the executive god part, stored up all admonitory experience and fitted things into a pattern and told the follower or person part what to do through an auditory hallucination.[27]

To Jaynes, consciousness depends on linguistic processes and the creation of an internal, metaphorical "I." Consciousness is a smaller part of our mental life than previously assumed. A great deal of our mental activity is not conscious but automatic: We do not think about it. This is one reason why it should not be so difficult to imagine ancient humans going through life without the "self-consciousness" we have developed. They may not have been able to view themselves at a distance or to imagine themselves doing something in the future.

> Consciousness is learned on the basis of language and taught to others. It is a cultural invention rather than a biological necessity. . . We know now that the brain is more plastic, more capable of being organized by the environment than we previously supposed. . . We can assume that the neurology of consciousness is plastic enough to allow the change from the bicameral mind to consciousness to be made largely on the basis of learning and culture.[28]

Although there is considerable controversy concerning Jaynes's theory, the idea of connecting the voices of gods in ancient times to a stage in the cultural development of language is fascinating. In addition to his view, there are other ways in which the development of language may have been responsible for some of the earlier beliefs of human beings. Instead of equating the voices of the gods with the right hemisphere's attempt to speak to the left, ancient men and women can be viewed as having misinterpreted internalized speech developing in the left hemisphere. It is possible that in the early phases of the evolution of language, humans were caught off guard by the fact that they could speak to themselves.

...

Some Alternative Opinions About the Role of Language in Conscious Thought

Jaynes's theory is a bold example of theories dealing with the topic of consciousness in terms of linguistic mechanisms. In our discussion of speculation about the implications of split-brain research so far, we mentioned several prominent investigators who felt that the left hemisphere was responsible for consciousness because it possessed the verbal skills "necessary" for consciousness. Not all current researchers and theorists believe that language is a prerequisite for consciousness, or for thought. Some writers have impressively refuted the idea that verbalization is necessary for thought.[29] One quoted a letter he received from Albert Einstein on the matter:

> The words or the language, as they are written or spoken, do not seem to play any role in my mechanism of thought. The psychical entities which seem to serve as elements of thought are certain signs and more or less clear images which can be 'voluntarily' reproduced and combined ... The above mentioned elements are, in my case, of visual and some muscular type. Conventional words or other signs have to be sought for laboriously only in a second stage, when the mentioned associative play is sufficiently established and can be reproduced at will.[30]

The eminent geneticist Francis Galton also wrote:

> It is a serious drawback to me in writing, and still more in explaining myself, that I do not think as easily in words as otherwise. It often happens that after being hard at work, and having arrived at results that are perfectly clear and satisfactory to myself, when I try to express them in language I feel that I must begin by putting myself upon quite another intellectual plane. I have to translate my thoughts into a language that does not run very evenly with them. I therefore waste a vast deal of time in seeking appropriate words and phrases, and am conscious, when required to speak on a sudden, of being often very obscure through mere verbal maladroitness, and not through want of clearness of perception. That is one of the small annoyances of my life.[31]

Others have also contended that words and verbal mechanisms cannot be equated with thought or consciousness. The mathematician Hadamard claimed that words were totally absent from his mind when he really thought and that every word he read or heard disappeared the moment he began to think it over.[32] The philosopher Schopenhauer probably expressed this general viewpoint most adamantly when he wrote, "thoughts die the moment they are embodied by words."[33]

...

The Right Hemisphere and the Unconscious

Arthur Koestler, a well-known writer, argued that the "creative act" usually occurs through other than conscious analytic intention. In his book *The Act of Creation,* Koestler mentioned the idea of incubation periods: putting a problem aside for a time in the hope of coming up with an insight later. He also suggested that the unconscious does a great deal of matchmaking or forming of analogies.

Several famous scientists have told how they found a solution to a problem during a dream. Otto Loewi, who won the 1936 Nobel Prize in Physiology or Medicine for showing that nerve impulses are transmitted by means of chemical agents, described how the critical experiment came to him in a near-sleep state. He had come up with the idea of chemical transmission 17 years earlier but had put it "aside" for lack of a way to test it. Fifteen years later he performed experiments (unrelated to his old idea) for which he had designed a technique to detect fluids secreted by a frog's heart. One night, two years later:

> I awoke, turned on the light, jotted down a few notes on a tiny slip of thin paper. Then I fell asleep again. It occurred to me at six o'clock in the morning that during the night I had written down something most important, but I was unable to decipher the scrawl. The next night, at three o'clock, the idea returned. It was the design of an experiment to determine whether or not the hypothesis of chemical transmission that I had uttered seventeen years ago was correct. I got up immediately, went to the laboratory, and performed a simple experiment on a frog heart according to the nocturnal design.[34]

Loewi isolated two frog hearts, the first with its nerves intact, the second without. He stimulated the vagus nerve of the first heart. The vagus nerve has an inhibitory effect on the heart, so its beat slowed down. He immediately removed some of the salt solution in which the heart was bathed and applied it to the second heart. It slowed down. By going a few steps further, Loewi unequivocally proved that nerves influence the heart (and most other tissue) by releasing specific chemical substances from their terminals.

A careful review of the chain of events leading to Loewi's experiment dispels any notion that it was an accidental or purely intuitive discovery. The background for it had been set by years of rigorous work. However, the act of connecting two critical ideas apparently came while he was in an unconscious or semiconscious state.

Koestler attributed a role to the unconscious in discovery, calling it the "type of thinking prevalent in childhood and in primitive societies, which has been superseded in the normal adult by techniques of thought which are more rational and realistic."[35] As for the incubation period (such as the 17-year period in Loewi's case), Koestler called it "thinking aside" or a rebellion against constraints that is "a temporary liberation from the tyranny of overprecise verbal concepts, of the axioms and prejudices ingrained in the very texture of specialized ways of thought."[36]

The temptation to reinterpret such ideas in terms of the laterality data is obviously great. Several investigators have suggested that dreaming is part of the realm of the right hemisphere. Some have proposed that the right hemisphere does all the dreaming; others proposed that the dream state allows the right hemisphere to express itself more freely than usual because the left hemisphere does not dominate or interfere. Sigmund Freud, the father of psychoanalysis, believed that the qualities of the unconscious mind are revealed through the logic of dreams.

Do the discoveries with split-brain patients have any consequences for Freud's theories? David Galin has suggested they do. According to Galin, they provide a neurological validation for Freud's notion of an unconscious mind. Galin pointed out that the right hemisphere's mode of thought is similar to Freud's description of the "unconscious," and he noted a parallel between the functioning of the isolated right hemisphere and mental processes that are repressed, unconscious, and unable to control behavior directly: "Certain aspects of right hemisphere functioning are congruent with the mode of cognition psychoanalysts have termed primary process, the form of thought that Freud originally assigned to the system Ucs (unconscious)."[37] These include the extensive use of images, lesser involvement in the perception of time and sequence, and a limited language of the sort that appears in dreams and slips of the tongue.

Galin believed that the two hemispheres usually operate in an integrated fashion, but at certain times they may be blocked from communicating with each other. As a result, a situation similar to what is found in split-brain patients may occur in a normal individual. Galin described several ways in which the two hemispheres of an ordinary person could function as if they had been surgically disconnected. In one interesting example, he talked of the inhibition of information transfer because of conflict: "Imagine the effect on a child when his mother presents one message verbally, but quite another with her facial expression and body language; 'I am doing it because I love you, dear' say the words, but 'I hate you and will destroy you,' says the face."[38]

Galin believed that although each hemisphere is exposed to the same sensory input, it effectively receives a different input because each emphasizes only one of the messages. The left will attend to the verbal cues, and the right will attend to the nonverbal cues. He continued with the following conjecture:

> In this situation, the two hemispheres might decide on opposite courses of action; the left to approach and the right to flee. . . The left hemisphere seems to win control of the output channels most of the time, but if the left is not able to "turn off" the right completely, it may settle for disconnecting the transfer of the conflicting information from the other side. . . Each hemisphere treats the weak contralateral input in the same way in which people in general treat the odd discrepant observation that does not fit with the mass of their beliefs; we first ignore it, and then if it is insistent, we actively avoid it.[39]

Galin believed that during such moments of disconnection, the left hemisphere alone governs consciousness. Mental events in the right hemisphere, however, continue a life of their own and act as a "Freudian" unconscious, as an "independent reservoir of inaccessible cognition," which may create uneasy emotional states in a person.

It is interesting to note that LeDoux and Gazzaniga made some anecdotal observations about their patient P.S. that seem psychodynamic in nature. They referred to the experiments where they addressed subjective questions to P.S.'s left and right hemispheres separately:

> The day that case P.S.'s left and right hemispheres equally valued himself, his friends, and other matters, he was a calm, tractable, and appealing adolescent. On the days that the right and left sides disagreed on these evaluations, case P.S. became difficult to manage behaviorally. Clearly, it is as if each mental system can read the emotional differences harbored by the other at any given time. When they are discordant, a feeling of anxiety, which is ultimately read out by hyperactivity and general overall aggression, is engendered. The crisp surgical instance of this dynamism raises the question of whether or not such processes are active in the normal brain, where different mental systems, using different neural codes, coexist within and between the cerebral hemispheres.[40]

...

From Split Brain to Normal Brain:
A Case for Mental Duality in Both

When the word *teacup* is projected tachistoscopically on a screen, with *tea* presented to the left and *cup* to the right of a fixation point, a split-brain patient cannot read the whole word. Instead, the patient will say the word was *cup,* because the verbal left hemisphere saw what was to the right of fixation (the right visual field). The patient's left hand, under control of the mute right hemisphere, will point to the word *tea* in an array of words that includes *cup* and *teacup.* Some theorists feel this situation is a convincing argument for the duality of mind in the split-brain patient. Roland Puccetti argued that the patient's responses indicate a true perceptual experience in each hemisphere. "So here it appears that what is going on in each hemisphere is not just an initial registration of the visual material but a reading out—verbally in one case, manually in the other—of what was actually seen."[41]

But Puccetti went beyond the issue of whether there are two minds in a split-brain patient to propose that, in fact, double consciousness is the normal situation in humans without the operation. In the intact human brain, under the same experimental conditions, the word *teacup* is seen at the same time in both hemispheres, one half of the word coming directly to each hemisphere and the other half coming indirectly via the corpus callosum (see description of the visual system in Chapter 2). Why then, Puccetti asked, does the subject not see *teacup teacup* instead of just *teacup,* if consciousness spans both hemispheres?

Some would answer that the duplication is only in the initial sensory registration of the stimulus that is not at a conscious level — the double sensory representations are fused in the processing that leads to our "seeing" the stimulus. Puccetti contended, however, that each hemisphere normally does "see" the whole visual field; that is, each hemisphere is conscious of *teacup* just as each hemisphere is conscious of half that word when the corpus callosum is split. Thus, cutting the corpus callosum does not in itself produce a divided mind but, rather, only deprives two existing minds of half their normal visual input (the ipsilateral half-field), subsequent to which the separate consciousnesses become evident. In the intact brain, neither half-brain has introspective access to the conscious contents of the other. The callosal connections do not provide this; rather, they provide transfer of more basic sensory information.

Puccetti explained his view of two separate centers of visual awareness by drawing an analogy with two side-by-side observers of a football game. Each observer sits in a booth that provides a direct window
view of half the field and a television view, similar in size and adjoining
the window, of the other half. The window-view half for each observer
is the television view for the other. If the television cables are cut, each
observer loses sight of the half of the football field that the other sees
directly through the window.

> Yet nothing in the visual experience of either of the viewers, before or
> after the cables are cut, provides any introspective evidence that there
> are really two of them, side by side. Indeed as Gazzaniga [1970] has
> pointed out, following split-brain surgery, the speaking viewer to the
> left initially does not even notice that half the field is gone.[42]

But why this duplication of conscious experience? Puccetti claimed,
as others have, that duplication has to occur at the sensory level, that
each half-brain must supply information about what it is seeing to the
other half. "How much more efficient it is if nature wires in a relay
system so that each half-brain sees the same visual target in the same
place in extrabodily space at almost the same time."[43] But at the same
time, he contended, conscious unity must be confined to each hemisphere; otherwise, there would be a doubling of the sensory field at a
conscious level, and this would be counterproductive when dealing with
any visual target. Thus, there is no overall mind spanning the two
half-brains.

Why is it that we are not aware of two separate conscious entities
within our heads? Why do the two half-brains seem to work so well
together? Puccetti felt that the cross-cuing phenomenon provides part
of the answer. Experiments with split-brain patients have shown that
the disconnected left (verbal) hemisphere will actually claim possession
of material presented to only the right hemisphere. A transcript from a
session with commissurotomy patient L.B., whose mute right hemisphere had just been shown a picture of his mother, helps illustrate this:

Examiner: "Do you know who it is?"

L.B.: "Uh-huh," in an affirmative tone.

Examiner: "Can you name it? Who is it?" When subject hadn't
answered after several seconds, examiner added, "Don't know who?"

L.B.: "I know who, but I can't verbalize it."

Examiner: "Can you give the name?"

L.B.: "I know I can spell it but you won't let me spell."[44]

L.B.'s left hand could spell out "Mom" under control of the mute right hemisphere, but the examiner did not allow this. The right hand could not do this, even though it is the talking left hemisphere that claims it can be done. What is significant is that "the verbal half brain insists it has this knowledge, under the surface somewhere, and implies that there is no other conscious center that has it."[45]

Puccetti also argued that the right hemisphere's continuing to faithfully cue the speaking hemisphere, as in a game of charades, under such experimental conditions attests to its lifetime role in a secondary position to the left hemisphere in most matters of communication with the outside world. Little is changed for the mute right hemisphere after commissurotomy. Occasionally it can undertake an independent action with the left arm or leg but on the whole has no way of expressing itself except through providing information to the left hemisphere.

Puccetti's hypothesis of duality of consciousness in the normal brain, as one may expect, has a large number of critics. Nevertheless, it is an interesting approach to questions brought to mind by split-brain research.

...

What Kind of "Selves" Are Hemispheres?

Philosopher Daniel Dennett has mocked the personalization attributed to brain parts:

> So what is it like to be the right hemisphere self in a split-brain patient? This is the most natural question in the world, and it conjures up a mind-boggling—and chilling—image: there you are, trapped in the right hemisphere of a body whose left side you know intimately and still control and whose right side is now as remote as the body of a passing stranger. You would like to tell the world what it is like to be you, but you can't! You're cut off from all verbal communication by the loss of your indirect phone lines to the radio station in the left hemisphere. You do your best to signal your existence to the outside world, tugging your half of the face into lopsided frowns and smiles, and occasionally (if you are a virtuoso right hemisphere self) scrawling a word or two with your left hand.[46]

Dennett goes on to say that this exercise in imagination simply is not the case because commissurotomy does not leave in its wake organizations both distinct and robust enough to support such a separate self. The conditions for accumulating the sort of narrative richness and independence that constitutes a "fully fledged" self are not present:

> For brief periods during carefully devised experimental procedures, a few of these patients bifurcate in their response to a predicament, temporarily creating a second center of narrative gravity...the life of the second rudimentary self lasts a few minutes at most, not much time to accrue the sort of autobiography of which fully fledged selves are made.[47]

Philosopher—psychologist Daniel N. Robinson of Georgetown University also argued that issues pertaining to the unity of consciousness are largely unaffected by split-brain data.[48] He pointed out that the issue is older and deeper than contemporary commentators generally acknowledge, and that examination of historical versions of the dispute reveal insights and confusions similar to those now filling the pages of contemporary journals. Much of the confusion has to do with questions of definition—words that have quite different meanings are used interchangeably, leading not only to confusion but to subtle deceptions.

Robinson acknowledged the scientific merit of new findings and theories regarding the lateralization of psychological processes. However, he saw only one consistent finding in research with split-brain patients that can be claimed to have relevance to issues of "split selves" or "double consciousness." This, he said, is the personal state of "epistemic contradiction," the contradictory knowledge-claims sometimes encountered in the testing of commissurotomized patients. The same patient, often at nearly the same time, will assert and deny a specific claim or fact of memory: "The left hand, as the expression goes, may not know what the right one is doing, or as today's commentator would say, the left brain doesn't know what the right one is saying, because the right one cannot speak." These contradictions "are used in defense of the notion of the disunity or multiplicity of self or," Robinson went on, "the duality of self, apparently because there happen to be two hemispheres."

The plain fact, Robinson argued, is that any number of experimental operations produce just this state in perfectly normal observers. For example, observers under certain cuing conditions will "recall" a number or a letter that, after it was initially presented briefly in an array, they could not recognize at all.[49] In certain psychophysical experiments observers will respond just as quickly to a flash they claim they do not "see" as to the same flash when it is presented alone.[50] Robinson mentioned other examples such as "hysterical" patients who adopt entirely distinct identities, sleep walkers who complete elaborate actions and do not recall anything about it afterward, and hypnotic subjects who deny what they know.

> For those who would use such findings as proof of a multiplicity of selves, there is an embarrassment of riches to which commissurotomies add very little, but for those committed to the duality thesis, the findings are actually too good for the thesis to be true. States of epistemic contradiction are, as it happens, not limited to two per person. Recall Eve's three faces, and Binet[51] turned up cases involving many more. Needless to say, however, none of these cases included any evidence of more than two hemispheres.[52]

The real problem, Robinson contended, has to do with meanings and interchangeable use of such words as "self," "self-identity," "personal identity," and "person." A person is a human being, often of unknown identity, possessing certain attributes not present to the same degree in the rest of the animal kingdom—a collection of attributes shared by many entities of a certain kind. One can answer "it is a person" to a what question.

To know who that person is we must go beyond the attributes that established personhood and establish the personal identity. If we inquire as to name, occupation, address, and details of a person's life, we may assert that we know the actual identity of the person — the personal identity. This is different from self-identity, however, because, for example, that specific person may be amnesic and therefore ignorant of the very identity we established. Nevertheless, the amnesic person is not doubtful of existing and "surely must be granted a self, and will claim as much whether we grant it or not."

Robinson contended that some of the effects observed in split-brain patients and the other examples of contradictory knowledge-claims may be taken as evidence of multiple personal identities and even multiple self-identities, but in no case are they evidence of multiple selves.*Robinson concluded:

> The separate personal identities and the different self-identities ascribed to and adopted by a person may be shocking to that person when subsequently discovered. But the basic fact of existence as a conscious entity cannot be shocking, for this is never news. As of now logic, language, and data leave the "moi" (me) intact and preserve the unity of self as an issue of continuing interest, and even of mystery.[53]

---

* *And, we add, it may be most reasonable to view them simply as laboratory manifestations of the many unconscious processes going on within a person's head that psychology and physiology have been attempting to document over the last hundred years.*

·········

IS THE MIND–BODY PROBLEM A DEAD ISSUE?

In the exciting rush of new discoveries and observations of brain–behavior relationships, the idea is sometimes fostered that "understanding" the mind (or at least some mental functions) is just around the corner. In addition, because it is often easy to refute naive or simplistic assignments of consciousness to either specific structures (as in earlier days) or to steps in information processing (as sometimes done in more recent times), there is a general impression fostered that philosophical and even psychological questions having to do with problems of relating mental events to physical events is nonsense, to be replaced by a new "neurophilosophy" that assumes mental events are completely relatable to neurophysiological events.

There are in fact still important conceptual and philosophical issues to be addressed in attempting to discover and explain the physiology underlying "cognitive operations." These are not dismissed by mocking Descartes's use of the pineal gland or by refuting John Eccles's pronouncement about where in physiology "consciousness" enters the scene. Unfortunately, the relative ease with which some attempts at dealing with consciousness have been attacked seems to have also trivialized serious questioning of the mind–brain "identity." As we mentioned in Chapter 4, a physiological correlate of some mental event is not identical to the event. Mental life may never be relatable to externally measured physiology - not because it does not arise from brain activity, but because what we experience inwardly is not explainable in terms of discretely measurable processes. Perhaps certain specific sensory aspects of the experience can be related in some causal manner to specific physiology, but the conscious experience as a whole probably has temporal and mechanistic background characteristics completely different from the time, structure, and process we are attempting to measure.

But will we measure "it" in the future? As physician and writer Jonathan Miller recently said:

> Indeed, the method by which we are acquainted with consciousness is so fundamentally different from the method by which we aquaint ourselves with brains that I suspect, as philosopher Colin McGinn does, that although we don't have to invoke anything other than brain—no magic that contravenes the laws of nature—we will never fully understand the connection.[54]

Miller concluded:

> There is obviously much more to be learned about the relationship between brains and minds, and it will be years, perhaps centuries, before we come up against the "cognitive closure" so courageously identified by Professor McGinn. The fact that such research is destined to describe an asymptotic curve, which approaches but never reaches the limit, does not preclude the necessity of our following it.[55]

·········

LEFT AND RIGHT IN BIOLOGY AND PHYSICS

French biologist Louis Pasteur discovered in the nineteenth century that molecules of tartaric acid could assume either of two mirror-image forms and that a certain plant mold could act on one, but not on the other, form of the acid. This meant that the plant mold, in effect, could tell left from right! Pasteur assumed that this implied that a fundamental asymmetry exists in the molecular structure of the plant mold itself and wrote, "This important criterion (of molecular asymmetry) constitutes perhaps the only sharply defined difference which can be drawn at the present time between the chemistry of dead or living matter." He went on to speculate that "life is dominated by asymmetrical actions. I can even imagine that all living species are primordially, in their structure, in their external forms, functions of cosmic asymmetry."[56]

Are the origins of asymmetry in humans and in certain other life forms to be found in more fundamental aspects of nature—in the fundamental forces operating in biology and physics? The forces of nature have long been assumed to preserve parity, a concept derived from physics that means, in its most general sense, that phenomena remain unchanged if reflected through a plane or viewed in a mirror; that is, natural interactions in the world look just as normal viewed in a mirror as they do viewed directly. It is only the presence of human artifacts (such as writing) or the knowledge of the exact arrangements of an original scene that can give away whether a picture is mirror-reversed or not. The laws governing a mirrored scene, including how objects interact, appear to be exactly the same as those governing the original. Pasteur's idea of a cosmic asymmetry, however, although perhaps not justified by the limited data on which it was based, was nevertheless prophetic of some recent developments in biology and physics.

...

Molecular Biology

The discovery of deoxyribonucleic acid (DNA) as the genetic material in cells and the discovery of DNA's helical structure was heralded as a major contribution to biology and genetics. The double strands of each DNA molecule encode genetic information in terms of the sequencing of component amino acids. The two long strands are wound around each other in a clockwise spiral; thus, the DNA molecule cannot be superimposed on its mirror reflection. Some investigators have speculated that this and other asymmetries at the molecular level underlie the gross asymmetry in some organisms, including the leftward displacement of the heart and, perhaps, handedness and cerebral lateralization in humans. They argue that these gross asymmetries must lie in the molecular mechanisms that control the development of the organism's structure.[57] Although each cell contains identical DNA molecules containing all of the information necessary to form the complete organism, the cells differentiate to form different kinds of tissue (muscle, bone, blood, neurons, etc.). It is thought that the genetic information in each cell interacts with some other source of "positional" information in the growing embryo that determines the cell type and ultimately the actual shape and structure of the organism.[58]

The mechanisms regulating the growth of structure and form are not known, and the existence of a positional code is only hypothesized. Psychologists Corballis and Beale suggested that any systematic differences in the formation of left and right would be part of this code and that genes themselves do not encode the direction of asymmetry. They argue that the positional code must consist of a structural asymmetry at the molecular level. Whether or not the asymmetries are expressed depends on interaction of the positional code with the genetic code. As noted in Chapter 9, Corballis and Beale proposed that in most people, handedness and cerebral lateralization are under the influence of a left–right gradient contained in the positional code that results in right-handedness and the left cerebral control of speech. In a small minority, however, this positional code gradient "is denied expression, and the directions of handedness and cerebral lateralization are assigned randomly and independently."[59]

...

Parity in Nuclear Physics

As previously mentioned, the forces of nature have long been assumed to preserve parity; that is, normal interactions in the world do not in any way define left and right in the sense that such concepts could be derived from asymmetries in the way things work (or forces operate). Even the deflection of a compass needle to the left or the right by a parallel current-carrying wire could not be used to define these directions, because the designations of the needle's "north" and "south" poles are essentially arbitrary. A mirror image of an experiment set up to deflect a compass needle with an electric current would look perfectly normal because the observer would assume the needle's poles were reversed.

In 1957, however, physicists discovered that some instances of the so-called weak nuclear force (or weak interaction) involving radioactive emissions from atoms did not conserve parity. The nucleus of the cobalt-60 atom was shown to emit electrons more frequently from one end than from the other. The north and south poles of a magnetic field, thus, could be defined in an absolute way by stating that if cobalt-60 nuclei are lined up in the field, then the south pole is that toward which the greater number of electrons are emitted.[60] This asymmetry would also allow one to distinguish between a compass needle's deflection (in the presence of a current-carrying wire) in the real world and in a mirror.

The issue of whether a fundamental distinction exists between left and right in the physical laws of the universe remains a debated one. Some physicists have appealed to "deeper" principles to argue that parity is still preserved, such as the essentially arbitrary nature in which "positive" and "negative" electric charge is defined, along with the consequent labeling of the direction of current flow. Even the direction of time flow is brought in as a factor to help preserve the sense of absolute symmetry in natural interactions. Nevertheless, there is a sense now that, at least at relatively fundamental levels of analysis of physical interactions, natural asymmetries do occur.

Are these more or less fundamental physical asymmetries the basis for the asymmetries evident at the level of molecular biology? At first glance it seems unlikely, because it is not evident how asymmetries at the level of weak nuclear interactions have any influence at the biochemical level, for chemical interactions depend on the electromagnetic force, a much stronger force than that associated with nuclear decay. It is thought that the influence of these asymmetries at the level of chemical interactions is negligible, yet some theorists have speculated that, given the time scale of biochemical evolution on Earth, the influence would be substantial.[61] In addition, there is some evidence that parity is not conserved at the level of electromagnetic and, therefore, chemical interactions.[62]

In reviewing these and other data for asymmetries in nature, Corballis and Beale concluded that "they do strengthen our conviction that the systematic asymmetries of morphology, molecular biology, and subatomic interactions are ultimately linked, and that there is, after all, an absolute, universal distinction between left and right."[63]

·········

POSTSCRIPT

In the process of reviewing the literature for this book and reflecting on our own direct involvement in the area of hemispheric specialization for many years, we have become increasingly aware of the "dichotomania" problem. One symptom of the problem is to exaggerate hemispheric differences and to ignore other forms of brain organization, such as the orderly differences within a hemisphere.

At the same time, we have become even more impressed with the reality of hemispheric differences and with their potential for helping us understand the brain mechanisms underlying higher mental functions. It is possible that some of the most profound human mental abilities are a result of nature's forfeiting, to an extent, a very old, stable, and successful method of changing the brain: bilaterally symmetric evolution. Why so much of nature involves mirror-symmetrical structure, and why the brain has for the most part evolved in a mirror-symmetrical fashion, is a theoretical issue that largely remains a subject of conjecture.

One suggestion is that a doubled structure is less subject to damage. Mechanisms in one side can easily take over functions lost in the other because they are basically doing the same thing. Once asymmetries developed, this advantage was lost. Substituting for this loss of redundancy, however, was the added survival value of language, sophisticated mental mapping capabilities, and whatever other talents the integrated action of the asymmetric components of the two hemispheres can generate.

In studying these asymmetries, researchers are going beyond what is different about the halves of the brain. They are uncovering ways in which the brain deals with different kinds of information in the environment and ways in which it generates some of our behavior. The discovery of different processes and mechanisms in the brain encourages the idea that mental abilities may be explained in these ways. Investigators have touched on issues of consciousness, emotion, and the unity of experience. Some of these may be premature attempts using insufficient data and inappropriate definitions, but they are steps, first steps, in the long endeavor to understand the brain and, perhaps, ourselves.

APPENDIX

·········

FUNCTIONAL NEUROANATOMY:
A Brief Review

The history of thought on the relationship between neuroanatomy and behavior has revolved around two opposing views. At one time, fanciful maps of the brain were drawn, allotting specific regions to "thrift," "love of family," "greed," "memory," and so on. At the other extreme was the view that the brain operates as a unit and that within the brain there are no relationships between particular regions and specific mental functions.

Brain researchers today have moved away from these extremes. The brain is now thought to be organized in both a focal and a diffuse manner, depending on what functions are being studied. Basic sensory and motor functions are controlled by very specific regions, whereas higher mental functions involve a constellation of regions across the brain.

In this Appendix we shall review some basic neuroanatomy, concentrating on the cortical regions of the cerebral hemispheres—the regions of the human brain involved in most of the debate about asymmetry of function. We have tried to present views that represent a consensus among brain researchers, although considerable controversy remains in many instances. Because of these uncertainties, it is necessary to consider the newest "maps" of the brain as a rough guide rather than as a definitive road atlas.

The central nervous system consists of the spinal cord and the brain. The brain is conventionally divided into three major regions: the hindbrain, the midbrain, and the forebrain. These areas and some of the structures within them are demarcated in Figure A.1.* The major divisions are made on an embryological basis. Each develops from a different embryonic layer and is roughly related to different evolutionary stages in the development of the vertebrate nervous system.

Hindbrain and midbrain structures have traditionally been thought to control the more automatic, unconscious aspects of behavior. These include basic functions essential to life, such as breathing, the sleep–wake cycle, and levels of arousal or degrees of responsiveness to external events. It is becoming more apparent that these deeper structures of the brain also contribute to the processing of information necessary for higher mental functions.

The forebrain is the largest and most highly developed section of the brain in humans and the higher animals. It consists of a complex of anatomically distinct groups of nerve-cell bodies called nuclei, which are surrounded by nerve fibers sheathed in myelin and covered by the cerebral cortex.** The cortex forms the familiar convoluted surface of the brain and consists of multiple layers of complexly interconnected neurons. It is the "newest" structure, in evolutionary terms, and is well developed only in mammals. The neocortex, as most of the human cortex is called, contains approximately 9 billion of the 12 billion neurons of the central nervous system. It is generally considered to be responsible for the highest functions of the human brain, such as abstract thought and language.

The entire central nervous system is essentially bisymmetric. A sagittal plane (front to back) through the middle of the human body will

---

* Reference is often made to the brain stem and to the cerebrum. The brain stem includes the hindbrain and midbrain structures, excluding the cerebellum. Some anatomists also include the very central nuclei of the forebrain (the thalamus), located immediately above the midbrain. The cerebrum refers to the forebrain.

** The nerve fibers sheathed in myelin are known as "white matter" because of their white appearance in fresh brain tissue. The cortex, which has a gray appearance, is known as "gray matter."

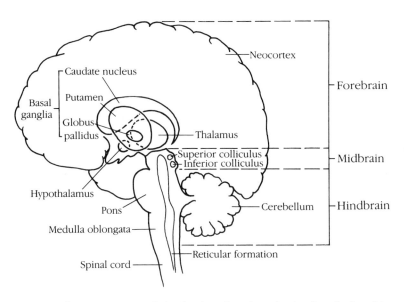

FIGURE A.1   Schematic view of the brain, showing the basic relationships of deep nuclear groups and brain-stem structures. [From Gazzaniga, Steen, and Volpe, *Functional Neuroscience*, Fig. 3.13, p. 61 (New York: Harper & Row Publishers, 1979).]

divide the nervous system into two mirror-image sections. The left and right halves of the brain stem do not physically separate until the thalamus of the forebrain. The forebrain looks like separate mirror-image halves connected by fiber bundles. These halves are the cerebral hemispheres.

...

Functional Areas of the Cortex

Almost the entire surface of each cerebral hemisphere consists of neocortex. Each hemisphere can be divided into four lobes, using the major folds of the cortex, called gyri (ridges) and sulci (valleys), as landmarks. Figure A.2 shows the divisions along the surface of one hemisphere. The central sulcus separates the frontal lobe from the parietal lobe. It also serves as the landmark for separating the anterior, or front, half of each hemisphere from the posterior areas.

The other major fissure, called the lateral sulcus (sylvian fissure), separates the temporal lobe from the frontal and parietal lobes. The most posterior portion of the cortex is called the occipital lobe.

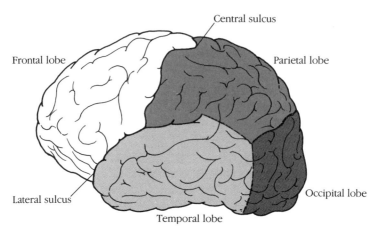

FIGURE A.2   Division of the cerebral hemisphere into lobes.

Each lobe is known to serve a different sensory or motor function. The occipital lobe is a visual center. Parts of the temporal lobe are involved with hearing. The anterior part of the parietal lobe is concerned with somatosensory function. The posterior part of the frontal lobe mediates motor function. Figure A.3 shows the areas involved.

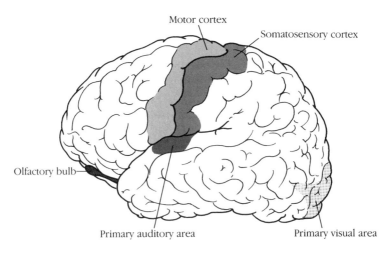

FIGURE A.3   Primary sensory and motor areas of the brain. The remaining areas (unshaded) are often termed "uncommitted" or "association" cortex.

The areas of the cortex receiving input from the sense organs or controlling the movements of particular body parts are called primary zones or primary projection areas. The primary motor areas of the frontal lobe control specific parts of the body (see Figure A.4). The

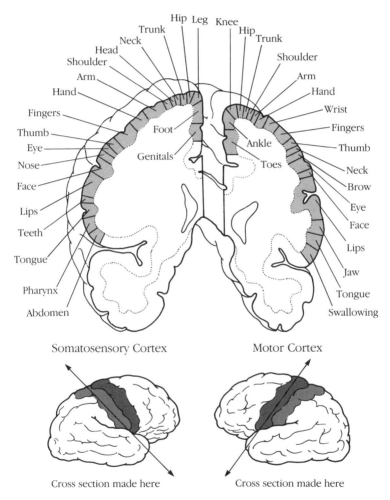

FIGURE A.4   The motor and somatosensory areas of the cortex are projections of areas of the body. Some areas, such as those representing the face, tongue, and fingers, are disproportionately large because the amount of cortical surface devoted to a given part of the body reflects the requirements of that body part. The lips take up more space in the motor cortex than they do in the somatosensory cortex, as the lips do more muscle-controlled moving than they do sensing. [From Lassen, Ingvar, and Skinhoj, "Brain Function and Blood Flow," Scientific American, Inc., 1978. All rights reserved.]

primary sensory areas in the parietal, temporal, and occipital lobes are said to possess high modal specificity: Each is active only when there is stimulation in its particular modality. In addition, within each primary sensory area, smaller areas respond only to highly specific properties or parts of its "sensory window."

All primary areas are topologically arranged so that there is a systematic, orderly representation in the cortex of different parts of the body, different auditory qualities, and specific parts of the visual field. Lesions in these areas lead to highly specific deficits, such as blindness in one part of the visual field, selective hearing loss, loss of sensation in one part of the body, or partial paralysis. The extent of the damage will determine the amount of the "sensory window" that is lost.

Figure A.5 shows the primary projection areas in the brains of five animal species, including human beings. In nonprimates most of the brain is devoted to sensory and motor functions; there is little else. In

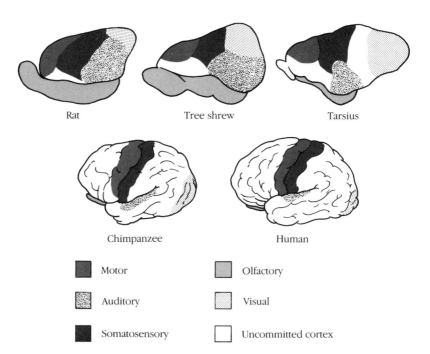

■ Motor	▦ Olfactory
▒ Auditory	░ Visual
■ Somatosensory	□ Uncommitted cortex

FIGURE A.5   The brains of five mammals, showing differences in the proportions of "uncommitted" cortex to areas devoted primarily to sensory and motor functions. [From Penfield, *Brain and Conscious Experience,* ed. J. C. Eccles (New York: Springer-Verlag, Inc., 1966), Pontifica Academia Scientiarum.]

primates a great deal of the cortex does not seem to be committed to the specific senses. These areas are known as "uncommitted" cortex or "association" areas.

...

The Association Areas of the Parietal, Occipital, and Temporal Lobes

Some investigators make a distinction between secondary and tertiary association cortex. Secondary zones are the areas adjacent to the primary projection areas and are still considered to have some modal specificity; that is, they are higher level processing centers for the specific sensory information coming into the primary area. Modality-specific information becomes integrated into meaningful wholes in secondary zones. Single sensory stimuli are combined and elaborated into progressively more complicated patterns. Damage to secondary zones gives rise to perceptual disorders restricted to a specific modality. In visual agnosia, for example, a patient can see but does not recognize or comprehend what is being looked at. There are also auditory and tactile agnosias.

Tertiary zones* lie at the borders of the parietal, temporal, and occipital secondary zones. In these association areas, or "zones of overlapping," modal specificity disappears. Neural activity does not seem to depend on stimulation of any single sensory modality. Various sensory fields overlap, and combinations of sensations become perceptions of a progressively higher order. Tactile and kinesthetic impulses are built up into perceptions of form and size and are associated with visual information from the same objects. It is thought that objects come to be represented ultimately by a constellation of memories compounded from several sensory channels. Damage to areas such as the parietal–occipital junction and parietal–temporal junction result in disorders transcending any single modality.

It is at this level that hemispheric asymmetries appear. Damage to the right hemisphere within these zones may produce disorders of manipulospatial abilities or the neglect syndrome, in which a patient ignores the left half of space. Damage within these zones in the left hemisphere may interfere with language comprehension or the ability to name objects. Thus, the association areas of the posterior of the brain seem to be

---

* *The definition of tertiary zones is from A. R. Luria,* Higher Cortical Functions in Man *(New York: Basic Books, 1966).*

concerned with high level perceptual processes and more abstract "manipulation" of these processes. The left and right hemispheres seem to differ in what processes they handle best.

···

The Association Areas of the Frontal Lobes

The rear of the frontal lobe is the primary motor area. The secondary motor area, analogous to the secondary sensory zones of the posterior of the brain, lies immediately in front of the motor strip and is called the premotor area. This area is involved in higher level motor organization. Damage to this region leads to disturbances in the organization of movements. (Damage to the motor strip itself leads to paralysis.) In the left hemisphere, damage to specific parts of the premotor area (Broca's area) leads to disorganization of speech—the expressive dysfunction known as Broca's aphasia.

The functions of the remaining areas of the frontal lobes seem more elusive. The areas in the anterior part of the frontal lobes (called prefrontal) are no longer directly tied in to motor control and are believed to serve higher integrative functions. This prefrontal area is often referred to as frontal granular cortex because of the characteristic "granular" neurons of which it is mostly composed. As shown in Figure A.6, these areas are particularly enlarged in the human brain. They account for humans' distinctively high forehead relative to that of other primates.

Damage to these prefrontal areas can result in both intellectual and personality changes. Although patients still seem capable of performing many different tasks, deficits in executing sequences of operations or solving complex problems becomes evident. A patient may have trouble shifting "set" and becomes stuck on a task. There is an inability to inhibit the first tendency aroused by a problem. Having done one step properly, the patient may continue to use the same strategy in totally inappropriate contexts. This is often referred to as perseveration. These syndromes suggest that the frontal lobes are involved in the planning and organization of actions.

The inflexibility seen in certain frontal lobe syndromes has often been called a deficit in abstract thinking, but this label is controversial. Some investigators claim a "dissociation between thought and action." The patient can verbalize what he or she should be doing yet is unable to carry it through.

The personality and emotional changes associated with damage to the frontal lobes are even more elusive than the intellectual deficits.

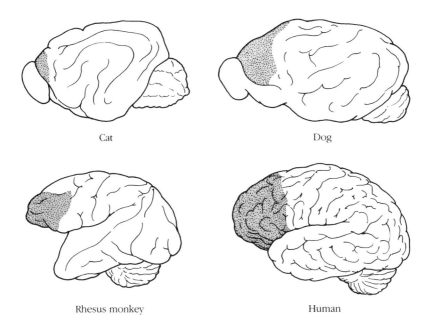

Cat

Dog

Rhesus monkey

Human

FIGURE A.6   The frontal granular cortex in the brains of four animal species (not drawn to scale). [From Walsh, *Neuropsychology—A Clinical Approach*, Fig. 4.1, p. 110 (Edinburgh: Churchill Livingstone Ltd., 1977).]

Earlier in this century, the frontal regions were the object of many experimental surgical procedures that attempted to control several forms of mental illness. Despite a great deal of literature on the subject, the question of how the frontal lobes function and the actual effects of the operations remain controversial.

In general, it appears that the frontal association areas not only play a major role in planning and controlling action but also may control or inhibit emotional tendencies. Luria has suggested that the frontal areas serve as a tertiary integrative zone for the motor system as well as for the limbic system, an older region deeper in the forebrain believed to play a major role in emotion.

NOTES

Chapter 1 Early Evidence from the Clinic: The Discovery of Asymmetry

[1]R. W. Sperry, "Brain Bisection and Consciousness," in *Brain and Conscious Experience*, ed. J. Eccles (New York: Springer-Verlag, 1966).

[2]R. Ornstein, *The Psychology of Consciousness*, 2nd Ed. (New York: Harcourt Brace Jovanovich, 1977).

[3]R. Ornstein, "The Split and Whole Brain," *Human Nature* 1 (1978): 76–83.

[4]P. Bakan, "The Eyes Have It," *Psychology Today* 4 (1971): 64–69.

[5]J. E. Bogen, "The Other Side of the Brain. VII: Some Educational Aspects of Hemispheric Specialization," *UCLA Educator* 17 (1975): 24–32.

[6]W. Gibson, "Pioneers in Localization of Brain Function," *Journal of the American Medical Association* 180 (1962): 944–951.

[7]P. Broca (1863), cited in R. J. Joynt, "Paul Pierre Broca: His Contribution to the Knowledge of Aphasia," *Cortex* 1 (1964): 206–213.

[8]P. Broca (1864), cited in M. Critchley, *Aphasiology and Other Aspects of Language* (London: Edward Arnold, 1970).

[9]P. Broca (1865), cited in S. Dimond, *The Double Brain* (London: Churchill-Livingstone, 1972).

[10]J. H. Jackson, *Selected Writings of John Hughlings Jackson*, ed. J. Taylor (New York: Basic Books, 1958).

[11]Ibid.

[12]Ibid.

[13]Ibid.

[14]T. Weisenberg and K. E. McBride, *Aphasia: A Clinical and Psychological Study* (New York: Commonwealth Fund, 1935).

[15]H. Hecaen and M. Albert, *Human Neuropsychology* (New York: Wiley, 1978).

[16]O. Dalin (1745), cited in A. L. Benton and R. J. Joynt, "Early Descriptions of Aphasia," *Archives of Neurology* 3 (1960): 205–222.

[17]A. Gates and J. Bradshaw, "The Role of the Cerebral Hemispheres in Music," *Brain and Language* 4 (1977): 403–431.

[18]J. Semmes, "Hemispheric Specialization, a Possible Clue to Mechanism," *Neuropsychologia* 6 (1968): 11–26.

[19]B. Bramwell, "On Crossed Aphasia," *Lancet* 8 (1899): 1473–1479.

[20]W. Penfield and L. Roberts, *Speech and Brain Mechanisms* (Princeton, N.J.: Princeton University Press, 1959).

[21]C. A. Mateer, R. L. Rapport, and D. D. Polly, "Electrical Stimulation of the Cerebral Cortex in Humans," in *Neuromethods*, ed. A. Boulton, G. Baker, and M. Hiscock (Clifton, N.J.: Humana Press, 1990).

[22]G. A. Ojemann, "Brain Organization for Language from the Perspective of Electrical Stimulation Mapping," *The Behavioral and Brain Sciences* 6 (1983): 235–238.

[23]J. A. Wada and T. Rasmussen, "Intracarotid Injection of Sodium Amytal for the Lateralization of Cerebral Speech Dominance: Experimental and Clinical Observations," *Journal of Neurosurgery* 17 (1960): 266–282.

[24]R. Rausch and M. Risinger, "Intracarotid Sodium Amobarbitol Procedure," in *Neuromethods*. Boulton, Baker, and Hiscock.

[25]T. Rasmussen and B. Milner, "The Role of Early Left-Brain Injury in Determining Lateralization of Cerebral Speech Functions," in *Evolution and Lateralization of the Brain*, ed. S. Dimond and D. Blizzard (New York: New York Academy of Sciences, 1977).

[26]D. W. Loring, K. Meador, G. Lee, A. Murro, J. Smith, H. Flanigin, B. Gallagher, and D. King, "Cerebral Language Lateralization: Evidence from Intracarotid Amobarbitol Testing," *Neuropsychologia* 28 (1990): 831–838.

[27]A. W. Ellis and A. W. Young, *Human Cognitive Neuropsychology* (London: Erlbaum, 1988).

[28]T. Shallice, *From Neuropsychology to Mental Structure* (Cambridge: Cambridge University Press, 1988).

[29]N. Geschwind, "Disconnection Syndromes in Animals and Man," *Brain* 88 (1965): 585–644.

[30]Ellis and Young, *Human Cognitive Neuropsychology*.

[31]Ibid.

[32]D. Marr, "Early Processing of Visual Information," *Philosophical Transactions of the Royal Society of London* B 275 (1976): 483–524.

Chapter 2   The Human Split Brain: Surgical Separation of the Hemispheres

[1]T. C. Erikson, "Spread of Epileptic Discharge," *Archives of Neurology and Psychiatry* 43 (1940): 429–452.

[2]W. Van Wagenen and R. Herren, "Surgical Division of Commissural Pathways in the Corpus Callosum," *Archives of Neurology and Psychiatry* 44 (1940): 740–759.

[3]G. Fechner (1860), cited in O. Zangwill, "Consciousness and the Cerebral Hemispheres," in *Hemispheric Function in the Human Brain*, ed. S. Dimond and G. Beaumont (New York: Halsted Press, 1974).

[4]A. J. Akelaitis, "Studies on the Corpus Callosum. II: The Higher Visual Functions in Each Homonymous Field Following Complete Section of the Corpus Callosum," *Archives of Neurology and Psychiatry* 45 (1941): 789–796; A. J. Akelaitis, "The Study of Gnosis, Praxis and Language Following Section of the Corpus Callosum and Anterior Commissure," *Journal of Neurosurgery* 1 (1944): 94–102.

[5]R. E. Myers, "Function of Corpus Callosum in Interocular Transfer," *Brain* 79 (1956): 358–363; R. E. Myers and R. W. Sperry, "Interhemispheric Communication Through the Corpus Callosum. Mnemonic Carry-Over Between the Hemispheres," *Archives of Neurology and Psychiatry* 80 (1958): 298–303.

[6]R. W. Sperry, "Hemisphere Deconnection and Unity in Conscious Awareness," *American Psychologist* 23 (1968): 723–733.

[7]M. S. Gazzaniga, *The Bisected Brain* (New York: Appleton-Century-Crofts, 1970).

[8]S. M. Ferguson, M. Rayport, and W. S. Corrie, "Neuropsychiatric Observations on Behavioral Consequences of Corpus Callosum Section for Seizure Control," in *Epilepsy and the Corpus Callosum*, ed. A. G. Reeves (New York: Plenum Press, 1985).

[9]F. Brémer, "An Aspect of the Physiology of Corpus Callosum," *Journal of Electroencephalography and Clinical Neurophysiology* 22 (1967): 391.

[10]C. B. Trevarthen, "Manipulative Strategies of Baboons, and the Origins of Cerebral Asymmetry," in *Hemispheric Asymmetry of Function*, ed. M. Kinsbourne (London: Tavistock, 1974).

[11]R. W. Doty, "Electrical Stimulation of the Brain in Behavioral Cortex," *Annual Review of Psychology* 20 (1969): 289–320.

[12]J. Levy, C. Trevarthen, and R. W. Sperry, "Perception of Bilateral Chimeric Figures Following Hemispheric Disconnection," *Brain* 95 (1972): 61–78.

[13]L. Franco and R. W. Sperry, "Hemisphere Lateralization for Cognitive Processing of Geometry," *Neuropsychologia* 15 (1977): 107–114.

[14]P. Greenwood, D. H. Wilson, and M. S. Gazzaniga, "Dream Report Following Commissurotomy," *Cortex* 13 (1977): 311–316.

[15]C. R. Clark and G. M. Geffen, "Corpus Callosum Surgery and Recent Memory," *Brain* 112 (1989): 165–175.

[16]E. Phelps, W. Hirst, and M. S. Gazzaniga, "Deficits in Recall Following Partial and Complete Commissurotomy," *Cerebral Cortex* 1 (1991): 492–498.

[17]M. S. Gazzaniga and S. A. Hillyard, "Language and Speech Capacity of the Right Hemisphere," *Neuropsychologia* 9 (1971): 273–280.

[18]E. Zaidel, "A Technique for Presenting Lateralized Visual Input with Prolonged Exposure," *Vision Research* 15 (1975): 283–289.

[19]E. Zaidel, "Auditory Language Comprehension in the Right Hemisphere Following Cerebral Commissurotomy and Hemispherectomy: A Comparison with Child Language and Aphasia," in *Language Acquisition and Language Breakdown*, ed. A. Caramazza and E. Zurif (Baltimore: Johns Hopkins University Press, 1978).

[20]M. S. Gazzaniga, "Right Hemisphere Language Following Brain Bisection: A 20 Year Perspective," *American Psychologist* 38 (1983): 525–537.

[21]E. Zaidel, "A Response to Gazzaniga: Language in the Right Hemisphere, Convergent Perspectives," *American Psychologist* 38 (1983): 342–346.

[22]E. Zaidel, "Language Functions in the Two Hemispheres Following Complete Cerebral Commissurotomy and Hemispherectomy," in *Handbook of Neuropsychology*, Vol 4, ed. F. Boller and J. Grafman (Amsterdam: Elsevier, 1990).

[23]N. Geschwind, "The Frequency of Callosal Syndromes in Neurological Practice," in *Epilepsy and the Corpus Callosum*, Reeves.

[24]R. D. Nebes, "Direct Examination of Cognitive Function in the Right and Left Hemispheres," in *Asymmetrical Function of the Brain*, ed. M. Kinsbourne (Cambridge: Cambridge University Press, 1978).

[25]L. Franco and R. W. Sperry, "Hemisphere Lateralization for Cognitive Processing of Geometry," *Neuropsychologia* 15 (1977): 107–111.

[26]R. Puccetti, "The Alleged Manipulospatiality Explanation of Right Hemisphere Visuospatial Superiority," *Behavioral and Brain Sciences* 4 (1981): 75–76.

[27]H. Erlichman and J. Barrett, "Right Hemisphere Specialization for Mental Imagery: A Review of the Evidence," *Brain and Cognition* 2 (1983): 55–76.

[28]M. J. Farah, M. S. Gazzaniga, J. D. Holtzman, and S. M. Kosslyn, "A Left Hemisphere Basis for Visual Imagery?" *Neuropsychologia* 23 (1985): 115–118.

[29]M. J. Farah, "The Neurological Basis of Mental Imagery," *Cognition* 18 (1984): 245–272.

[30]S. M. Kosslyn, "Seeing and Imagining in the Cerebral Hemispheres," *Psychological Review* 94 (1987): 148–175.

[31]J. Sergent, "The Neuropsychology of Visual Image Generation: Data, Method, and Theory," *Brain and Cognition* 13 (1990): 98–129.

[32]Ibid.

[33]W. F. McKeever, K. F. Sullivan, S. M. Ferguson, and M. Rayport, "Hemispheric Disconnection Effects in Patients with Corpus Callosum Section," in *Epilepsy and the Corpus Callosum*, Reeves.

[34]J. Levy-Agresti and R. W. Sperry, "Differential Perceptual Capacities in Major and Minor Hemispheres," *Proceedings of the National Academy of Science, U.S.A.* 61 (1968): 115.

[35]J. Levy, "Psychobiological Implications of Bilateral Asymmetry," in *Hemispheric Function in the Human Brain*, Dimond and Beaumont.

[36]C. Trevarthen, and M. Kinsbourne, cited in J. Levy, "Cerebral Asymmetries as Manifested in Split Brain Man," in *Hemispheric Disconnection and Cerebral Function*, ed. M. Kinsbourne and W. L. Smith (Springfield, Ill.: Charles C. Thomas, 1974).

[37]J. Levy and C. Trevarthen, "Metacontrol of Hemispheric Function in Human Split Brain Patients," *Journal of Experimental Psychology: Human Perception and Performance* 2 (1976): 299–312.

[38]Ibid.

[39]J. Levy, "The Regulation and Generation of Perception in the Asymmetric Brain," in *Brain Circuits and Functions of the Mind—Essays in Honor of Roger Sperry*, ed. C. Trevarthen (Cambridge: Cambridge University Press, 1990).

[40]R. W. Sperry, "Lateral Specialization in the Surgically Separated Hemispheres," in *The Neurosciences Third Study Program*, ed. F. O. Schmitt and F. C. Worden (Cambridge, Mass.: MIT Press, 1974).

[41]J. D. Holtzman, J. J. Sidtis, B. T. Volpe, D. H. Wilson, and M. S. Gazzaniga, "Dissociation of Spatial Information for Stimulus Localization and the Control of Attention," *Brain* 104 (1981): 861–872.

[42]J. Sergent, "Furtive Incursions into Bicameral Minds," *Brain* 113 (1990): 537–568.

[43]S. E. Seymour, P. A. Reuter-Lorenz, and M. S. Gazzaniga, "The Disconnection Syndrome: Basic Findings Reaffirmed," in press.

[44]Gazzaniga and LeDoux, *The Integrated Mind*.

Chapter 3   Asymmetries in the Normal Brain

[1]M. Mishkin and D. G. Forgays, "Word Recognition as a Function of Retinal Locus," *Journal of Experimental Psychology* 43 (1952): 43–48.

[2]M. I. Barton, H. Goodglass, and A. Shai, "Differential Recognition of Tachistoscopically Presented English and Hebrew Words in Right and Left Visual Fields," *Perceptual and Motor Skills* 21 (1965): 431–437.

[3]E. L. Schwartz, R. Desimone, T. D. Albright, and C. G. Gross, "Shape Recognition and Inferior Temporal Neurons," *Proceedings of the National Academy of Sciences, U.S.A.* 80 (1984): 5776–5778.

[4]G. Geffen, J. L. Bradshaw, and G. Wallace, "Interhemispheric Effects on Reaction Time to Verbal and Nonverbal Visual Stimuli," *Journal of Experimental Psychology* 87 (1971): 415–422; G. Rizzolatti, C. Umilta, and G. Berlucchi, "Opposite Superiorities of the Right and Left Cerebral Hemispheres in Discriminative Reaction Time to Physiognomical and Alphabetic Material," *Brain* 94 (1971): 431–442.

[5]D. Kimura, "Spatial Localization in Left and Right Visual Fields," *Canadian Journal of Psychology* 23 (1969): 445–458.

[6]M. P. Bryden and C. Rainey, "Left–Right Differences in Tachistoscopic Recognition," *Journal of Experimental Psychology* 66 (1963): 568–571; H. L. Dee and D. Fontenot, "Cerebral Dominance and Lateral Differences in Perception and Memory," *Neuropsychologia* 11 (1973): 167–173; D. Kimura, "Dual Functional Asymmetry of the Brain in Visual Perception," *Neuropsychologia* 4 (1966): 275–285.

[7]D. Kimura, "Some Effects of Temporal Lobe Damage on Auditory Perception," *Canadian Journal of Psychology* 15 (1961): 156–165.

[8]M. R. Rosenzweig, "Representation of the Two Ears at the Auditory Cortex," *American Journal of Physiology* 167 (1951): 147–158.

[9]D. Dirks, "Perception of Dichotic and Monaural Verbal Material and Cerebral Dominance in Speech," *Acta Otolaryngologica* 58 (1964): 73–80.

[10]B. Milner, L. Taylor, and R. W. Sperry, "Lateralized Suppression of Dichotically Presented Digits After Commissural Section in Man," *Science* 161 (1968): 184–185; S. P. Springer and M. S. Gazzaniga, "Dichotic Listening in Partial and Complete Split Brain Patients," *Neuropsychologia* 13 (1975): 341–346.

[11]R. Zatorre, "Perceptual Asymmetry in the Dichotic Fused Words Test and Cerebral Speech Lateralization Determined by the Carotid Amytal Test," *Neuropsychologia* 27 (1989): 1207–1219.

[12]G. Geffen and R. Caudrey, "Reliability and Validity of the Dichotic Monitoring Test for Language Laterality," *Neuropsychologia* 19 (1981): 413–423.

[13]H. W. Gordon, "Degree of Ear Asymmetries for Perception of Dichotic Chords and for Illusory Chord Localization in Musicians of Different Levels of Competence," *Journal of Experimental Psychology: Human Perception and Performance* 6 (1980): 516–527; B. Bartholomeus, "Effects of Task Requirements on Ear Superiority for Sung Speech," *Cortex* 10 (1974): 215–223.

[14]M. P. Bryden, "Tachistoscopic Recognition, Handedness, and Cerebral Dominance," *Neuropsychologia* 3 (1965): 1–8.

[15]D. Kimura, "Functional Asymmetry of the Brain in Dichotic Listening," *Cortex* 3 (1967): 163–178.

[16]D. Kimura and S. Folb, "Neural Processing of Backwards Speech Sounds," *Science* 161 (1968): 395–396; M. Studdert-Kennedy and D. Shankweiler, "Hemispheric Specialization for Speech Perception," *Journal of the Acoustical Society of America* 48 (1970): 579–594.

[17]D. Kimura, "Left-Right Differences in the Perception of Melodies," *Quarterly Journal of Experimental Psychology* 16 (1964): 355–358.

[18]F. W. K. Curry, "A Comparison of Left-Handed and Right-Handed Subjects on Verbal and Nonverbal Dichotic Listening Tasks," *Cortex* 3 (1967): 343–352.

[19]R. Klatzky and R. Atkinson, "Specialization of the Cerebral Hemispheres in Scanning for Information in Short-Term Memory," *Perception and Psychophysics* 10 (1971): 335–338.

[20]M. H. VanKleeck, "Hemispheric Differences in Global Versus Local Processing of Hierarchical Visual Stimuli by Normal Subjects: New Data and a Meta-Analysis of Previous Studies," *Neuropsychologia* 27 (1989): 1165–1178.

[21]J. G. Seamon and M. S. Gazzaniga, "Coding Strategies in Cerebral Laterality Effects," *Cognitive Psychology* 5 (1973): 249–256.

[22]S. Sasanuma, "Kana and Kanji Processing in Japanese Aphasics," *Brain and Language* 2 (1975): 369–383.

[23]S. Sasanuma and O. Fujimura, "Selective Impairment of Phonetic and Non-Phonetic Transcription of Words in Japanese Aphasic Patients: Kana vs. Kanji in Visual Recognition and Writing," *Cortex* 7 (1971): 1–18.

[24]S. Sasanuma, M. Itoh, K. Mori, and Y. Kobayashi, "Tachistoscopic Recognition of Kana and Kanji Words," *Neuropsychologia* 15 (1977): 547–553.

[25]J. Sergent and J. B. Hellige, "Role of Input Factors in Visual-Field Asymmetries," *Brain and Cognition* 5 (1986): 174–199.

[26]S. Christman, "Perceptual Characteristics in Visual Field Research," *Brain and Language* 11 (1989): 238–257.

[27]F. L. Kitterle and R. S. Kaye, "Hemispheric Symmetry in Contrast and Orientation Sensitivity," *Perception and Psychophysics* 37 (1985): 391–396; M. Rebai, L. Mecacci, J. D. Bagot, and C. Bonnet, "Hemispheric Asymmetries in the Visual Evoked Potentials to Temporal Frequency: Preliminary Evidence," *Perception* 15 (1986): 589–594.

[28] J. L. Bradshaw, *Hemispheric Specialization and Psychological Functions* (New York: Wiley, 1989).

[29] J. B. Hellige, "Hemispheric Asymmetry," *Annual Review of Psychology* 41 (1990): 55–80.

[30] M. P. Bryden, "Strategy Effects in the Assessment of Hemispheric Asymmetry," in *Strategies of Information Processing*, ed. G. Underwood (London: Academic Press, 1978).

[31] M. P. Bryden, "An Overview of the Dichotic Listening Procedure and Its Relation to Cerebral Organization," in *Handbook of Dichotic Listening*, ed. K. Hugdahl (Chichester: Wiley, 1988).

[32] T. A. Montor and M. P. Bryden, "On the Relationship Between Visual Spatial Attention and Visual Field Asymmetries," *Quarterly Journal of Experimental Psychology* 44 (1992): 529–555; M. P. Bryden and T. A. Montor, "Attentional Factors in Visual Field Asymmetries," *Canadian Journal of Psychology* 45 (1991): 427–447.

[33] D. Hines and P. Satz, "Cross-Modal Asymmetries in Perception Related to Asymmetry in Cerebral Function," *Neuropsychologia* 12 (1974): 239–247; E. B. Zurif and M. P. Bryden, "Familial Handedness and Left–Right Difference in Auditory and Visual Perception," *Neuropsychologia* 7 (1969): 179–187.

[34] S. Blumstein, H. Goodglass, and V. Tarter, "The Reliability of Ear Advantage in Dichotic Listening," *Brain and Language* 2 (1975): 226–236; Hines and Satz, "Cross-Modal Asymmetries in Perception."

[35] J. Levy and C. Trevarthen, "Metacontrol of Hemispheric Function in Human Split Brain Patients," *Journal of Experimental Psychology: Human Perception and Performance* 2 (1976): 299–312.

[36] J. B. Hellige, "Cerebral Laterality and Metacontrol," in *Recent Advances in Laterality*, ed. F. Kitterle (Hillsdale, N.J.: Erlbaum, 1991).

[37] J. B. Hellige, "Interhemispheric Interaction When Both Hemispheres Have Access to the Same Stimulus Information," *Journal of Experimental Psychology: Human Perception and Performance* 15 (1989): 711–722.

[38] J. B. Hellige, "Cerebral Laterality and Metacontrol."

[39] M. Kinsbourne, "The Mechanisms of Hemisphere Asymmetry in Man," in *Hemispheric Disconnection and Cerebral Function*, ed. M. Kinsbourne and W. L. Smith (Springfield, Ill.: Charles C. Thomas, 1974).

[40] M. Kinsbourne, "The Control of Attention by Interaction Between the Cerebral Hemispheres," in *Attention and Performance IV*, ed. S. Kornblum (New York: Academic Press, 1973).

[41] J. Morais and M. Landercy, "Listening to Speech While Retaining Music: What Happens to the Right Ear Advantage?" *Brain and Language* 4 (1977): 295–308.

[42] P. A. Reuter-Lorenz, M. Kinsbourne, and M. Moscovitch, "Hemispheric Control of Spatial Attention," *Brain and Cognition* 12 (1990): 240–266.

[43] M. Moscovitch, "Information Processing," in *Handbook of Neurobiology-Neuropsychology*, ed. M. S. Gazzaniga (New York: Plenum Press, 1979).

[44] M. E. Day, "An Eye Movement Phenomenon Relating to Attention, Thought, and Anxiety," *Perceptual and Motor Skills* 19 (1964): 443–446.

[45] P. Bakan, "Hypnotizability, Laterality of Eye Movement and Functional Brain Asymmetry," *Perceptual and Motor Skills* 28 (1969): 927–932.

[46] M. Kinsbourne, "Eye and Head Turning Indicates Cerebral Lateralization," *Science* 176 (1972): 539–541.

[47] D. Galin and R. Ornstein, "Individual Differences in Cognitive Style. 1: Reflexive Eye Movements," *Neuropsychologia* 12 (1974): 367–376; K. Kocel, D. Galin, R. Ornstein, and E. Merrin, "Lateral Eye Movement and Cognitive Mode," *Psychonomic Science* 27 (1972): 223–224.

[48] H. Ehrlichman and A. Weinberger, "Lateral Eye Movements and Hemispheric Asymmetry: A Critical Review," *Psychological Bulletin* 85 (1979): 1080–1101.

[49] S. Carlton, P. Bakan, and M. Moretti, "Conjugate Lateral Eye Movements: A Second Look," *International Journal of Neuroscience* 48 (1989): 1–18.

[50] M. Kinsbourne and R. E. Hicks,

"Mapping Cerebral Functional Space: Competition and Collaboration in Human Performance," in *Asymmetrical Function of the Brain,* ed. M. Kinsbourne (Cambridge: Cambridge University Press, 1978).

[51]M. Kinsbourne and J. Cook, "Generalized and Lateralized Effects of Concurrent Verbalization on a Unimanual Skill," *Quarterly Journal of Experimental Psychology* 23 (1971): 341–345.

[52]R. E. Hicks, "Intrahemispheric Response Competition Between Vocal and Unimanual Performance in Normal Adult Human Male," *Journal of Comparative and Physiological Psychology* 89 (1975): 50–60.

[53]D. W. Kee and B. Cherry, "Lateralized Interference in Finger Tapping: Initial Value Differences Do Not Affect the Outcome," *Neuropsychologia* 28 (1990): 313–316.

Chapter 4   Measuring the Brain and Its Activity: Some Physiological Correlates of Asymmetry

[1]N. Geschwind and W. Levitsky, "Human Brain: Left–Right Asymmetries in Temporal Speech Region," *Science* 161 (1968): 186–187.

[2]J. A. Wada, R. Clark, and A. Hamm, "Cerebral Hemispheric Asymmetry in Humans," *Archives of Neurology* 32 (1975): 239–246; S. F. Witelson and W. Pallie, "Left Hemisphere Specialization for Language in the Newborn: Anatomical Evidence of Asymmetry," *Brain* 96 (1973): 641–646.

[3]A. M. Galaburda, J. Corsiglia, G. D. Rosen, and G. F. Sherman, "Planum Temporale Asymmetry, Reappraisal Since Geschwind and Levitsky," *Neuropsychologia* 25 (1987): 853–868.

[4]M. LeMay and A. Culebras, "Human Brain-Morphologic Differences in the Hemispheres Demonstrable by Carotid Anteriography," *New England Journal of Medicine* 287 (1972): 168–170.

[5]M. LeMay and N. Geschwind, "Asymmetries of the Human Cerebral Hemispheres," in *Language Acquisition and Language Breakdown,* ed. A. Caramazza and E. Zurif (Baltimore: Johns Hopkins University Press, 1978).

[6]W. H. Oldendorf, "Principles of Imaging Structure by Nuclear Magnetic Resonance," *Archives of Neurology* 32 (1983): 239–246.

[7]A. M. Galaburda, M. LeMay, T. Kemper, and N. Geschwind, "Right–Left Asymmetries in the Brain," *Science* 199 (1978): 852–856.

[8]D. Galin and R. Ornstein, "Lateral Specialization of Cognitive Mode: An EEG Study," *Psychophysiology* 9 (1972): 412–418.

[9]D. L. Molfese, R. B. Freeman, Jr., and D. S. Palermo, "The Ontogeny of the Brain Lateralization for Speech and Nonspeech Stimuli," *Brain and Language* 2 (1975): 356–368.

[10]C. C. Wood, W. R. Goff, and R. S. Day, "Auditory Evoked Potentials During Speech Perception," *Science* 173 (1971): 1248–1251.

[11]A. C. Papanicolaou, A. L. Schmidt, B. D. Moore, and H. M. Eisenberg, "Cerebral Activation Patterns in an Arithmetic and a Visuospatial Processing Task," *International Journal of Neuroscience* 20 (1983): 283–288.

[12]A. C. Papanicolaou, H. S. Levin, H. M. Eisenberg, and B. D. Moore, "Evoked Potential Indices of Selective Hemispheric Engagement in Affective and Phonetic Tasks," *Neuropsychologia* 21 (1983): 401–405.

[13]A. S. Gevins, N. H. Morgan, S. L. Bressler, B. A. Cutillo, R. M. White, J. Illes, D. S. Greer, J. C. Doyle, and G. M. Zeitlin, "Human Neuroelectric Patterns Predict Performance Accuracy," *Science* 235 (1987): 580–585; A. S. Gevins and J. Illes, "Neurocognitive Networks of the Human Brain," in *Windows on the Brain,* ed. R. A. Zappulla, F. F. LeFever, J. Jaeger, and R. Bilder, *Annals of the New York Academy of Sciences* 620 (1991).

[14]D. S. Barth, W. Sutherling, J. Engel, Jr., and J. Beatty, "Neuromagnetic Localization of Epileptiform Spike Activity in the Human Brain," *Science* 218 (1982): 891–894.

[15]G. L. Romani, S. J. Williamson, and L. Kaufman, "Characterization

of the Human Auditory Cortex by the Neuromagnetic Method," *Experimental Brain Research* 47 (1982): 381–393.

[16]A. C. Papanicolaou, S. Baumann, R. L. Rogers, C. Saydjari, E. G. Amparo, and H. M. Eisenberg, "Localization of Auditory Response Sources Using Magnetoencephalography and Magnetic Resonance Imaging," *Archives of Neurology* 47 (1990): 33–37.

[17]N. A. Lassen and D. H. Ingvar, "Radioisotopic Assessment of Regional Cerebral Blood Flows," in *Progress in Nuclear Medicine*, Vol. 1 (Baltimore: University Park Press, 1972).

[18]N. A. Lassen, D. H. Ingvar, and E. Skinhoj, "Brain Function and Blood Flow," *Scientific American* 239 (1978): 62–71.

[19]J. Risberg, J. H. Halsey, E. L. Wills, and E. M. Wilson, "Hemispheric Specialization in Normal Man Studied by Bilateral Measurements of the Regional Cerebral Blood Flow: A Study with the ^{133}Xe Inhalation Technique," *Brain* 98 (1975): 511–524.

[20]G. Deutsch, W. T. Bourbon, A. C. Papanicolaou, and H. M. Eisenberg, "Visuospatial Tasks Compared via Activation of Regional Cerebral Blood Flow," *Neuropsychologia* 26 (1988): 445–452.

[21]G. Deutsch, A. C. Papanicolaou, W. T. Bourbon, and H. M. Eisenberg, "Cerebral Blood Flow Evidence of Right Frontal Activation in Attention Demanding Tasks," *International Journal of Neuroscience* 36 (1987): 23–28.

[22]R. Kuzniecky, J. M. Mountz, and F. Thomas, "Ictal ^{99m}Tc-HMPAO Brain SPECT and EEG Nonlocalizable Partial Seizures," *Journal of Neuroimaging*, in press.

[23]J. M. Mountz and G. Deutsch, "^{99m}Tc-HMPAO SPECT Measures of a Mental Rotation Task," *Journal of Nuclear Medicine*, in press.

[24]P. T. Fox, S. E. Peterson, M. I. Posner, and M. E. Raichle, "Language-Related Brain Activation Measured with PET: Comparison of Auditory and Visual Word Presentations," *Journal of*

Cerebral Blood Flow and Metabolism 7, Supplement 1 (1987): S294.

[25]J. Sergent, S. Ohta, and B. MacDonald, "Functional Neuroanatomy of Face and Object Processing," *Brain* 115 (1992): 15–36.

[26]Ibid.

[27]J. V. Haxby, C. L. Grady, B. Horwitz, L. G. Ungerleider, M. Mishkin, R. E. Carson, P. Herscovitch, M. B. Schapiro, and S. I. Rapoport, "Dissociation of Object and Spatial Visual Processing Pathways in Human Extrastriate Cortex," *Proceedings of the National Academy of Sciences* U.S.A 88 (1991): 1621–1625; B. Horwitz, C. L. Grady, J. V. Haxby, L. G. Ungerleider, M. B. Schapiro, M. Mishkin, and S. I. Rapoport, "Functional Associations Among Human Posterior Extrastriate Brain Regions During Object and Spatial Vision," *Journal of Cognitive Neuroscience* 4 (1992): 311–322.

[28]J. den Hollander, H. Hetherington, D. Twieg, and G. Pohost, "^{31}P NMR Metabolite Mapping of Human Brain at 4.1T Using Time Domain Analysis," *Magnetic Resonance in Medicine*, in press; M. A. Thomas, H. P. Hetherington, D. J. Meyerhoff, and D. B. Twieg, "Localized Double Quantum Filtered ^{1}H NMR Spectroscopy," -*Journal of Magnetic Resonance* 93 (1991): 485–496.

[29]S. Ogawa, T.-M. Lee, A. R. Kay, and D. W. Tank, "Brain Magnetic Resonance Imaging with Contrast Dependent on Blood Oxygenation," *Proceedings of the National Academy of Sciences,* U.S.A 97 (1990): 9868–9872.

[30]G. Deutsch, "A Critical Overview of the Contributions of Functional Neuroimaging to Neuropsychology," *Journal of Experimental and Clinical Neuropsychology* 14 (1992): 86–87.

[31]A. Oke, R. Keller, I. Mefford, and R. N. Adams, "Lateralization of Norepinephrine in the Human Thalamus," *Science* 200 (1978): 1411–1413.

[32]L. Amaducci, S. Sorbi, A. Albanese, and G. Gainotti, "Choline-acetyl transferase (CHAT) Activity Differs in Right and Left Human Temporal Lobes," *Neurology* 31 (1981): 799–805.

[33]S. D. Glick, D. A. Ross, and L. B.

Hough, "Lateral Asymmetry of Neuro-transmitters in Human Brain," *Brain Research* 234 (1982): 53–63.

[34]K. H. Pribram and D. McGuinness, "Arousal, Activation, and Effort in the Control of Attention," *Psychological Review* 82 (1975): 116–149.

[35]D. M. Tucker and P. A. Williamson, "Asymmetric Neural Control Systems in Human Self-Regulation," *Psychological Review* 91 (1984): 185–215.

[36]M. E. Phelps, "Electron Generator Produced Labeled Precursors and Compounds for Positron Emission Tomography," presented at Functional Neuroimaging: Looking at the Mind, November 5–6, Back Bay Hilton, Boston, Massachusetts (1992).

[37]D. N. Robinson, *The Enlightened Machine* (New York: Columbia University Press, 1980).

Chapter 5   The Puzzle of the Left-Hander

[1]W. Dennis, "Early Graphic Evidence of Dextrality in Man," *Perceptual and Motor Skills* 8 (1958): 147–149; R. A. Dart, "The Predatory Implement Technique of Australopithecus," *American Journal of Physical Anthropology* 7 (1949): 1–38; R. S. Uhrbrock, "Laterality in Art," *Journal of Aesthetics and Art Criticism* 32 (1973): 27–35; S. Coren and C. Porac, "Fifty Centuries of Right Handedness: The Historical Record," *Science* 198 (1977): 631–632.

[2]M. C. Corballis, "The Origins and Evolution of Human Laterality," in *Neuropsychology and Cognition*, Vol. 1, ed. R. N. Malateska and L. C. Hartlage (The Hague: Martinus Nijhoff Publishers, 1982).

[3]M. Barsley, *Left Handed People* (North Hollywood, Calif.: Wilshire Book Co., 1979).

[4]C. Sagan, *The Dragons of Eden* (New York: Random House, 1977).

[5]J. A. Froude, *Thomas Carlyle in London, 1834–1881* (London: Longmans, Green, 1884)

[6]D. J. Cunningham, "Right Handedness and Left Handedness," *Journal of the Royal Anthropological Institute of Great Britain and Ireland* 32 (1902): 273–196.

[7]R. C. Oldfield, "The Assessment and Analysis of Handedness: The Edinburgh Inventory," *Neuropsychologia* 9 (1971): 97–114.

[8]S. Coren and C. Porac, *Lateral Preferences and Human Behavior* (New York: Springer-Verlag, 1981); S. Coren and C. Porac, "Effects of Simulated Refractive Asymmetries on Eye Dominance,"

Bulletin of the Psychonomic Society 9 (1977): 269 -271.

[9]Ibid.

[10]Ibid.

[11]H. D. Chamberlain, "The Inheritance of Left Handedness," *Journal of Heredity* 19 (1928): 557–559.

[12]R. L. Collins, "The Sound of One Paw Clapping: An Inquiry Into the Origins of Left Handedness," in *Contributions to Behavior-Genetic Analysis—The Mouse as Prototype,* ed. G. Lindzey and D. B. Thiessen (New York: The Meredith Corporation, 1970).

[13]R. L. Collins, "When Left Handed Mice Live in Right Handed Worlds," *Science* 187 (1975): 181–184.

[14]A. Blau, *The Master Hand* (New York: American Ortho-Psychiatric Association, 1946).

[15]M. Annett, "A Model of the Inheritance of Handedness and Cerebral Dominance," *Nature* 204 (1964): 59–60.

[16]M. Annett, *Left, Right, Hand and Brain* (London: Erlbaum, 1985).

[17]R. G. Howard and A. M. Brown, "Twinning: A Marker for Biological Insults," *Child Development* 41 (1970): 519–530.

[18]H. Gordon, "Left-Handedness and Mirror Writing Especially Among Defective Children," *Brain* 43 (1920): 313–368.

[19]T. Rasmussen and B. Milner, "The Role of Early Left-Brain Injury in Determining Lateralization of Cerebral Speech Functions," in *Evolution and Lateralization of the Brain*, ed. S. Dimond and D. Blizzard (New York: New York Academy of Sciences, 1977).

[20]P. Bakan, G. Dibb, and P. Reed, "Handedness and Birth Stress," *Neuropsychologia* 11 (1973): 363–366.

[21]A. Searleman, C. Porac, S. Coren, "Relationship Between Birth Order, Birth Stress, and Lateral Preference: A Critical Review," *Psychological Bulletin* 105 (1989): 397–408.

[22]M. Schwartz, "Discrepancy Between Maternal Report and Hospital Records," *Developmental Neuropsychology* 4 (1988): 303–304; M. Schwartz, "Handedness, Prenatal Stress, and Pregnancy Complications," *Neuropsychologia* 26 (1988): 925–929; M. Schwartz, "Left Handedness and Prenatal Complications" in *Left Handedness: Behavioral Implications and Anomalies,* ed. S. Coren (Amsterdam: Elsevier, 1990).

[23]P. Satz, "Pathological Left-Handedness: An Explanatory Model," *Cortex* 8 (1972): 121–135.

[24]P. Satz, D. L. Orsini, E. Saslow, and R. Henry, "The Pathological Left-Handedness Syndrome," *Brain and Cognition* 4 (1985): 27–46; P. Satz, D. L. Orsini, E. Saslow, and R. Henry, "Early Brain Injury and Pathological Left-Handedness: Clues to a Syndrome," in *The Dual Brain,* ed. E. Zaidel (New York: Guilford Press, 1985).

[25]H. Lansdell, "Verbal and Nonverbal Factors in Right-Hemisphere Speech: Relation to Early Neurological History," *Journal of Comparative and Physiological Psychology* 69 (1969): 734–738.

[26]Rasmussen and Milner, "The Role of Early Left-Brain Injury."

[27]D. W. Loring, K. Meador, G. Lee, A. Murro, J. Smith, H. Flanigin, B. Gallagher, and D. King, "Cerebral Language Lateralization: Evidence from Intracarotid Amobarbitol Testing," *Neuropsychologia* 28 (1990): 831–838.

[28]A. R. Luria, *Traumatic Aphasia* (The Hague: Mouton, 1970). A. Subirana, "The Prognosis in Aphasia in Relation to Cerebral Dominance and Handedness," *Brain* 81 (1958): 415–425.

[29]M. P. Bryden, "Tachistoscopic Recognition, Handedness, and Cerebral Dominance," *Neuropsychologia* 3 (1965): 1–8; P. Satz, K. Achenbach, E. Patteshall, and E. Fennell, "Order of Report, Ear Asymmetry, and Handedness in Dichotic Listening," *Cortex* 1 (1965): 377–396.

[30]H. Hecaen and J. Sauget, "Cerebral Dominance in Left Handed Subjects," *Cortex* 7 (1971): 19–48.

[31]D. L. Orsini, P. Satz, H. V. Soper, and R. K. Light, "The Role of Familial Sinistrality in Cerebral Organization," *Neuropsychologia* 23 (1985): 223–232.

[32]J. Levy and M. Reid. "Variations in Writing Posture and Cerebral Organization," *Science* 194 (1976): 337.

[33]A. M. Weber and J. L. Bradshaw, "Levy and Reid's Neurological Model in Relation to Writing Hand/Posture: An Evaluation," *Psychological Bulletin* 90 (1981): 74–78; J. Levy, "Handwriting Posture and Cerebral Organization: How Are They Related?" *Psychological Bulletin* 91 (1982): 589–608.

[34]J. H. Halsey, V. W. Blauenstein, E. M. Wilson, and E. L. Wills, "Brain Activation in the Presence of Brain Damage," *Brain and Language* 9 (1980): 47–60.

[35]E. Strauss, J. Wada, and B. Kosaka, "Writing Posture and Cerebral Dominance for Speech," *Cortex* 20 (1984): 143–147.

[36]C. Hardyck and L. Petrinovich, "Left Handedness," *Psychological Bulletin* 84 (1977): 385–404.

[37]J. Levy, "Possible Basis for the Evolution of Lateral Specialization of the Human Brain," *Nature* 224 (1969): 614–615.

[38]E. Miller, "Handedness and the Pattern of Human Ability," *British Journal of Psychology* 62 (1971): 111–112; F. Newcombe and G. Ratcliff, "Handedness, Speech Lateralization, and Ability," *Neuropsychologia* 11 (1973): 339–407.

[39]C. Mebert and G. Michel, "Handedness in Artists," in *Neuropsychology of Left Handedness,* ed. J. Herron (New York: Academic Press, 1980).

[40]N. Geschwind and P. Behan, "Left Handedness: Association with Immune Disease, Migraine, and Developmental Learning Disorders," *Proceedings of the National Academy of Sciences,* U.S.A. 79 (1982): 5097–5100.

[41]N. Geschwind and P. Behan,

"Laterality, Hormones, and Immunity," in *Cerebral Dominance: The Biological Foundations,* ed. N. Geschwind and A. M. Galaburda (Cambridge, Mass.: Harvard University Press, 1984).

[42]N. Geschwind and N. Galaburda, *Cerebral Lateralization: Biological Mechanisms, Associations and Pathology* (Cambridge, Mass.: MIT Press, 1987).

[43]C. P. Benbow and J. C. Stanley, "Sex Differences in Mathematical Ability: Fact or Artifact?", *Science* 210 (1983): 1262–1264.

[44]M. P. Bryden, I. C. McManus, R. E. Steenhuis, "Handedness is Not Related to Self-Reported Disease Incidence," *Cortex* 27 (1991): 605–611; W. F. McKeever and D. A. Rich, "Left Handedness and Immune Disorders," *Cortex* 26 (1990): 33–40; B. D. Smith, M. B. Meyers, and R. Kline, "For Better or Worse: Left Handedness, Pathology, and Talent," *Journal of Clinical and Experimental Neuropsychology* 11 (1989): 944–958.

[45]I. C. McManus and M. P. Bryden, "Geschwind's Theory of Cerebral Lateralization: Developing a Formal,

Causal Model," *Psychological Bulletin* 110 (1991): 237–253.

[46]D. F. Halpern and S. Coren, "Do Right Handers Live Longer?" *Nature* 333 (1988): 213.

[47]D. H. Halpern and S. Coren, "Hand Preference and Life Span," *New England Journal of Medicine* 324 (1991): 998.

[48]S. Coren, "Left Handedness and Accident-Related Injury Risk," *American Journal of Public Health* 79 (1989): 1–2; S. Coren and D. F. Halpern, "Left Handedness—A Marker for Decreased Survival Fitness," *Psychological Bulletin* 109 (1991): 90–106.

[49]D. M. Morens and A. R. Katz, "Left-handedness and Life Expectancy," *New England Journal of Medicine* 325 (1991): 1041.

[50]M. E. Salive, J. M. Guralnik, R. J. Glynn, "Left-handedness and Mortality," *American Journal of Public Health* 83 (1993): 265–267.

[51]K. Hugdahl, P. Satz, M. Mitrushina, and E. N. Miller, "Left-handedness and Old Age: Do Left-handers Die Earlier?" *Neuropsychologia* 31 (1993): 325–333.

Chapter 6   Further Evidence from the Clinic: Aphasia, Apraxia, Agnosia

[1]A. W. Ellis and A. W. Young, *Human Cognitive Neuropsychology* (London: Lawrence Erlbaum, 1988).

[2]Ibid.

[3]H. Hecaen and M. L. Albert, *Human Neuropsychology* (New York: Wiley, 1978); A. R. Luria, *Higher Cortical Functions* (New York: Basic Books, 1966).

[4]K. W. Walsh, *Neuropsychology—A Clinical Approach* (London: Churchill-Livingston, 1978); K. M. Heilman and E. Valenstein, *Clinical Neuropsychology* (New York: Oxford University Press, 1979).

[5]E. B. Zurif, "Language Mechanisms: A Neuropsychological Perspective," *American Scientist* 68 (1980): 305–311.

[6]A. Kreindler, C. Calavrezo, and L. Mihailescu, "Linguistic Analysis of One Case of Jargon Aphasia,"

Revue Roumaine de Neurologic 8 (1971): 209–228.

[7]J. W. Brown, *Aphasia, Apraxia and Agnosia* (Springfield, Ill.: Charles C. Thomas, 1972).

[8]A. K. Coughlan, and E. K. Warrington, "Word-Comprehension and Word-Retrieval in Patients with Localized Cerebral Lesions," *Brain* 101 (1978): 163–185; S. J. Dimond, *Neuropsychology: A Textbook of Systems and Psychological Functions of the Human Brain* (London: Butterworths, 1980).

[9]N. Geschwind, "Disconnexion Syndromes in Animals and Man," *Brain* 88 (1965): 237–294; N. Geschwind, "The Organization of Language and the Brain," *Science* 170 (1970): 940–944.

[10]Dimond, *Neuropsychology.*

[11]Geschwind, "Disconnexion Syndromes in Animals and Man."

[12]J. C. Marshall, "On the Biology of Language Acquisition," in *Biological Studies of Mental Processes*, ed. D. Caplan (Cambridge, Mass.: MIT Press, 1980).

[13]T. Shallice, *From Neuropsychology to Mental Structure* (Cambridge: Cambridge University Press, 1988); Ellis and Young, *Human Cognitive Neuropsychology.*

[14]J. W. Brown, *Mind, Brain, and Consciousness* (New York: Academic Press, 1977).

[15]P. MacLean, "Cerebral Evolution and Emotional Processes: New Findings on the Striatal Complex," *Annals of the New York Academy of Science* 193 (1972): 137–149; G. Coghill, *Anatomy and the Problem of Behavior* (New York: Cambridge University Press, 1929).

[16]Dimond, *Neuropsychology.*

[17]G. A. Ojemann, "Subcortical Language Mechanisms," in *Studies in Neurolinguistics*, Vol. 1, ed. H. Whitaker and H. A. Whitaker (New York: Academic Press, 1976); G. A. Ojemann, "Asymmetric Function of the Thalamus in Man," *Annals of the New York Academy of Science* 299 (1977): 380–396.

[18]A. Smith, "Speech and Other Functions After Left (Dominant) Hemispherectomy," *Journal of Neurology, Neurosurgery and Psychiatry* 29 (1966): 467–471; C. W. Burkland and A. Smith, "Language and the Cerebral Hemispheres," *Neurology* 27 (1977): 627–633.

[19]A. Smith, "Nondominant Hemispherectomy," *Neurology* 19 (1969): 442–445.

[20]Geschwind, "Disconnexion Syndromes in Animals and Man."

[21]M. Coltheart, "Deep Dyslexia: A Right-Hemisphere Hypothesis," in *Deep Dyslexia*, ed. M. Coltheart, K. Patterson, and J. C. Marshall (London: Routledge and Kegan Paul, 1980).

[22]D. Hines, "Differences in Tachistoscopic Recognition Between Abstract and Concrete Words as a Function of Visual Half-Field and Frequency," *Cortex* 13 (1977): 66–73.

[23]M. Danly and B. Shapiro, "Speech Prosody in Broca's Aphasia," *Brain and Language* 16 (1982): 171–190.

[24]K. M. Heilman, R. Scholes, and R. T. Watson, "Auditory Affective Agnosia: Disturbed Comprehension of Affective Speech," *Journal of Neurology, Neurosurgery and Psychiatry* 38 (1975): 69–72.

[25]E. D. Ross and M. M. Mesulam, "Dominant Language Functions of the Right Hemisphere?" *Archives of Neurology* 36 (1979): 144–148.

[26]E. D. Ross, "The Aprosodias:Functional-Anatomic Organization of the Affective Components of Language in the Right Hemisphere," *Annals of Neurology* 38 (1981): 561–589.

[27]M. L. Albert, R. W. Sparks, and N. A. Helm, "Melodic Intonation Therapy for Aphasia," *Archives of Neurology* 29 (1973): 130–131.

[28]E. Winner and H. Gardner, "The Comprehension of Metaphor in Brain-Damaged Patients," *Brain* 100 (1977): 717–729.

[29]N. S. Foldi, M. Cicone, and H. Gardner, "Pragmatic Aspects of Communication in Brain Damaged Patients," in *Language Functions and Brain Organization*, ed. S. J. Segalowitz (New York: Academic Press, 1983).

[30]W. R. Gowers, *A Manual of Diseases of the Nervous System* (London: J & A Churchill, 1893).

[31]M. Kinsbourne, "The Minor Cerebral Hemisphere as a Source of Aphasic Speech," *Archives of Neurology* 25 (1971): 302–306.

[32]J. L. Cummings, D. F. Benson, M. J. Walsh, and H. L. Levine, "Left-to-Right Transfer of Language Dominance: A Case Study," *Neurology* 29 (1979): 1547–1550.

[33]A. C. Papanicolaou, B. D. Moore, H. S. Levin, and H. M. Eisenberg, "Evoked Potential Correlates of Right Hemisphere Involvement in Language Recovery Following Stroke," *Archives of Neurology* 44 (1987): 521–524.

[34]G. Deutsch, A. C. Papanicolaou, and H. M. Eisenberg, "CBF During Tasks Intended to Differentially Activate the Cerebral Hemispheres: New Normative Data and Preliminary Applications in Recovering Stroke Patients," *Journal of*

Cerebral Blood Flow and Metabolism 7 Supplement (1987): S306.

[35]M. Fiorelli, J. Blin, S. Bakchine, D. Laplane, and J. C. Baron, "PET Studies of Cortical Diaschisis in Patients with Motor Hemi-Neglect," *Journal of Neurological Sciences* 104 (1991): 135–142.

[36]E. K. Warrington, "Constructional Apraxia," in *Handbook of Clinical Neurology,* Vol. 4, ed. P. J. Vinken and G. W. Bruyn (Amsterdam: Elsevier/North-Holland Biomedical Press, 1969).

[37]A. L. Benton, "Visuoperceptive, Visuospatial and Visuoconstructive Disorders," in *Clinical Neuropsychology,* ed. K. M. Heilman and E. Valenstein (Oxford: Oxford University Press, 1979).

[38]E. DeRenzi, P. Faglioni, and G. Scotti, "Hemispheric Contribution to Exploration of Space Through Visual and Tactile Modality," *Cortex* 6 (1970): 191–203; D. J. Fontenot and A. L. Benton, "Tactile Perception of Direction in Relation to Hemispheric Locus of Lesion," *Neuropsychologia* 9 (1971): 83–88.

[39]A. L. Benton, "The Neuropsychology of Facial Recognition," *American Psychologist* 35 (1980): 176–186; Benton, "Visuoperceptive, Visuospatial, and Visuoconstructive Disorders."

[40]J. Sergent, S. Ohta, and B. MacDonald, "Functional Neuroanatomy of Face and Object Recognition," *Brain* 115 (1992): 15–36.

[41]J. Sergent and J. L. Signoret, "Outstanding Issues in the Study of Prosopagnosia," *Journal of Clinical and Experimental Neuropsychology* 13 (1991): 34.

[42]E. Goldberg, "Associative Agnosias and the Functions of the Left Hemisphere," *Journal of Clinical and Experimental Neuropsychology* 12 (1990): 467–484.

[43]Ibid.

[44]Ellis and Young, *Human Cognitive Neuropsychology.*

[45]D. Marr, *Vision* (San Francisco: W. H. Freeman, 1982).

[46]Ellis and Young, *Human Cognitive Neuropsychology.*

Chapter 7   Further Evidence from the Clinic: Neglect, Memory, Music, and Emotion

[1]K. Heilman and S. Watson, "The Neglect Syndrome-A Unilateral Defect of the Orienting Response," in *Lateralization in the Nervous System,* ed. S. Harnad, R. Doty, L. Goldstein, J. Jaynes, and G. Krauthamer (New York: Academic Press, 1977).

[2]B. T. Volpe, J. E. LeDoux, and M. S. Gazzaniga, "Information Processing of Visual Stimuli in an 'Extinguished' Field," *Nature* 282 (1979): 122–124.

[3]G. Deutsch, J. Tweedy, and B. Lorinstein, "Some Temporal and Spatial Factors Affecting Visual Neglect," *International Journal of Neuroscience* 12 (1981): 271.

[4]R. D. Nebes, "Direct Examination of Cognitive Function in the Right and Left Hemispheres, " in *Asymmetrical Function of the Brain,* ed. M. Kinsbourne (Cambridge: Cambridge University Press, 1978); M. S. Gazzaniga and J. E. LeDoux, *The Integrated Mind* (New York: Plenum Press, 1978).

[5]M. Kinsbourne, "Mechanisms of Unilateral Neglect," in *Neurophysiological and Neuropsychological Aspects of Spatial Neglect,* ed. M. Jeannerod (New York: North Holland Publishing Co., 1987), p. 69–86.

[6]K. Heilman and T. Van Den Abell, "Right Hemisphere Dominance for Attention: the Mechanisms Underlying Hemispheric Asymmetries of Inattention (Neglect)," *Neurology* 30 (1980): 327–330

[7]S. Weintraub and M.-M. Mesulam, "Right Cerebral Dominance in Spatial Attention: Further Evidence Based on Ipsilateral Neglect," *Archives of Neurology* 44 (1987):621–625.

[8]E. Bisiach, "Understanding Consciousness: Clues from Unilateral Neglect and Related Disorders," in *The Neuropsychology of Consciousness,* ed. A. Mil-

ner and M. Rugg (London: Academic Press, 1992).

[9]E. Bisiach and C. Luzatti, "Unilateral Neglect of Representational Space," *Cortex* 14 (1978): 129–133.

[10]K. S. Lashley, "In Search of the Engram," in *Symposium of the Society for Experimental Biology,* No. 4 (London: Cambridge University Press, 1950).

[11]W. Penfield and P. Perot, "The Brain's Record of Auditory and Visual Experience. A Final Summary and Discussion," *Brain* 86 (1963): 595–696. W. Penfield and L. Roberts, *Speech and Brain Mechanisms* (Princeton, N.J.: Princeton University Press, 1959).

[12]G. Deutsch and J. R. Tweedy, "Cerebral Blood Flow in Severity Matched Alzheimer and Multi-infarct Patients," *Neurology* 37 (1987): 431–438.

[13]G. A. Miller,"The Magical Number Seven, Plus or Minus Two: Some Limits on Our Capacity for Processing Information," *Psychological Review* 63 (1956): 81–97.

[14]S. M. Kosslyn and O. Koenig, *Wet Mind: The New Cognitive Neuroscience* (New York: Free Press-Macmillan, 1992).

[15]Ibid.

[16]R. P. Kesner, "Mnemonic Functions of the Hippocampus: Correspondence Between Animals and Humans," in *Conditioning Representation of Neural Function,* ed. C. D. Woody (New York: Plenum Press, 1983); B. Milner, "Hemispheric Specialization: Scope and Limits," in *The Neurosciences: Third Research Program,* ed. F. O. Schmitt and F. G. Warden (Cambridge, Mass.: MIT Press, 1974).

[17]M. Moscovitch and C. Umilta, "Conscious and Nonconscious Aspects of Memory: A Neuropsychological Framework of Modules and Central Systems," in *Perspectives on Cognitive Neuroscience,* ed. R. G. Lister and H. J. Weingartner (Oxford: Oxford University Press, 1991); M. Moscovitch, "Memory and Working-with-Memory: A Component Process Model Based on Modules and Central Systems," *Journal of Cognitive neuroscience,* 4 (1992): 257–267.

[18]Ibid.

[19]M. Moscovitch, "Confabulation and the Frontal System: Strategic vs Associative Retrieval in Neuropsychological Theories of Memory," in *Varieties of Memory and Consciousness: Essays in Honor of Endel Tulving,* ed. H. L. Roediger and F. I. M. Craik (Hillsdale, N.J.: Erlbaum, 1989).

[20]Kosslyn and Koenig, *Wet Mind: The New Cognitive Neuroscience.*

[21]C. B. Blakemore and M. A. Falconer, "Long Term Effects of Anterior Temporal Lobectomy on Certain Cognitive Functions," *Journal of Neurology, Neurosurgery and Psychiatry* 30 (1967): 364–367; B. Milner and H. L. Teuber, "Alteration of Perception and Memory in Man: Reflections on Methods," in *Analysis of Behavioral Change,* ed. L. Wieskrantz (New York: Harper & Row, 1968).

[22]B. Milner, "Visual Recognition and Recall After Right Temporal-Lobe Excision in Man," *Neuropsychologia* 6 (1968): 191–209.

[23]B. Milner, "Visually Guided Maze Learning in Man: Effects of Bilateral Hippocampal, Bilateral Frontal, and Unilateral Cerebral Lesions," *Neuropsychologia* 3 (1965): 317–338.

[24]N. Geschwind, "The Organization of Language and the Brain," *Science* 170 (1970): 940–944; M. S. Gazzaniga and J. E. LeDoux, *The Integrated Mind* (New York: Plenum Press, 1978).

[25]G. Deutsch, A. C. Papanicolaou, H. M. Eisenberg, D. W. Loring, and H. S. Levin, "CBF Gradient Changes Elicited by Visual Stimulation and Visual Memory tasks," *Neuropsychologia* 24 (1986): 283–287.

[26]T. Shallice and G. Vallar, "The Impairment of Auditory-Verbal Short-Term Storage," in *Neuropsychological Impairments of Short-Term Memory,* ed. G. Vallar and T. Shallice (Cambridge: Cambridge University Press, 1990).

[27]E. DeRenzi and P. Nichelli, "Verbal and Non-Verbal Short-Term Memory Impairment Following Hemispheric Damage," *Cortex* 11 (1975): 341–354.

[28]C. J. Marsolek, S. M. Kosslyn, and L. R. Squire, "Form-Specific Visual Priming in the Right Cerebral Hemisphere," *Journal of Experimental*

Psychology: Learning, Memory and Cognition 18 (1992): 492–508.

[29]Ibid.

[30]K. A. Paller, "Recall and Stem-Completion Priming Have Different Electrophysiological Correlates and Are Modified Differentially by Directed Forgetting," *Journal of Experimental Psychology: Learning, Memory and Cognition* 16 (1990): 1021–1032; K. A. Paller and M. Kutas, "Brain Potentials During Memory Retrieval: Neurophysiological Support for the Distinction Between Conscious Recollection and Priming," *Journal of Cognitive Neuroscience* (1993): in press.

[31]L. R. Squire, "Declarative and Non-declarative Memory: Multiple Brain Systems Supporting Learning and Memory," *Journal of Cognitive Neuroscience* 4 (1992): 232–243.

[32]J. Kinoshita, "Mapping the Mind," *New York Times Magazine,* October 18 (1992): 44–54.

[33]M. Mishkin, "A Memory System in the Monkey," *Philosophical Transactions Review Society of London,* Series Biological 298 (1982): 85–92; L. R. Squire, *Memory and Brain* (New York: Oxford University Press, 1987).

[34]R. Desimone, "The Physiology of Memory: Recordings of Things Past," *Science* 258 (1992): 245–246.

[35]Mishkin, "A Memory System in the Monkey."

[36]M. Colombo, M. R. D'Amato, H. R. Rodman, and C. G. Gross, "Auditory Association Cortex Lesions Impair Auditory Short-Term Memory in Monkeys," *Science* 247 (1990): 336.

[37]G. Goldenberg, I. Podreka, M. Steiner, and K. Wilmes, "Regional Cerebral Blood Flow Patterns in Imagery Tasks - Results of Single Photon Emission Computed Tomography," in *Cognitive and Neuropsychological Approaches to Mental Imagery,* ed. D. M. Engelkamp and J. T. E. Richardson (Dordrecht: Martinus Nijhoff, 1988).

[38]A. R. Damasio, "Category-Related Recognition Defects as a Clue to the Neural Substrates of Knowledge," *Trends in Neuroscience* 13 (1990): 95–98.

[39]Kinoshita, "Mapping the Mind."

[40]B. Milner, "Laterality Effects in Audition," in *Interhemispheric Relations and Cerebral Dominance,* ed. V. Mountcastle (Baltimore: Johns Hopkins University Press, 1962).

[41]J. E. Bogen and H. W. Gordon, "Musical Tests of Functional Lateralization with Intracarotid Amobarbital," *Nature* 230 (1971): 524–525.

[42]H. W. Gordon and J. E. Bogen, "Hemispheric Lateralization of Singing After Intracarotid Sodium Amobarbitone," *Journal of Neurology, Neurosurgery, and Psychiatry* 37 (1974): 727–738.

[43]R. J. Zatorre, "Musical Perception and Cerebral Function: A Critical Review," *Music Perception* 2 (1984): 196–221.

[44]T. Alajouanine, "Aphasia and Artistic Realization," *Brain* 71 (1948): 229–241.

[45]A. Gates and J. Bradshaw, "The Role of the Cerebral Hemispheres in Music," *Brain and Language* 4 (1977): 403–431.

[46]T. Bever and R. Chiarello, "Cerebral Dominance in Musicians and Non-musicians," *Science* 185 (1974): 137–139.

[47]R. J. Zatorre, "Recognition of Dichotic Melodies by Musicians and Nonmusicians," *Neuropsychologia* 17 (1979): 607–617.

[48]J. Sergent, E. Zuck, S. Terriah, and B. MacDonald, "Distributed Neural Network Underlying Musical Sight-Reading and Keyboard Performance," *Science* 257 (1992): 106–109.

[49]Ibid.

[50]W. James, *The Principles of Psychology* (New York: Holt, 1890).

[51]P. Eckman, R. W. Levenson, and W. V. Friesen, "Autonomic Nervous System Activity Distinguishes Emotions," *Science* 221 (1983): 1208–1210.

[52]K. M. Heilman and R. T. Watson, "Arousal and Emotions," in *Handbook of Neuropsychology,* Vol. 3, ed. F. Boller and J. Grafman (Amsterdam: Elsevier, 1989).

[53]G. Hohmann, "Some Effects of Spinal Cord Lesions on Experimental Emotional Feelings," *Psychophysiology* 3 (1966): 143–156.

[54]S. Schachter, "The Interaction of Cognitive and Physiological Determinants

of Emotional State," in *Advances in Experimental Social Psychology,* Vol. 1, ed. L. Berkowitz (New York: Academic Press, 1970).

[55]Ibid.

[56]A. C. Papanicolaou, *Emotion: A Reconsideration of the Somatic Theory* (New York: Gordon and Breach, 1989).

[57]W. B. Cannon, "The James-Lange Theory of Emotion: A Critical Examination and an Alternative Theory," *American Journal of Psychology* 39 (1927): 106–124.

[58]P. Bard, "Emotion. I: The Neuro-Humoral Basis of Emotional Reactions," in *Handbook of General Experimental Psychology,* ed. C. Murchison (Worcester, Mass.: Clark University Press, 1934).

[59]J. W. Papez, "A Proposed Mechanism of Emotion," *Archives of Neurology and Psychiatry* 38 (1937): 725–743.

[60]G. Gainotti, "Reactions 'Catastrophiques' et Manifestations d'-Indifference au Cours des Atteintes Cerebrales," *Neuropsychologia* 7 (1969): 195–204.

[61]G. F. Rossi and G. Rosadini, "Experimental Analysis of Cerebral Dominance in Man," in *Brain Mechanisms Underlying Speech and Language,* ed. C. H. Milikan and F. L. Danley (New York: Grune & Stratton, 1967); H. Terzian, "Behavioral and EEG Effects of Intracarotid Sodium Amytal Injection," *Acta Neurochirurgia (Wein)* 12 (1964): 230–239.

[62]Terzian, "Behavioral and EEG Effects."

[63]Ibid.

[64]B. Milner, "Comments of Rossi and Rosadini," in B*rain Mechanisms Underlying Speech and Language,* ed. Milikan and Danley; T. Tsunoda and M. Oka, "Lateralization for Emotion in the Human Brain and Auditory Cerebral Dominance," *Proceedings of the Japanese Academy* 52 (1976): 528–531.

[65]H. A. Sackheim, M. S. Greenberg, A. L. Weiman, R. C. Gur, J. P. Hunger-buhler, and N. Geschwind, "Hemispheric Asymmetry in the Expression of Positive and Negative Emotions: Neurological Evidence," *Archives of Neurology* 39 (1982): 210–218.

[66]K. M. Heilman, R. Scholes, and R. T. Watson, "Auditory Affective Agnosia: Disturbed Comprehension of Affective Speech," *Journal of Neurology, Neurosurgery and Psychiatry* 38 (1975): 69–72.

[67]D. M. Tucker, R. T. Watson, and K. M. Heilman, "Affective Discrimination and Evocation in Patients with Right Parietal Disease," *Neurology* 27 (1977): 947–950.

[68]J. C. Borod, F. Andelman, L. K. Obler, J. R. Tweedy, and J. Welkowitz, "Right Hemisphere Specialization for the Appreciation of Emotional Words and Sentences: Evidence from Stroke Patients," *Neuropsychologia* 30 (1992): 827–844.

[69]D. Van Lancker and J. J. Sidtis, "Identification of Affective-Prosodic Stimuli by Left and Right Hemisphere Damaged Subjects: All Errors Are Not Created Equal," *Journal of Speech and Hearing Research* 35 (1992): 963–970.

[70]J. C. Borod, "Interhemispheric and Intrahemispheric Control of Emotion: A Focus on Unilateral Brain Damage," *Journal of Consulting and Clinical Psychology* 60 (1992): 339–348.

[71]H. A. Sackheim, R. C. Gur, and M. Saucy, "Emotions Are Expressed More Intensely on the Left Side of the Face," *Science* 202 (1978): 434–436.

[72]J. C. Borod and H. S. Caron, "Facedness and Emotion Related to Lateral Dominance, Sex, and Expression Type," *Neuropsychologia* 18 (1980): 237–242.

[73]J. Borod, E. Koff, and B. White, "Facial Asymmetry in Posed and Spontaneous Expressions of Emotion," *Brain and Cognition* 2 (1983): 165–175.

[74]B. B. Schiff and B. MacDonald, "Facial Asymmetries in the Spontaneous Response to Positive and Negative Emotional Arousal," *Neuropsychologia* 28 (1990): 777–785.

[75]F. L. King and D. Kimura, "Left Ear Superiority in Dichotic Perception of Vocal Nonverbal Sounds," *Canadian Journal of Psychology* 26 (1972): 111–116; M. P. Haggard and A. M. Parkinson, "Stimulus and Task Factors as Determinants of Ear Advantages,"

Quarterly Journal of Experimental Psychology 23 (1971): 168–177.

[76]R. G. Ley and M. P. Bryden, "Hemispheric Differences in Recognizing Faces and Emotions," *Brain and Language* 7 (1979): 127–138.

[77]Borod, "Interhemispheric and Intrahemispheric Control of Emotion."

[78]H. Gardner, H. H. Brownell, W. Wapner, and D. Michelow, "Missing the Point: The Role of the Right Hemisphere in the Processing of Complex Linguistic Materials," in *Cognitive Processing in the Right Hemisphere,* ed. E. Perecman (New York: Academic Press, 1983).

[79]Borod, "Interhemispheric and Intrahemispheric Control of Emotion."

[80]K. Yokoyama, R. Jennings, P. Ackles, B. S. Hood, and F. Boller, "Lack of Heart Rate Changes During an Attention-Demanding Task after Right Hemisphere Lesions," *Neurology* 37 (1987): 624–630; P. Zoccolotti, D. Scabini, and C. Violani, "Electrodermal Responses in Patients with Unilateral Brain Damage," *Journal of Clinical Neuropsychology* 4 (1982): 143–150.

[81]K. M. Heilman and R. T. Watson, "Arousal and Emotions," in *Handbook of Neuropsychology,* Vol. 3, ed. F. Boller and J. Grafman (Amsterdam: Elsevier, 1989).

[82]K. M. Heilman, H. D. Schwartz, and R. T. Watson, "Hypoarousal in Patients with the Neglect Syndrome and Emotional Indifference," *Neurology* 28 (1978): 229–232.

Chapter 8   Sex and Asymmetry

[1]M. Coltheart, E, Hull, and D. Slater, "Sex Differences in Imagery and Reading," *Nature* 253 (1975): 438–440.

[2]D. F. Halpern, *Sex Differences in Cognitive Abilities* (New York: Erlbaum, 1992).

[3]H. Lansdell, "A Sex Difference in Effect of Temporal Lobe Neurosurgery on Design Preference," *Nature* 194 (1962): 852–854.

[4]J. McGlone, "Sex Differences in Functional Brain Asymmetry," *Cortex* 14 (1978): 122–128.

[5]J. Inglis and J. S. Lawson, "Sex Differences in the Effects of Unilateral Brain Damage on Intelligence," *Science* 212 (1981): 693–695.

[6]J. A. Wada, R. Clark, and A. Hamm, "Cerebral Hemisphere Asymmetry in Humans," *Archives of Neurology* 32 (1975): 239–246.

[7]M. Diamond, "Age Sex, and Environmental Influences on Anatomical Asymmetry in Rat Forebrain," in *Cerebral Dominance: The Biological Foundations,* ed. N. Geschwind and A. M. Galaburda (Cambridge, Mass.: Harvard University Press, 1984).

[8]A. S. Berreb, R. H. Fitch, D. L. Ralphe, and J. O. Denenberg, "Corpus Callosum: Region Specific Effects of Sex, Early Experience, and Age." *Brain Research* 438 (1988): 216–224.

[9]L. Allen, M. Richey, Y. Chai, and R. Gorski, "Sex Differences in the Corpus Callosum of the Living Human Being," *Journal of Neuroscience* 11 (1991): 933–942.

[10]M. C. Linn and A. C. Petersen, "Emergence and Characterization of Sex Differences in Spatial Ability: A Meta-Analysis," *Child Development* 56 (1985): 1479–1498.

[11]G. Deutsch and J. H. Halsey, Jr., "Cortical Blood Flow Indicates Frontal Asymmetries Dominate in Males but not in Females During Task Performance," *Journal of Cerebral Blood Flow and Metabolism* 11 (1991): S787.

[12]K. Podell, E. Goldberg, R. Harner, and S. Riggio, "Lateralization of Frontal Lobe Functions in Human Males," *Society for Neuroscience Abstracts* 17 (1991): 340.3.

[13]E. Goldberg and K. Podell, "Sex Differences in the Lateralization of Frontal Lobe Functions," *Society for Neuroscience Abstracts* 19 (1993): in press.

[14]D. A. Lake and M. P. Bryden, "Handedness and Sex Differences in Hemispheric Asymmetry," *Brain and Language* 3 (1976): 266–282.

[15]D. M. Piazza, "The Influence of Sex

and Handedness in the Hemispheric Specialization of Verbal and Nonverbal Tasks," *Neuropsychologia* 18 (1980): 163–176.

[16]M. P. Bryden, *Laterality: Functional Asymmetry in the Intact Brain* (New York: Academic Press, 1982).

[17]S. F. Witelson, "Sex and the Single Hemisphere: Specialization of the Right Hemisphere for Spatial Processing," *Science* 193 (1976): 425–427.

[18]D. P. Waber, "The Search for Biological Correlates of Behavioral Sex Differences in Humans," in *Human Sexual Dimorphism,* ed. J. Ghesquiere, R. D. Martin, and F. Newcombe (London: Taylor and Francis, 1985).

[19]J. Levy, "Lateral Differences in the Human Brain in Cognition and Behavioral Control," in *Cerebral Correlates of Conscious Experience,* ed. P. Buser and A. Rougeul-Buser (New York: North Holland Publishing Co., 1978).

[20]J. B. Becker, S. M. Breedlove, and D. Crews, *Behavioral Endocrinology* (Cambridge, Mass.: MIT Press, 1992).

[21]J. M. Reinisch and S. A. Sanders, "Effects of Prenatal Exposure to Diethylstilbestrol (DES) on Hemispheric

Laterality and Spatial Ability in Human Males," *Hormones and Behavior* 26 (1992): 62–75.

[22]S. M. Resnick, S. A. Berenbaum, I. I. Gottesman, and T. J. Bouchard, "Early Hormonal Influences of Cognitive Functioning in Congenital Adrenal Hyperplasia," *Developmental Psychology* 22 (1986): 191–198.

[23]V. Schute, cited in D. Kimura, "Sex Differences in the Brain," *Scientific American* (1992): 118–122.

[24]E. Hamson, "Variations in Sex-Related Cognitive Abilities Across the Menstrual Cycle," *Brain and Cognition* 14 (1990): 26–43.

[25]D. Kimura, cited in D. Kimura, "Sex Differences in the Brain," *Scientific American* (1992): 118–122.

[26]C. P. Benbow, "Mathematical Ability: Is Sex a Factor?" *Science* 212 (1981): 118–119.

[27]C. P. Benbow, "Sex Differences in Mathematical Reasoning Ability in Intellectually Talented Preadolescents: Their Nature, Effects, and Possible Causes," *Behavioral and Brain Sciences* 11 (1988): 169–232.

[28]Ibid.

Chapter 9   Phylogeny and Ontogeny: The Evolution and Development of Asymmetry

[1]R. L. Collins, "On the Inheritance of Handedness. I: Laterality in Inbred Mice," *Journal of Heredity* 59 (1968): 9–12; J. M. Warren, J. M. Abplanalp, and H. B. Warren, "The Development of Handedness in Cats and Rhesus Monkeys," in *Early Behavior: Comparative and Developmental Approaches,* ed. H. W. Stevenson, E. H. Hess, and H. L. Reingold (New York: Wiley, 1967).

[2]R. L. Collins, "On the Inheritance of Handedness II: Selection for Sinistrality in Mice," *Journal of Heredity* 60 (1969): 117–119.

[3]P. F. MacNeilage, M. G. Studdert-Kennedy, and B. Lindblom, "Primate Handedness Reconsidered," *Behavioral and Brain Sciences* 10 (1987): 247–303.

[4]Ibid.

[5]J. Fagot and J. Vauclair, "Manual

Laterality in Non-Human Primates: A Distinction Between Handedness and Manual Specialization," *Psychological Bulletin* 109 (1991): 76–89.

[6]R. Steenhuis and M. P. Bryden, "Different Dimensions of Hand Preference That Relate to Skilled and Unskilled Activities," *Cortex* 25 (1989): 289–304.

[7]W. D. Hopkins, D. A. Washburn, and D. M. Rumbaugh, "Note on Hand Use in the Manipulation of Joysticks by Rhesus Monkeys and Chimpanzees," *Journal of Comparative Psychology* 104 (1989): 91–94.

[8]G. Ettlinger and D. Gautrin, "Visual Discrimination Performance in the Monkey: The Effect of Unilateral Removal of Temporal Cortex," *Cortex* 7 (1971): 315–331; J. M. Warren and A. J. Nonneman, "The Search for Cerebral Dominance in Monkeys," in

Origins and Evolution of Language and Speech, ed. S. Harnad, H. Steklis, and J. Lancaster (New York: New York Academy of Sciences, 1976).

9J. H. Dewson, A. Cowey, and L. Weiskrantz, "Disruptions of Auditory Sequence Discrimination by Unilateral and Bilateral Cortical Ablations of Superior Temporal Gyrus in the Monkey," *Experimental Neurology* 28 (1970): 529–548.

10H. E. Heffner and R. S. Heffner, "Temporal Lobe Lesions and Perception of Species-Specific Vocalizations by Macaques," *Science* 226 (1984): 75–76.

11F. F. Ebner and R. E. Myers, "The Corpus Callosum and Interhemispheric Transmission of Tactual Learning," *Journal of Neurophysiology* 25 (1962): 380–391.

12J. S. Stamm and R. W. Sperry, "Function of Corpus Callosum in Contralateral Transfer of Somesthetic Discrimination in Cats," *Journal of Comparative and Physiological Psychology* 50 (1957): 138–143; H. Gulliksen and T. Voneida, "An Attempt to Obtain Replicate Learning Curves in the Split Brain Cat," *Physiological Psychology* 3 (1975): 77–85; S. Robinson and T. J. Voneida, "Hemisphere Differences in Cognitive Capacity in the Split Brain Cat," *Experimental Neurology* 38 (1973): 123–134.

13C. R. Hamilton, "Hemispheric Specialization in Monkeys," in *Brain Circuits and Functions of the Mind,* ed. C. B. Trevarthen (Cambridge: Cambridge University Press, 1990); C. R. Hamilton, "Functional Lateralization in Monkeys," in *Recent Advances in Laterality,* ed. F. Kitterle (Hillsdale: Erlbaum, 1991).

14Hamilton, "Functional Lateralization in Monkeys."

15G. H. Yeni-Komshian and D. Benson, "Anatomical Study of Cerebral Asymmetry in the Temporal Lobe of Humans, Chimpanzees, and Rhesus Monkeys," *Science* 192 (1976): 387–389.

16M. Lemay and N. Geschwind, "Hemispheric Differences in the Brains of

Great Apes," *Brain, Behavior, and Evolution* 11 (1975): 48–52.

17C. P. Groves and N. K. Humphrey, "Asymmetry in Gorilla Skulls: Evidence of Lateralized Brain Function?" *Nature* 244 (1973): 53–54.

18M. Diamond, "Age, Sex, and Environmental Influences on Anatomical Asymmetry in Rat Forebrain," in *Cerebral Dominance: The Biological Foundations,* ed. N. Geschwind and A. M. Galaburda (Cambridge, Mass.: Harvard University Press, 1984).

19S. D. Glick, J. N. Carlson, K. L. Drew, and R. M. Shapiro, "Functional and Neurochemical Asymmetry in the Corpus Striatum," in *Duality and Unity of the Brain,* ed. D. Ottoson (New York: Plenum Press, 1987).

20E. Mach (1885), cited in S. D. Glick and D. Ross, "Lateralization of Function in the Rat Brain. Basic Mechanism May Be Operative in Humans," *Trends in the Neurosciences* 12 (1981): 196–199.

21M. R. Petersen, M. D. Beecher, S. R. Zoloth, D. B. Moody, and W. C. Stebbins, "Neural Lateralization of Species-Specific Vocalizations by Japanese Macaques," *Science* 202 (1978): 324–326.

22W. D. Hopkins, K. D. Morris, S. Savage-Rumbaugh, and D. Rumbaugh, "Hemispheric Priming by Meaningful and Nonmeaningful Symbols in Language Trained Chimpanzees: Further Evidence of a Left Hemisphere Advantage," *Behavioral Neuroscience* 106 (1992): 575–582.

23Ibid.

24F. Nottebohm, "Brain Pathways for Vocal Learning in Birds: A Review of the First Ten Years," *Progress in Psychobiology and Physiological Psychology* 9 (1980): 86–124; F. Nottebohm, "Learning, Forgetting, and Brain Repair," in *Cerebral Dominance: The Biological Foundations,* Geschwind and Galaburda.

25J. S. McCasland, "Neuronal Control of Bird Song Production," *Journal of Neuroscience* 7 (1987): 23–39.

26J. Cynx, H. Williams, and F. Nottebohm, "Hemispheric Differences in Avian Song Discrimination," *Pro-*

ceedings of the National Academy of Sciences, U.S.A. 89 (1992): 1372–1375.

[27]N. Geschwind, "Implications for Evolution, Genetics, and Clinical Syndromes" in *Cerebral Lateralization in Nonhuman Species,* ed. S. Glick (Orlando: Academic Press, 1985).

[28]Ibid.

[29]E. H. Lenneberg, *Biological Foundations of Language* (New York: Wiley, 1967).

[30]L. S. Basser, "Hemiplegia of Early Onset and the Faculty of Speech with Special Reference to the Effects of Hemispherectomy," *Brain* 85 (1962): 427–460.

[31]S. Krashen, "Lateralization, Language Learning, and the Critical Period: Some New Evidence," *Language Learning* 23 (1973): 63–74.

[32]M. Kinsbourne, "The Ontogeny of Cerebral Dominance," in *Developmental Psycholinguistics and Communication Disorders,* ed. D. Aaronson and R. W. Reiber (New York: New York Academy of Sciences, 1975).

[33]B. T. Woods and H. L. Teuber, "Changing Patterns of Childhood Aphasia," *Annals of Neurology* 3 (1978): 273–280.

[34]A. Smith, "Speech and Other Functions After Left (Dominant) Hemispherectomy," *Journal of Neurology, Neurosurgery, and Psychiatry* 29 (1966): 467–471; A. Smith and C. W. Burkland, "Dominant Hemispherectomy," *Science* 153 (1966): 1280–1282.

[35]M. Dennis and H. Whitaker, "Language Acquisition Following Hemidecortication: Linguistic Superiority of the Left Over the Right Hemisphere," *Brain and Language* 3 (1976): 404–433.

[36]D. V. M. Bishop, "Linguistic Impairment After Left Hemidecortication for Infantile Hemiplegia? A Reappraisal," *Quarterly Journal of Experimental Psychology* 35 (1983): 199–207.

[37]J. Chi, E. Dooling, and F. Giles, "Left–Right Asymmetries of the Temporal Speech Areas of the Human Fetus," *Archives of Neurology* 34 (1972): 346–348.

[38]J. A. Wada, R. Clark, and A. Hamm, "Cerebral Hemispheric Asymmetry in Humans," *Archives of Neurology* 32 (1975): 239–246.

[39]G. Turkewitz and S. Creighton, "Changes in Lateral Differentiation of Head Posture in the Human Neonate," *Developmental Psychology* 8 (1974): 85–89; J. Liederman and M. Kinsbourne, "The Mechanism of Neonatal Rightward Turning Bias: A Sensory or Motor Asymmetry?" *Infant Behavior and Development* 5 (1980): 223–238.

[40]J. Viviani, G. Turkewitz, and E. Karp, "A Relationship Between Laterality of Functioning at 2 Days and at 7 Years of Age," *Bulletin of the Psychonomic Society* 12 (1978): 189–192.

[41]D. L. Molfese, R. B. Freeman, Jr., and D. S. Palermo, "The Ontogeny of Brain Lateralization for Speech and Nonspeech Stimuli," *Brain and Language* 2 (1975): 356–368.

[42]J. A. Wada and A. Davis, "Fundamental Nature of Human Infants' Brain Asymmetry," *Canadian Journal of Neurological Sciences* 4 (1977): 203–207.

[43]M. Nagafuchi, "Development of Dichotic and Monaural Hearing Abilities in Young Children," *Acta Otolaryngologica* 69 (1970): 409–414.

[44]A. K. Entus, "Hemispheric Asymmetry in Processing of Dichotically Presented Speech and Nonspeech Stimuli by Infants," in *Language Development and Neurological Theory,* ed. S. J. Segalowitz and F. Gruber (New York: Academic Press, 1977).

[45]F. Vargha-Khadem and M. C. Corballis, "Cerebral Asymmetry in Infants," *Brain and Language* 8 (1979): 1–9.

[46]C. Berlin, L. Hughes, S. Lowe-Bell, and H. Berlin, "Right Ear Advantage in Children 5 to 13," *Cortex* 9 (1973): 394–402; P. Satz, D. J. Bakker, J. Tenunissen, R. Goebel, and H. Van der Vlugt, "Developmental Parameters of the Ear Asymmetry: A Multivariate Approach," *Brain and Language* 2 (1975): 171–185.

[47]Satz et al., "Developmental Parameters of the Ear Asymmetry."

[48]Ibid.

[49]Molfese et al., "The Ontogeny of Brain Lateralization."

[50]Wada et al., "Cerebral Hemispheric Asymmetry in Humans."

[51]S. Witelson and D. L. Kigar, "Anatomical Development of the Corpus Callosum in Humans: A Review With Reference to Sex and Cognition," in *Brain Lateralization in Children*, ed. D. L. Molfese and S. J. Segalowitz (New York: Gilford, 1988).

[52]C. Chiarello, "A House Divided? Cognitive Functioning with Callosal Agenesis," *Brain and Language* 11 (1980): 128–158; M. Lassonde, M. P. Bryden, and P. Demers, "The Corpus Callosum and Cerebral Speech Lateralization," *Brain and Language* 38 (1990): 195–206.

[53]H. C. Sauerwein, P. Nolin, and M. Lassonde, "Cognitive Functioning in Callosal Agenesis," in *Callosal Agenesis: The Natural Split Brain*, ed. M. Lassonde and M. Jeeves (New York: Plenum Press, 1993).

[54]C. Temple and J. Ilsley, "Sounds and Shapes: Language and Spatial Cognition in Callosal Agenesis," in *Callosal Agenesis*, Lassonde and Jeeves.

[55]Ibid.

[56]Ibid.

[57]M. Morgan, "Embryology and Inheritance of Asymmetry," in *Lateralization in the Nervous System*, ed. S. Harnad, R. Doty, L. Goldstein, J. Jaynes, and G. Krauthamer (New York: Academic Press, 1977).

[58]M. Corballis and M. J. Morgan, "On the Biological Basis of Human Laterality: I. Evidence for a Maturational Left-Right Gradient," *Behavioral and Brain Sciences* 2 (1978): 261–336.

[59]Krashen, "Lateralization, Language Learning, and the Critical Period: Some New Evidence."

[60]H. J. Neville, "Whence the Specialization of the Language Hemisphere?" in *Modularity and the Motor Theory of Speech Perception*, ed. I. G. Mattingly and M. Studdert-Kennedy (Hillsdale, N.J.: Erlbaum, 1991).

[61]H. Poizner, U. Bellugi, and E. Klima, "Brain Function for Language: Perspectives from Another Modality," in *Modularity and the Motor Theory of Speech Perception*, Mattingly and Studdert-Kennedy.

[62]L. Obler, R. Zattore, L. Galloway, and J. Vaid, "Cerebral Lateralization in Bilinguals: Methodological Issues," *Brain and Language* 15 (1982): 40–54.

[63]M. Paradis, "Language Lateralization in Bilinguals—Enough Already," *Brain and Language* 39 (1990): 576–586.

[64]A. Berquier and R. Ashton, "Language Lateralization in Bilinguals: More Not Less Is Needed: A Reply to Paradis," *Brain and Language* 43 (1992): 528–533.

Chapter 10   Asymmetry's Role in Developmental Disabilities and Psychiatric Illness

[1]S. T. Orton, *Reading, Writing, and Speech Problems in Children* (New York: Norton, 1937).

[2]J. M. Rumsey, "Biology of Developmental Dyslexia," *Journal of the American Medical Association* 268 (1992): 912–915; D. D. Duane and D. B. Gray, ed. *The Reading Brain: The Biological Basis of Dyslexia* (Parkland, M.D.: York Press, 1991).

[3]Rumsey, "Biology of Developmental Dyslexia."

[4]M. P. Bryden, "Does Laterality Make Any Difference? Thoughts on the Relation Between Cerebral Asymmetry and Reading," in *Brain Lateralization in Children* ed. D. Molfese and S. Segalowitz (New York: Guilford Press, 1988).

[5]Ibid.

[6]A. M. Galaburda, G. P. Sherman, G. D. Rosen, F. Aboitiz, and N. Geschwind, "Developmental Dyslexia: Four Consecutive Patients with Cortical Anomalies," *Annals of Neurology* 18 (1985): 222–233.

[7]P. Humphreys, W. E. Kaufmann, and A. Galaburda, "Developmental Dyslexia in Women: Neuropathological Findings in Three Cases," *Annals of Neurology* 28 (1990): 727–738.

[8]E. W. Hynd, M. Semrud-Clikeman, A. R. Lorys, E. S. Novey, and D. Elipulos, "Brain Morphology in Develop-

mental Dyslexia and Attention Deficit Disorder/Hyperactivity," *Archives of Neurology* 47 (1990): 919–926; J. P. Larsen, T. Hoien, I. Lundberg, and H. Odegaard, "MRI Evaluation of the Size and Symmetry of the Planum Temporale in Adolescents with Developmental Dyslexia," *Brain and Language* 39 (1990): 289–301.

[9]R. Duara, A. Kusch, K. Gross-Glenn, W. Barker, B. Jullad, and S. Pascal, "Neuroanatomic Differences Between Dyslexic and Normal Readers on Magnetic Resonance Imaging Scans," *Archives of Neurology* 48 (1991): 410–416.

[10]D. L. Flowers, F. D. Wood, and C. Naylor, "Regional Cerebral Blood Flow Correlates of Language Processing in Reading Disability," *Archives of Neurology* 48 (1991): 637–643; J. M. Rumsey, P. Andreason, A. Zametkin, T. Aquino, A. C. King, S. D. Hamburger, A. Pikus, J. L. Rapoport, R. M. Cohen, "Failure to Activate Left Tempoparietal Cortex in Dyslexia: A [15]O PET Study," *Archives of Neurology* 49 (1992): 527–534.

[11]J. G. Sheenan, *Stuttering: Research and Therapy* (New York: Harper & Row, 1970).

[12]F. K. Curry and H. H. Gregory, "The Performance of Stutterers on Dichotic Listening Tasks Thought to Reflect Cerebral Dominance," *Journal of Speech and Hearing Research* 12 (1969): 73–82.

[13]P. Quinn, "Stuttering, Cerebral Dominance, and the Dichotic Word Test," *Medical Journal of Australia* 2 (1972): 639–643; N. Slorach and B. Noehr, "Dichotic Listening in Stuttering and Dyslalic Children," *Cortex* 9 (1973): 295–300.

[14]R. K. Jones, "Observations on Stammering After Localized Cerebral Injury," *Journal of Neurology, Neurosurgery, and Psychiatry* 29 (1966): 192–195.

[15]G. Andrews, P. T. Quinn, and W. A. Sorby, "Stuttering: An Investigation into Verbal Dominance for Speech," *Journal of Neurology, Neurosurgery, and Psychiatry* 35 (1972): 414–418.

[16]H. Sussman and P. MacNeilage,

"Studies of Hemispheric Specialization for Speech Production," *Brain and Language* 2 (1975): 131–151.

[17]H. Sussman and P. MacNeilage, "Hemispheric Specialization for Speech Production in Stutterers," *Neuropsychologia* 13 (1975): 19–26.

[18]F. Wood, D. Stump, A. McKeehan, S. Sheldon, and J. Proctor, "Patterns of Regional Cerebral Blood Flow During Attempted Reading Aloud by Stutterers Both On and Off Haloperidol Medication," *Brain and Language* 9 (1980): 141–144.

[19]K. D. Pool, M. D. Devous, F. J. Freeman, B. C. Watson, and T. Finitzo, "Regional Cerebral Blood Flow in Developmental Stutterers," *Archives of Neurology* 48 (1991): 509–512.

[20]I. Rapin, "Autistic Children: Diagnosis and Clinical Features," *Pediatrics* 87 Supplement (1991): 751–761.

[21]L. Selfe, *Nadia: A Case of Extraordinary Drawing Ability in an Autistic Child* (New York: Academic Press, 1977).

[22]D. Fein, M. Humes, E. Kaplan, D. Lucci, and L. Waterhouse, "The Question of Left Hemisphere Dysfunction in Infantile Autism," *Psychological Bulletin* 95 (1984): 258–281.

[23]G. Dawson, "Cerebral Lateralization in Autism: Clues to the Role in Language and Affective Development," in *Brain Lateralization in Children*, Molfese and Segalowitz.

[24]G. Dawson, S. Warrenburg, and P. Fuller, "Cerebral Lateralization in Individuals Diagnosed as Autistic in Early Childhood," *Brain and Language* 15 (1982): 353–368.

[25]G. Dawson, C. Phillips, L. Galpert, "Hemispheric Specialization and the Language Abilities of Autistic Children," *Child Development* 57 (1986): 1440–1453.

[26]K. Aiken, "Examining the Evidence for a Common Structural Basis to Autism," *Developmental Medicine and Child Neurology* 33 (1991): 930–938.

[27]E. Courchesne, "Neuroanatomic Imaging in Autism," *Pediatrics* 87 Supplement (1991): 781–790.

[28]M. Zilbovicius, B. Garreau, N. Tzourio, B. Mazoyer, B. Bruck, J.-L. Martinot,

C. Raynaud, Y. Samson, A. Syrota, and G. Lelord, "Regional Cerebral Blood Flow in Childhood Autism," *American Journal of Psychiatry* 149 (1992): 924–930.

[29]N. A. Akshoomoff, E. Courchesne, G. A. Press, and V. Iragui, "Contribution of the Cerebellum to Neuropsychological Functioning: Evidence from a Case of Cerebellar Degenerative Disorder," *Neuropsychologia* 30 (1992): 315–328.

[30]M. R. Prior and J. L. Bradshaw, "Hemispheric Functioning in Autistic Children," *Cortex* 15 (1979): 73–81.

[31]P. Flor-Henry, "Schizophrenic-like Reactions and Affective Psychoses Associated with Temporal Lobe Epilepsy: Etiological Factors," *American Journal of Psychiatry* 26 (1969): 400–403.

[32]K. Davison and L. R. Bagley, "Schizophrenia-like Psychosis Associated with Organic Disorder of the Central Nervous System: A Review of the Literature," *British Journal of Psychiatry Special Publication* 4 (1969): 113–150.

[33]D. Galin, "Implications for Psychiatry of Left and Right Cerebral Specialization," *Archives of General Psychiatry* 31 (1974): 572–583.

[34]J. Gruzelier and N. Hammond, "Schizophrenia—A Dominant Hemisphere Temporal Lobe Disorder?" *Research Communications in Psychology, Psychiatry, and Behavior* 1 (1976): 33–72.

[35]G. Beaumont and S. Dimond, "Brain Disconnection and Schizophrenia," *British Journal of Psychiatry* 123 (1972): 661–662.

[36]R. W. Coger and E. A. Serefetinides, "Schizophrenia, Corpus Callosum, and Interhemispheric Communication: A Review," *Psychiatry Research* 34 (1990): 163—184.

[37]W. C. Drevets, T. O. Videen, J. L. Price, S. H. Preskorn, S. T. Carmichael, and M. E. Raichle, "A Functional Anatomical Study of Unipolar Depression," *Journal of Neuroscience* 12 (1992): 3628–3641.

[38]J. H. Gruzelier, "Hemispheric Imbalance Syndromes of Schizophrenia, Premorbid Personalities, and Neurodevelopmental Influences," *Handbook of Schizophrenia*, Vol. 5, 1991.

Chapter 11   Hemisphericity, Education, and Altered States

[1]S. Aurobindo, quoted in J. E. Bogen, "The Other Side of the Brain. VII: Some Educational Aspects of Hemispheric Specialization," *UCLA Educator* 17 (1975): 24–32.

[2]R. Ornstein, *The Psychology of Consciousness* (New York: Harcourt Brace Jovanovich, 1977).

[3]A. Harrington and O. Godehard, "Whole Brain Politics and Brain Laterality Research," *European Archives of Psychiatry and Neurological Sciences* 239 (1989): 141–143.

[4]H. Gardner, "What We Know (and Don't Know) about the Two Halves of the Brain," *Harvard Magazine* 80 (1978): 24–27.

[5]J. A. Paredes and M. J. Hepburn, "The Split Brain and the Culture-and-Cognition Paradox," *Current Anthropology* 17 (1976): 121–127.

[6]J. E. Bogen, R. DeZare, W. D. Ten-Houten, and J. F. Marsh, "The Other Side of the Brain. IV: The A/P Ratio," *Bulletin of the Los Angeles Neurological Societies* 37 (1972): 49–61.

[7]J. A. Zook and J. H. Dwyer, "Cultural Differences in Hemisphericity: A Critique," *Bulletin of the Los Angeles Neurological Societies* 41 (1976): 87–90.

[8]R. Ornstein, "The Split and Whole Brain," *Human Nature* 1 (1978): 76–83; J. Dabbs, "Left–Right Differences in Cerebral Blood Flow and Cognition," *Psychophysiology* 17 (1980): 548–551.

[9]A. McGee-Cooper, *You Don't Have to Go Home from Work Exhausted* (New York: Bantam, 1992).

[10]E. P. Torrance and C. Reynolds, *Norms-Technical Manual for "Your Style of Learning and Thinking,"* (Athens, Ga.: Department of Educational Psychology, University of Georgia, 1980).

[11]E. P. Torrance, C. P. Reynolds, T. Riegel, and O. Ball, "Your Style of Learning and Thinking; Forms A and B: Preliminary Norms, Abbreviated Notes, Scoring Keys, and Selected References," *Gifted Child Quarterly* 21 (1977): 563–573.

[12]N. Herrmann, *The Creative Brain,* (Lake Lure, N.C.: Brain Books, 1991).

[13]M. E. Humphrey and O. L. Zangwill, "Cessation of Dreaming After Brain Injury," *Journal of Neurology, Neurosurgery, and Psychiatry* 14 (1951): 322–325.

[14]P. Greenwood, D. H. Wilson, and M. S. Gazzaniga, "Dream Report Following Commissurotomy," *Cortex* 13 (1977): 311–316.

[15]K. D. Hoppe, "Split Brains and Psychoanalysis," *The Psychoanalytic Quarterly* 46 (1977): 220–224.

[16]P. Bakan, "Hypnotizability, Laterality of Eye Movements, and Functional Brain Asymmetry," *Perceptual and Motor Skills* 28 (1969): 927–932.

[17]C. MacLeod and L. Lack, "Hemispheric Specificity: A Physiological Concomitant of Hypnotizability," *Psychophysiology* 19 (1982): 687–699.

[18]P. Bakan, "Handedness and Hypnotizability," *International Journal of Clinical and Experimental Hypnosis* 18 (1970): 99–104.

[19]L. Frumkin, H. Ripley, and G. Cox, "Changes in Cerebral Hemisphere Lateralization with Hypnosis," *Biological Psychiatry* 13 (1978): 741–750.

[20]J. E. Bogen, "The Other Side of the Brain. VII: Some Educational Aspects of Hemispheric Specialization," *UCLA Educator* 17 (1975): 24–32.

[21]G. Prince, "Putting the Other Half of the Brain to Work," *Training. The Magazine of Human Resources Development* 15 (1978): 57–61.

[22]I. Sonnier (ed.) *Methods and Techniques of Holistic Education* (Springfield, Ill.: Charles C. Thomas, 1985); I. Sonnier (ed.) *Hemisphericity as a Key to Understanding Individual Differences* (Springfield, Ill.: Charles C. Thomas, 1992); L. J. Harris, "Right Brain Training: Some Reflections on the Application of Research on Cerebral Hemispheric Specialization to Education," in *Brain Lateralization in Children,* ed. D. L. Molfese and S. J. Segalowitz (New York: Guilford Press, 1988).

[23]B. Edwards, *Drawing on the Right Side of the Brain* (Los Angeles, J. P. Tarcher, 1989).

[24]E. K. Warrington, "Constructional Apraxia," in *Handbook of Clinical Neurology,* Vol. 4, ed. P. J. Vinken and G. W. Bruyn (Amsterdam: Elservier North Holland, 1986).

[25]Harris, "Right Brain Training."

[26]C. H. Delacato, *The Treatment and Prevention of Reading Problems (The Neuropsychological Approach)* (Springfield, Ill.: Charles C. Thomas, 1959).

[27]H. J. Cohen, H. G. Birch, and L. T. Taft, "Some Considerations for Evaluating the Doman-Delacato 'Patterning' Method," *Pediatrics* 45 (1970): 302–314.

[28]American Academy of Pediatrics, "The Doman–Delacato Treatment of Neurologically Handicapped Children," *Journal of Pediatrics* 72 (1968): 750.

[29]Cohen et al., "Some Considerations for Evaluating the Doman–Delacato 'Patterning' Method."

[30]C. Sagan, *The Dragons of Eden* (New York: Random House, 1977).

[31]Ibid.

[32]Ibid.

[33]Ibid.

Chapter 12   Concluding Hypotheses and Speculations

[1]D. Kimura and Y. Archibald, "Motor Functions of the Left Hemisphere," *Brain* 97 (1974): 337–350.

[2]Ibid.

[3]M. Studdert-Kennedy and D. Shankweiler, "Hemispheric Specialization for Speech Perception," *Journal of the* *Acoustical Society of America* 48 (1970): 579–594.

[4]J. Schwartz and P. Tallal, "Rate of Acoustic Change May Underlie Hemispheric Specialization for Speech Perception," *Science* 207 (1980): 1380–1381.

[5]A. M. Liberman, F. S. Cooper, D. Shankweiler, and M. Studdert-Kennedy, "Perceptions of the Speech Code," Psychological Review 74 (1967): 431–461.

[6]G. Deutsch and J. H. Halsey, Jr., "Cortical Blood Flow Indicates Active Motor Component During Speech Sound Discrimination Task," Journal of Clinical and Experimental Neuropsychology 12 (1990): 416.

[7]R. J. Zatorre, A. C. Evans, E. Meyer, and A. Gjedde, "Lateralization of Phonetic and Pitch Discrimination in Speech Processing," Science 256 (1992): 846–849.

[8]D. P. Corina, J. Vaid, and U. Bellugi, "The Linguistic Basis of Left Hemisphere Specialization," Science 255 (1992): 1258–1260.

[9]E. Goldberg and L. D. Costa, "Hemispheric Differences in the Acquisition and Use of Descriptive Systems," Brain and Language 14 (1981): 144–173.

[10]E. Goldberg, H. G. Vaughan, Jr., and L. J. Gerstman, "Nonverbal Descriptive Systems and Hemispheric Asymmetry: Shape versus Texture Discrimination," Brain and Language 5 (1978): 249–257.

[11]Ibid.

[12]C. J. Connoly, External Morphology of the Primate Brain (Springfield, Ill.: Charles C. Thomas, 1950); M. LeMay and A. Culebras, "Human Brain-Morphologic Differences in the Hemispheres Demonstrable by Carotid Arteriography," New England Journal of Medicine 287 (1972): 168–170; A. M. Galaburda, M. LeMay, T. L. Kemper, and N. Geschwind, "Right–Left Asymmetries in the Brain," Science 199 (1978): 852–856.

[13]M. LeMay, "Morphological Cerebral Asymmetries of Modern Man, Fossil Man, and Nonhuman Primate," in Origins and Evolution of Language and Speech, ed. S. R. Harnad, H. D. Steklis, and J. Lancaster, Annals of the New York Academy of Sciences 280 (1976): 349–366; J. A. Wada, R. Clarke, and A. Hamm, "Cerebral Hemispheric Asymmetry in Humans," Archives of Neurology 32 (1975): 239–246.

[14]H. A. Whitaker and G. A. Ojemann, "Lateralization of the Higher Cortical Functions: A Critique," in Evolution and Lateralization of the Brain, ed. S. J. Dimond and D. A. Blizard, Annals of the New York Academy of Sciences 299 (1977): 459–473.

[15]R. C. Gur, I. K. Packer, J. P. Hungerbuhler, M. Reivich, W. D. Obrist, W. S. Amarnek, and H. A. Sackheim, "Differences in the Distribution of Gray and White Matter in Human Cerebral Hemispheres," Science 207 (1980): 1226–1228.

[16]J. Semmes, "Hemispheric Specialization: A Possible Clue to Mechanism," Neuropsychologia 6 (1968): 11–26.

[17]J. Levy, "Interhemispheric Collaboration: Single Mindedness in the Asymmetrical Brain," in Hemispheric Function and Collaboration in the Child, ed. C. T. Best (New York: Academic Press, 1985).

[18]N. D. Cook, "The Transmission of Information in Natural Systems," Journal of Theoretical Biology 108 (1984): 349–367; N. D. Cook, "Callosal Inhibition: The Key to the Brain Code," Behavioral Science 29 (1984): 98–110.

[19]Ibid.

[20]S. H. Woodward, "An Anatomical Model of Hemispheric Asymmetry," Journal of Clinical and Experimental Neuropsychology 10 (1988): 68.

[21]G. Hinton, J. L. McClelland, and D. E. Rumelhart, "Distributed Representations," in Parallel Distributed Processing. Explorations in the Microstructure of Cognition, Vol. 1, ed. D. E. Rumelhart, J. L. McClelland, and the PDP Research Group (Cambridge, Mass.: MIT Press, 1986).

[22]Woodward, "An Anatomical Model of Hemispheric Asymmetry."

[23]R. W. Sperry, "Brain Bisection and Consciousness," in Brain and Conscious Experience, ed. J. Eccles (New York: Springer-Verlag, 1966).

[24]J. Eccles, The Brain and Unity of Conscious Experience: The 19th Arthur Stanley Eddington Memorial Lecture (Cambridge: Cambridge University Press, 1965).

[25]J. E. LeDoux, D. H. Wilson, and

M. S. Gazzaniga, "A Divided Mind: Observation on the Conscious Properties of the Separated Hemispheres," *Annals of Neurology* 2 (1977): 417–421.

[26]Ibid.

[27]J. Jaynes, cited in S. Keen, "Reflections on the Dawn of Consciousness," *Psychology Today* 11 (1977): 58.

[28]Ibid.

[29]J. Hadamard, *The Psychology of Invention in the Mathematical Field* (Princeton University Press, 1945); R. Penrose, *The Emperor's New Mind* (New York: Oxford University Press, 1989).

[30]Hadamard, *The Psychology of Invention in the Mathematical Field.*

[31]Penrose, *The Emperor's New Mind.*

[32]Hadamard, *The Psychology of Invention in the Mathematical Field.*

[33]Ibid.

[34]O. Loewi, *Perspectives in Biology and Medicine* 4 (Chicago: University of Chicago Press, 1960).

[35]A. Koestler, *The Act of Creation* (New York: Dell, 1964).

[36]Ibid.

[37]D. Galin, "Implications for Psychiatry of Left and Right Cerebral Specialization," *Archives of General Psychiatry* 31 (1974): 572–583.

[38]Ibid.

[39]Ibid.

[40]LeDoux et al., "A Divided Mind."

[41]R. Puccetti, "The Case for Mental Duality: Evidence from Split Brain Data and Other Considerations," *The Behavioral and Brain Sciences* 4 (1981): 93–123.

[42]Ibid.

[43]Ibid.

[44]R. W. Sperry, E. Zaidel, and D. Zaidel, "Self Recognition and Social Awareness in the Disconnected Minor Hemisphere," *Neuropsychologia* 17 (1979): 153–166.

[45]Ibid.

[46]D. C. Dennett, *Consciousness Explained* (Boston: Little Brown, 1991).

[47]Ibid.

[48]D. N. Robinson, "Cerebral Plurality and the Unity of Self," *American Psychologist* 37 (1982): 904–910.

[49]G. Sperling, "The Information Available in Brief Visual Presentations," *Psychological Monographs* 74 (1960): (11, Whole No. 498).

[50]D. H. Raab, "Backward Masking," *Psychological Bulletin* 60 (1963): 118–129.

[51]A. Binet, *Alterations of Personality* (H. Baldwin, trans.) (New York: Appleton, 1896).

[52]Robinson, "Cerebral Plurality and the Unity of Self."

[53]Ibid.

[54]J. Miller, "Trouble in Mind," *Scientific American,* September (1992): p 180.

[55]Ibid.

[56]R. Dubos, *Pasteur and Modern Science* (London: Heinemann, 1960).

[57]M. C. Corballis and I. L. Beale, *The Ambivalent Mind* (Chicago: Nelson-Hall, 1983).

[58]L. Wolpert, "Pattern Formation in Biological Development," *Scientific American* 239 (1978): 124–137.

[59]Corballis and Beale, *The Ambivalent Mind.*

[60]Ibid.

[61]B. Norden, "The Asymmetry of Life," *Journal of Molecular Evolution* 11 (1978): 313–332.

[62]E. M. Henley, "Parity and Time-Reversal Invariance in Nuclear Physics," *Annual Review of Nuclear Science* 19 (1969): 367–427.

[63]Corballis and Beale, *The Ambivalent Mind.*

INDEX